Comments on *Stop that heart attack!* from readers

'An excellent read. This book is a must for absolutely anyone interested in
heart health – as a reference, an inspiration, a good laugh and a new old
friend!'
The Family Heart Digest

'The style is easy to read and there are plenty of humorous and personal
anecdotes and some wonderful cartoons to make a serious issue an enjoyable
read.'
Sara Stanner, British Nutrition Foundation

'Clear and readable, this book would be most suited to the well-motivated
individual who is ready to make lifestyle changes.'
Sister Caroline Brennan, Cardiology News

'Dr Cutting writes well and the text is interesting.'
Dr Richard Wray, Consultant Physician,
Department of Cardiology, Conquest Hospital, St Leonards-on-Sea

'It was a pleasure to read! I'm now going to put all the useful information to
the test . . . I'll be keeping it with me for inspiration.'
Suzanna Stuart

'The doctor offers hope for many healthy years to come if we use his knowledge and common sense and set ourselves attainable goals in exercise and
adjusted diet. Thank you Dr Cutting for helping me to *Stop that heart attack!*'
Reviewed by Julia Westall, BCPA Journal

'I think that this book is really well set out and easy to read and has a mine of
useful information.'
Prof Philip James,
Rowett Research Institute, Aberdeen

'Concepts are well explained for the layman without being patronising and
unusually for this type of book it is medically sound and gets the balance
right.'
Professor Paul Durrington, Professor of Medicine,
Manchester Royal Infirmary

'This is one of those books that once you start reading you really cannot put
down. It ought to be on the reading list for every secondary school
student . . .'
British Cardiac Patients' Association

I'm sure the general public will find it enlightening, humourous and educational. I am impressed with his nutritional knowledge.'
Azmina Govindji BSc, SRD, Consultant Nutritionist and Dietitian

'It is the best written book I have ever read . . . It is magnificent in every way.'
Dr Thomas White MD, retired General Practitioner

'Thank you for asking me to read this excellent book, I really enjoyed it! I too share the author's enthusiasm for healthy eating to stop heart disease. The book is easy to read for the motivated member of the public but also scientifically sound for the interested health professional . . . It is well written and is a pleasure to read with plenty of humour, common sense and personal anecdotes. I would highly recommend this book.'
Jacqui Lynas BSc, SRD, Specialist Lipid Dietitian

'This is an excellent book for those who are interested in unclogging their arteries, or getting down to their ideal weight for good, or controlling their blood pressure, or discovering a new vitality.'
The Family Heart Digest

'. . . an excellent, comprehensive book . . .'
Dr Chris Steele, TV Quick

'This is a brilliant book! I've found it invaluable. The clear explanations and humour make it such light reading, and so interesting. I can't speak too highly of this book.'
Rosemary A. May

'As a bus driver I have been trying for some time to get fit, unsuccessfully. I found this book both informative and easy to read. As a person who doesn't normally read, I found the humourous angle helped me to read on and finish the book.'
Stewart Holt

'I found myself wide awake at 3am and unable to put the book down . . . This book should be compulsory reading at an early age.'
British Journal of Cardiology

'. . . thank heavens for Dr Derrick Cutting . . . recipes that won't take a week to prepare and are ideally suited to your average burger-loving Brit.'
Amanda Ursell, The Sunday Times

'This is an exceptional book . . .it does exactly what it says on the cover and provides successful and medically accurate strategies for a healthy and fulfilled life.'
Cardiology News

'. . . enjoyable, informative and can be highly recommended.'
Diabetes Research & Wellness Foundation

Comments from people who have put Dr Cutting's plan to the test

Stop that HEART ATTACK!

DR DERRICK CUTTING

with cartoons by *MADDOCKS*

'Packed with information on how to live
a longer, healthier life.' *Slimming Magazine*

THIRD EDITION
fully revised and updated

CLASS PUBLISHING

Printing history
First published 1998
Reprinted with revisions 1999
Second edition 2001
Third edition 2004
Reprinted 2004

Published by
Class Publishing (London) Ltd,
Barb House, Barb Mews, London W6 7PA
Tel: 020 7371 2119 [International +4420]
Fax: 020 7371 2878
Email: post@class.co.uk
Visit our website at: www.class.co.uk

A CIP catalogue record for this book is available from the British Library

ISBN 1 85959 096 9

The information presented in this book is accurate and current
to the best of the author's knowledge. The author and publisher,
however, make no guarantee as to, and assume no responsibility for,
the correctness, sufficiency or completeness of such information or
recommendation. The reader is advised to consult a doctor
regarding all aspects of individual health care.

Designed and typeset by Martin Bristow
Editorial team: Michèle Clarke (2nd and 3rd editions); Sally Critchlow,
Bridget Jones, Mary Korndorffer (1st and 2nd editions)
Indexed by Valerie Elliston
Cartoons by Peter Maddocks
Line illustrations by David Woodroffe

Printed and bound in Finland by WS Bookwell, Juva

Contents

Preface to Third Edition

It seems such a short time ago that I was writing a preface to the second edition and explaining that any doubts about the need for this book had been swept away by the response to the first edition. The call for a third edition confirms that, in the face of so many confusing and conflicting messages about health, the demand for a medically accurate guide that's easy to read is as strong as ever.

Stop that heart attack! is much more about health than disease. Inevitably, some of its most enthusiastic readers are those who have already had a heart attack, but I can only agree with the reviewers who said it should be compulsory reading for young people!

This edition has been fully revised to take account of the latest developments. The section on hormone replacement therapy has been rewritten to clear up the confusion caused by media coverage of recent research. New evidence for the benefits of fish oil is explained. You can read about advances since the first edition sounded the alarm on salt, and find out what action you need to take. Should you lower your cholesterol level even if it's normal? When should you take drugs as well as changing your lifestyle? These questions are answered in the light of the latest research. There is a completely new section on South Asian diets, and practical advice on avoiding the slippery slope to weight gain, diabetes, high blood pressure and heart disease.

Acknowledgements

I am indebted to Professor Paul Durrington, Azmina Govindji, Professor Philip James, Jacqui Lynas, Sue Phipps and Dr Richard Wray who read the manuscripts. Baldeesh Rai of *Heart UK* kindly provided information on South Asian diets.

Readers have been a tremendous encouragement, and it's thanks to them that this book is now in its third edition.

Proper writing is something I do with a pencil, carefully crafting each sentence to the aroma of real wood pencil shavings. (You may mock, but I really do care about every clause and comma.) So I am forever grateful to my wife, Heather, who faithfully and efficiently converts my manuscripts into electronic data. Our two daughters, Serena and Christabel, are a constant reminder that health is precious – even though writing about it so often deprives me of their company.

Derrick Cutting
www.stha.ndirect.co.uk

Copyright

Notes

Calories

Reference to the number of 'calories' in food always means kilo-calories (kcal). Strictly speaking, this should be written as 'Calories' with a capital C, but for easy reading we refer to kilocalories as 'calories'.

1 kcal = 1 Calorie = 1000 calories

1 megajoule (MJ) = 1000 kilojoules (kJ) = 239 kilocalories (kcal).

Abbreviations

g = grams; mmol/l = millimoles per litre;
oz = ounce; ml = millilitre; lb = pound weight.

Registered Trade Marks

Trade names are used in this book as examples only and do not imply any particular recommendation.

All Bran, Crunchy Nut Corn Flakes, Frosties, and Rice Krispies
    are registered trade marks of The Kellogg Company
Benecol is a registered trademark and produced for McNeil Consumer
    Nutritionals Ltd
Cheerios, Golden Grahams, Nesquik, Shredded Wheat and Shreddies
    are registered trade marks of Société des Produits Nestlé S.A.,
    Vevey, Switzerland
Dolmio is a registered trade mark of Master Foods
Flora pro.activ is a trademark of Van den Bergh Foods Ltd
Jordans is a registered trade mark of W Jordan (Cereals) Ltd
Kwai is a registered trade mark of Biocare
LoSalt is a trade mark of Klinge Foods Ltd
Olestra is made by Proctor and Gamble
Omacor is a registered trade mark of Solvay Healthcare
Polydextrose is made by Pfizer
Quorn is a registered trade mark of ICI Ltd
Simplesse is made by Nutrasweet
Solo is a registered trademark of the Low Sodium Sea Salt Co.
Sugar Puffs is a registered trade mark of Quaker Trading Ltd
Weetabix is a registered trade mark of Weetabix Ltd, Kettering, UK

Introduction

If you want to feel good and look good, you have to get healthy from the inside out. And your circulation is at the heart of your wellbeing. Our epidemics of heart disease, high blood pressure, obesity and diabetes are just outward signs indicating that so many of us do not have this inner health.

Half the adults in the Western world are overweight and, when you're fat, it shows. But the heart and arteries are out of sight and, all too often, out of mind. If we had windows into our bodies, we would see the fatty deposits that lead to strokes and heart attacks starting to form in the arteries of pre-school children!

In the UK, 275,000 people have a heart attack each year and one person in four dies of heart disease. It's the modern plague – and it's not just a plague of middle-aged men: *five times more women die of heart disease than of breast cancer.*

The great news is: there are simple steps that you can take to restore your inner health. By making the right changes, *you can feel better, look better* and *help your heart and arteries.* Not only that, *you will be cutting your risk of cancer* and *protecting yourself against premature ageing.*

Who wants to get old? In Western societies, arteries fur up and blood pressure rises as people get older. It doesn't have to be that way. We can learn from cultures in which people reach old age with unclogged arteries and lovely low blood pressures – completely free of heart disease. The lifestyle plan in this book can truly keep you young at heart.

Recent research has revolutionised our understanding of the way the body digests carbohydrate foods. Did you know that baked potatoes and wholemeal bread push up blood glucose faster than table sugar does? Now you can read the latest on the glycaemic index (GI number) of foods and use it to control body weight, diabetes and energy levels!

If you have diabetes, your risk of heart disease is hugely increased. Apart from controlling blood glucose, there are lots of vitally important ways to improve your health and protect your arteries. This book is full of them.

Of course, you may have heart disease already. Perhaps the first you knew about it was an unexpected heart attack or it may be that you suffer from angina. Either way, it's all the more important to slash your chances of having a heart attack in future. These pages tell you how to do just that.

It gets better. Doctors used to think that, once arteries had been narrowed by a build-up of fatty deposits, there wasn't much you could do about it. Oh, you might slow down the artery-clogging process, but the idea of actually stopping it was wildly optimistic; to reverse the process would clearly be impossible. I bring good news! Several scientific studies have now shown that you can indeed start unblocking arteries again; when big enough changes are made, heart disease can be sent into reverse!

Research has also discovered more about free radicals – those unstable chemicals that go round damaging cells in your body. Over the years, free radicals on the rampage cause ageing, cancer and heart disease. But we have also learnt more about special substances in our diet – antioxidants – that can protect against free radical attack. You can't stop the clock, but you can slow it down – and keep your ticker happy.

New evidence has exposed an epidemic that few have even heard of! There's a high chance that raised homocysteine levels are putting you at risk of a heart attack. You can find out how to keep your level down. It's simple!

Do you have a hearty appetite for life? This isn't a book about giving up all the things you enjoy; it's about living life to the full. Too much of the advice about diet just tells you to cut down your favourite foods. But science has uncovered the fact that some foods are positively helpful when it comes to protecting your heart and circulation, and even avoiding cancer. You can discover here the secret of getting the right balance of helpful foods. Eating to your heart's content could give you a longer life, and more energy to enjoy it.

Should we be eating a low-fat diet, or is it more important to eat the right kind of fat? Do the new fat spreads really lower cholesterol or are they just gimmicks? What's the difference between soluble and insoluble fibre? Does fibre lower cholesterol? Is salt essential or dangerous? OK, so fish does you a power of good, but what if you hate fish? Is it true that garlic's good for you, or is that just an old wives' tale? Can alcohol protect your heart, and is red wine really better than other drinks? These are just a few of the basic questions about food that you will find answered here. This book is about scientific evidence, not unfounded theories.

No matter how compelling the evidence, it's of no use to you unless you can translate it into everyday eating and living. This is a practical book. You'll find tips on making a shopping list, understanding food labels, eating on a budget, and feeding children. You can find out how to eat out without doing yourself in. Essential kitchen skills are covered too. Whether it's simple white sauce or rich fruit cake, I'll show you how to make it without fat.

Are you fed up with miracle diets that don't work? Perhaps *permanent* weight control is your heart's desire. Nutritional science can come to your rescue, and this book shows you how.

Have you been told you should reduce your cholesterol level? Perhaps you have tried to get your cholesterol down and been disappointed with the result. My book gives you a plan that will succeed where so many are failing – a plan to cut the 'bad' kind of cholesterol while looking after the 'good' sort.

Is there really any evidence that exercise prevents heart disease and, if so, what sort of exercise and how much of it is needed? Or could exercise bring on a heart attack? What's the best way to enjoy exercise if you're not a fitness fanatic? I'll sort out the facts from the fiction and show you how simply you can invigorate your life.

There is essential information for smokers here – and for non-smokers (who often find themselves smoking passively). If you're a smoker but would rather not be, why not make use of the plan in this book that's helped so many to become ex-smokers?

Like smoking, high blood pressure significantly raises your risk of heart disease. Some people need drugs to reduce blood pressure, but many could avoid the need for drugs if only they knew how. I explain a four-point plan to bring that pressure down.

Research shows a link between some forms of stress and increased rates of heart disease. Stress is a part of life, but it needn't be the death of you. You can put stress in its place with my simple stress-busting kit.

Weighing up risks can be tricky. You may have thought about taking hormone replacement therapy to cut your risk of heart disease, but been worried and confused by recent reports about the dangers of HRT. This is an understandable dilemma – especially if you're a woman. Help is at hand with this straightforward guide to the latest findings of research.

Some risks are so big that urgent action is needed, while others are too small to bother about. You can get things in perspective with my ABC of assessing your risk. There's a ready reckoner of risk so you can check your chances of having a heart attack in the next ten years, and there's clear advice on how to get that risk right down!

If you already have heart disease, you urgently need this programme to cut the risk of a future heart attack. You may need drug treatment too. You'll find some essential information in Chapter 25, including the latest research findings on drugs used to lower cholesterol levels.

How to use this book

If you read this book from cover to cover, the picture will unfold in a logical sequence until it is complete. But I realise you may not want to read it like that. I won't be in the least offended if you focus on the parts you find most interesting.

Key messages and action points are highlighted throughout the book. These will make it easier to skim sections without losing the thread. And, even if you do read every word, the panels will help a great deal when you want to go back and revise.

The **Fat** chapter contains a lot of information. It's important information, but if it all seems a bit much at first, don't worry: let the key-message panels help you through; you can always come back for more detail later. And, if you don't really like words at all, at least there are the cartoons to look at!

The **Action Plan** in Chapter 28 makes it easy to convert your new understanding into everyday living. You can see at a glance where action is needed – and reward yourself for the progress you've made. Useful books and addresses are listed in the appendix and the glossary provides a reminder of technical terms explained in the text.

I'd love to hear how successful you've been at changing your life and reducing your risk. Any suggestions for improving future editions would also be most welcome. You can write to me c/o Class Publishing, Barb House, Barb Mews, London, W6 7PA.

Are you interested in unclogging your arteries, or getting down to your ideal weight for good, or controlling your blood pressure and cholesterol, or discovering a new vitality? If you are, read on . . .

Chapter 1

What is heart disease?

LETHAL EPIDEMIC SWEEPS WESTERN WORLD

This sensational headline is no exaggeration. Heart disease is epidemic in Western civilisation.

Coronary heart disease is the single biggest killer in the UK. "Hang on!" you may be saying. "You're a bit out of date: cancer is the biggest killer now." Perhaps you heard recently that, for the first time in many years, deaths from heart disease have dipped a little below cancer deaths. But 'cancer' is not a single disease; it's lots of different diseases all lumped together. So coronary heart disease is still the single biggest killer. And if you add other diseases of the heart and circulation (which would include strokes) to coronary heart disease, this group of 'cardiovascular diseases' claims far more lives than all the cancers put together.

The good news is that deaths from heart disease have dropped a little; it seems that some messages about healthy living are starting to get through. But this has only scratched the surface. We still have a lethal epidemic on our hands.

Heart disease is not a male disease: it kills almost a quarter of our women too. OK, you have to die of something, but many are struck down in the prime of life. And statistics for deaths are only part of the story: many are living with heart disease.

'I feel as I always have, except for an occasional heart attack.'

Robert Benchley (1889–1945)
Groucho Marx Grouchofile, 1976

When it really happens, it's not funny, is it?

Don's story

It was 4.00am. Don had been dreaming. It was a nightmare. He was trying to get up – trying to escape from a huge brute of a man who was sitting on his chest. He woke and realised it was just a dream. Or was it? It felt as though an elephant was on his chest. The pain got more intense as he came to. It was a crushing, endless pain; he could hardly breathe.

Don woke his wife, June. She could see at once that he was ill – very ill. He was pale, almost grey, and beads of sweat were running down his face. She called an ambulance. Don felt sick. He was afraid. He couldn't stand the pain a moment longer. The ambulance was there in minutes. The paramedics were very efficient; they set up a drip, put Don on a monitor, and knew exactly what to do. Soon, Don was being wheeled on a trolley into the hospital. June waited anxiously outside the treatment room. Everyone was very busy. A doctor confirmed it was a heart attack and that they were doing everything they could. Then, more doctors in white coats ran into the treatment room.

Forty minutes later, a doctor came out and June feared the worst. The doctor's strained face broke into a faint smile. It had been a close call, but Don must be a fighter, the doctor explained. The following hours would be critical. They were going to move Don to the coronary care unit where he would be in the best possible hands.

Don went on to make a full recovery from his heart attack, but it took Don and June a long time to come to terms with what had happened. Don had always been so well before this; there had never been any hint of heart disease. This had come totally out of the blue.

Gradually, Don came to understand what had happened to him. He realised that, unless he made some changes, it was all too likely to happen again – perhaps with a more tragic outcome. He had heart disease, but he didn't want another heart attack.

June was a great support. She didn't just help Don change his lifestyle: she changed hers as well. At first she did this to encourage Don, but then she learnt that it was vital for her too; she learnt that far more women were dying of heart disease than of breast cancer. Not only that, she discovered to her surprise that eating and living better gave her a new vitality and made life more enjoyable.

*Don was heartened to find out that making the right changes could halt the progress of his heart disease and reduce his chances of another attack. He was delighted when he went on to discover a plan of action that could actually **undo** some damage – a plan to send heart disease into reverse!*

What is a heart attack and why does it happen?

A sudden, unexpected heart attack is one of the commonest ways that heart disease shows up. But, although the attack is sudden, the run-up to it has taken years.

Figure 1 shows a human heart. The heart is made of a marvellous muscle that just keeps pumping blood round the body, day in, day out (and even while the rest of you is asleep, of course). To do this marathon task, it needs a constant supply of blood itself.

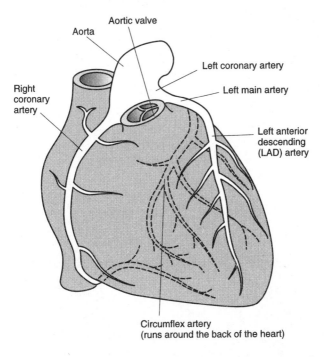

Figure 1 The human heart. The coronary arteries surround the heart muscle and send branches into the muscle, delivering blood containing oxygen. They start from the aorta, just above the aortic valve. Dotted lines indicate the arteries running around the back of the heart.

Blood is delivered to the heart muscle by the coronary arteries. In Western societies, because of our faulty diet and lifestyle, it is normal for arteries to become narrower as the years go by. The process starts in childhood.

This narrowing of arteries is the result of fatty, cholesterol-laden deposits (often called 'atheroma', which means 'porridge') forming on the smooth artery lining. The hardening ('sclerosis') of these fatty deposits of atheroma produces tough 'plaques' inside arteries. You can see why the gradual hardening and furring up of arteries is called 'atherosclerosis'.

Coronary atherosclerosis – the formation of fatty plaques in the heart's vital coronary arteries – builds up silently for years before it makes itself felt.

Figure 2 shows how atherosclerosis constricts the passage inside a coronary artery. Obviously, this reduces the rate at which blood can be delivered to the working heart muscle. Perhaps you remember Poiseuille's formula from your school physics, which indicated that the rate at which liquid flows in a tube depends on the fourth power of the radius – although it doesn't apply where there's turbulence. But if you neither remember nor care, suffice it to say that a little narrowing causes a huge increase in resistance to flow – a little constriction but a lot of friction.

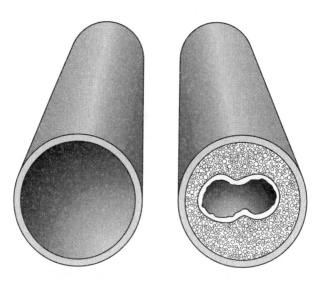

Figure 2 Build up of atheroma deposits in the arteries gradually blocks the flow of blood.

That's not all. And don't worry, we don't need any physics for this next bit. The craggy surface of an atherosclerotic plaque is liable to become damaged; when this happens, the damaged area is plugged by the smallest blood cells (platelets), setting off a clot (or thrombus). A small clot could merely add to the size of the plaque – accelerating the process of atherosclerosis. But a bigger clot can completely block the artery and this is called coronary thrombosis – one of the names for a heart attack.

Sudden blockage of a coronary artery is the immediate cause of a heart attack. This is normally the result of coronary thrombosis; occasionally a lump of clot or plaque may break off and move downstream until it lodges at a narrow section, causing a total obstruction.

Of course, the sudden blockage of a coronary artery means that the part of the heart muscle that was supplied by that artery is at once deprived of blood and oxygen. That hurts! But, because the heart is an internal organ, you don't feel the pain where the heart is; pain is referred, usually to the chest, but sometimes to the shoulder, arm, neck or jaw. Small heart attacks can be painless ('silent').

Muscle can't survive without blood and the affected area of heart muscle dies. If this is only a small area, the victim has a good chance of a full recovery; the damaged part heals with a small scar that doesn't interfere with the work of the heart. When more heart muscle is knocked off, it causes sudden death in some cases and, in others, an incomplete recovery because the heart has lost some pumping power.

So this is what a heart attack is: the death of a bit of heart muscle – big or small. As you know, we doctors don't like using simple words (in case our patients think we're simple too). Another name for heart muscle is 'myocardium' and another term for the death of a tissue deprived of blood is 'infarction'. So we prefer to call a heart attack a 'myocardial infarction' (MI).

Sometimes a heart attack is followed by an abnormal rhythm to the heartbeat (arrhythmia), or a cardiac arrest, in which the heart stops altogether.

What's angina?

You now understand how the narrowing of coronary arteries by atherosclerosis restricts the flow of oxygen-rich blood to the working heart muscle. If the heart muscle doesn't get enough oxygen to fuel the work it's doing, it hurts. This pain is called angina (sometimes 'angina pectoris', which means in the chest).

Angina, like the pain of a heart attack, is usually a heavy or tight pain but it's much less intense than most heart attacks. Mind you, the intensity of angina varies enormously from a dull ache to a severe pain 'like a vice round the chest' and some heart attacks are written off as 'indigestion'. Not surprisingly, because it's coming from the heart muscle, angina pain is felt in the same areas as the pain of a heart attack – typically across the front of the chest, but sometimes in the shoulder, arm or jaw. Of course, angina is the pain of unhappy heart muscle – not dying heart muscle.

The harder the heart is working, the more oxygen it needs, and angina is usually provoked by exercise and relieved by rest. It can also be brought on by strong emotions, eating a heavy meal, or going out on a cold day. Sometimes angina comes on for no apparent reason – when someone is sitting in a chair or lying in bed. Occasionally, spasm of the muscular wall in a coronary artery can be the trigger.

Are there different kinds of heart disease?

Yes. There are various forms of heart disease – some very rare, others not so rare. You can be born with faulty heart valves. Some older folk have damaged heart-valves because of rheumatic fever in childhood. Then there are several forms of cardiomyopathy, in which the heart muscle is abnormal.

But the only kind of heart disease most people need worry about is coronary heart disease, which causes heart attacks, sudden death, and angina. When people speak of 'heart disease', this is what they mean because everything else is uncommon by comparison. This is the epidemic that grips the Western world.

How can I escape the epidemic?

That's what this book is all about. Don's heart attack struck after years of silent atherosclerosis. You will learn how properly balanced nutrition, without deprivation, can put paid to that. But thrombosis is just as important; without that crucial clot, Don's heart attack would not have happened. It's not just a question of luck. You'll discover how the way you live and eat can stop those clots cropping up where they're not wanted. More remarkable still, you will find out how putting all parts of this plan into action can actually start unclogging arteries that have been clogging up for years – something doctors once took to be impossible.

And it goes well beyond your heart. When clogging and clots get to the arteries of the brain, rather than the coronary arteries, the result is a stroke. When the legs are affected, pain on walking (claudication), and even amputation, can follow. The plan in this book to help your coronary arteries will also benefit the arteries that supply your brain and your legs.

A healthy circulation is the lifeblood of a vital body. Looking after your arteries could give you a new lease of life.

◆ Heart attacks strike unexpectedly

◆ Arteries have been clogging up for years before a heart attack

◆ The narrowing and hardening of arteries is called atherosclerosis

◆ Atherosclerosis in coronary arteries reduces blood flow to heart muscle

◆ When the heart muscle goes short of blood, angina results

◆ A heart attack occurs when a blood clot (thrombosis) blocks a coronary artery

◆ This book reveals how to stop atherosclerosis and thrombosis

Chapter 2

Why do we get heart disease?

The epidemic

Almost a quarter of all deaths in the United Kingdom are caused by coronary heart disease. No other single disease claims so many of our lives. It kills about 130,000 Britons each year.

And yet, in rural areas of developing countries you would be hard pressed to find a single case of coronary heart disease; it is virtually unknown. But when groups of people adopt westernised diets and lifestyles, heart disease appears.

You don't have to live the life of a rural African to escape heart disease; in some industrialised countries it is much less of a problem than in the UK.

Why are some groups of people plagued by an epidemic of heart disease and others not? Why does one person die from a heart attack at 40 and another live to 95? Scientists investigating these questions have identified certain characteristics that increase your chances of getting heart disease. These characteristics are called 'risk factors'. Here are some important risk factors:

- High blood cholesterol;
- High blood pressure;
- Smoking;

- Diabetes;

- Being overweight;

- Lack of exercise.

Every one of these risk factors can be reduced or, in some cases, completely overcome. Here are some more:

- Age – the older you are, the greater the risk;

- Male sex – women are at lower risk before the menopause;

- Family history – heart disease in a close relative under 60.

These are risk factors you cannot change. (There is no evidence that a sex change will reduce your risk.)

In the Seven Countries Study (1980), Professor Ancel Keys investigated the diets and cholesterol levels of men aged between 40 and 59 from Japan, Greece, Yugoslavia, Italy, the Netherlands, the United States and Finland. The 111,579 men were studied for 15 years; during this time there had been 2288 deaths and there were big differences between the countries. Important findings were:

- Groups of people with low cholesterols had low rates of heart disease;

- High death rates were linked with high intakes of saturated fat;

- Low death rates were linked with consumption of olive oil.

Other studies around the world have confirmed that all groups of people with very low average cholesterol levels have low rates of heart disease.

The three most important risk factors for coronary heart disease are:

- Raised blood cholesterol;

- High blood pressure;

- Smoking.

But in South Japan, largely because of their diet, the average cholesterol level is very low. As a result, heart disease is rare even though smoking and high blood pressure are common. (Of course, smoking is still very damaging to the health of the Japanese smoker.) In this sense, raised cholesterol is the 'essential' risk factor; without this, a population is not plagued by heart disease even if other risk factors are present.

When the Japanese migrate and eat Western diets, their cholesterols rise and they start getting heart disease. So bang goes the theory that it's all down to genetics.

- ◆ Heart disease kills more Britons than any other single disease
- ◆ Third world countries are free of heart disease until they adopt Western ways
- ◆ Countries with low cholesterols have low rates of heart disease
- ◆ The top three risk factors are cholesterol, blood pressure, and smoking
- ◆ When the Japanese migrate and eat Western diets, they get heart disease
- ◆ 'Normal' UK cholesterols would be high in Japan

Does that mean I needn't bother if my cholesterol's OK?

No. In a country with a very low average cholesterol level, heart disease is uncommon. Assessing the risk in an individual person is different – especially an individual from a country plagued by heart disease. For a start, a 'normal' cholesterol level in the UK would be relatively high in, say, Japan. Also, as you read this book, you will learn about lots of ways that a good diet can protect you apart from bringing down your cholesterol level.

Your personal risk of heart disease is influenced enormously by other risk factors such as smoking and blood pressure. Your cholesterol level is of fundamental importance but you cannot judge your risk by looking at cholesterol on its own.

You cannot judge risk by cholesterol alone

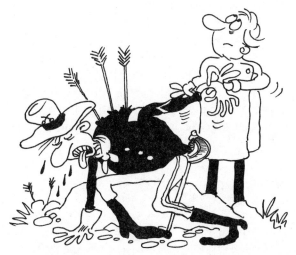

"That's odd ... his cholesterol was fine."

Chapter 3

Cholesterol and lipids explained

'. . . Explaining metaphysics to the nation –
I wish he would explain his explanation.'

Lord Byron (George Gordon, 6th Baron Byron), (1788–1824)
Don Juan, 1819–24 canto 1, dedication st. 2

What is cholesterol?

Cholesterol is a glistening white fatty or waxy substance. Chemically speaking, it is a sterol. It is found in people and animals but not in plants (so when the label on a vegetable margarine says, 'Contains no cholesterol', this is a statement of the obvious and would be equally true of any purely vegetable product).

We could not survive without a certain amount of cholesterol because we need it to make cell membranes and various hormones, as well as bile salts and vitamin D. But we don't need any in our food – otherwise vegans would be in trouble – because the body makes its own cholesterol.

What do you mean by 'lipids'?

'Lipids' is really a posh word for fats – and fat-like substances such as waxes. The key thing about lipids is that they cannot be dissolved in water; it takes an organic solvent, like dry-cleaning fluid, to shift that duck fat from your dinner jacket.

When a doctor talks about your lipids, he is referring to the levels of cholesterol and triglycerides in your blood. A triglyceride is a naturally occurring fat (formed by the combination of one molecule of glycerol with three fatty acid molecules). Most of the fat we eat is in the form of triglycerides and this is also the form in which fat is stored in our bodies.

Cholesterol on the move

Of course, cholesterol has to be transported in the bloodstream from where it is made (the liver and small intestine) to the places where it is needed. This presents the body with a problem; big lumps of fatty cholesterol, which don't mix with water, would soon gum up the works and bring the circulation to a standstill.

To get round this, lipids are carried in tiny particles called lipoproteins. These lipoproteins act like a detergent, surrounding minute globules of cholesterol with a wetting agent and preventing them from clumping together.

The good, the bad and the ugly

Having a high blood cholesterol level increases your risk of getting heart disease. But some of the cholesterol in the blood is not harmful at all. Cholesterol carried in high-density lipoprotein (HDL) is being taken away from body tissues, including artery walls, and back to the liver. In fact the higher your level of this HDL-cholesterol, the lower your risk of heart disease. That's why HDL-cholesterol is sometimes called 'the good cholesterol'.

Most of the blood cholesterol is carried by low-density lipoprotein (LDL). This LDL-cholesterol is being transported the other way – from the liver to other parts of the body. Having a high level of LDL-cholesterol in your blood increases your risk of heart disease because it leads to the formation of fatty deposits in arteries. No surprise, then, that LDL-cholesterol is often called 'the bad cholesterol'.

And the ugly? Believe me, the fatty lumps of atheroma that block up arteries and lead to heart attacks and strokes are very ugly. So, remember:

LOW-density lipoprotein (LDL) cholesterol should be LOW;
HIGH-density lipoprotein (HDL) cholesterol should be HIGH.

What should the total cholesterol level be?

In 1986, the American Multiple Risk Factor Intervention Trial (MR
FIT) studied over 361,000 men and showed that, throughout the
range 3.9–7.8 mmol/l, the higher the cholesterol level, the higher
the death rate from coronary heart disease.

Table 1 Serum cholesterol levels in England

Total cholesterol (mmol/l)	Men %	Women %
<5.2 (normal)	31	29
5.2–6.5	41	39
6.5–7.8	21	22
>7.8	7	10
mean	5.8	6.0 mmol/l

Data from *Health Survey for England*, 1994. © Crown copyright.

On this basis the lower your cholesterol, the better. The value of
5.2 mmol/l was chosen as the ideal maximum because above this
level the rise in heart disease becomes noticeably steeper (Figure 3).

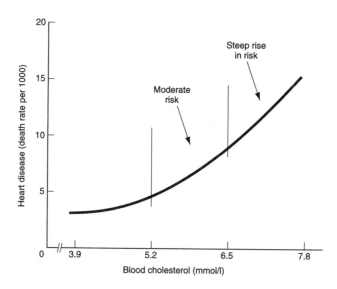

Figure 3 Cholesterol levels and death rates for coronary heart disease. The MR FIT study showed that, as cholesterol levels rose, so did the death rate. ©1996, The Lancet Ltd.

Dangerously low?

It's worth mentioning that in the MR FIT study the total mortality – deaths from all causes – began to rise again as the cholesterol level dropped below 4.14 mmol/l, even though deaths from heart disease continued to fall. Some other studies have shown the same trend. In fact, there is an increased incidence of cancer among groups with very low cholesterols.

This alarming observation naturally led to the fear that very low cholesterol levels might be dangerous. Don't worry. We now know that cancers can cause the low cholesterol level – not vice versa. Rapidly growing cancers use up cholesterol. In any study of several thousand people with very low cholesterol levels, inevitably some will already have cancer; this will increase the total mortality of the group. But a low cholesterol level cannot cause cancer. And, if you are lucky enough to find your cholesterol is very low, it is most unlikely to be due to cancer! As you would expect, people (such as the Chinese and Japanese) who have average cholesterol levels around 4 mmol/l do not have higher overall cancer rates than groups of people with higher cholesterols (even though different groups of people have more of one type of cancer and less of another).

There have been many studies demonstrating that when cholesterol levels are lowered, either by diet or by drugs, the rates of coronary heart disease fall. Some of these appeared to show extra deaths from other causes, including violence, among those treated with drugs. This was a niggling concern until recently but in the last few years several major trials using the drugs simvastatin and pravastatin have been published. In these, lowering cholesterol achieved big reductions both in coronary deaths and in deaths from all causes.

An important test of the drugs

The West of Scotland Coronary Prevention Study (WOSCOPS) published in 1995 included 6595 men aged 45–64 with raised cholesterol levels (average 7.0 mmol/l) but no past history of a heart attack. Each man was randomly allocated to one or the other of two groups (just as if a coin had been tossed). Half the men were given the cholesterol-lowering drug pravastatin and the other half were given placebo (dummy) tablets so that neither the men nor their doctors knew who was taking the active drug and who wasn't until the code was broken at the end of the five-year trial. (This 'randomised, placebo-controlled, double-blind' design is a standard way of eliminating bias in clinical trials.)

Giving pravastatin for five years had reduced the risk of:

- Heart attack by 31%;

- Death from any cause by 22%.

◆ A 'fasting lipid' test measures your cholesterol and triglycerides

◆ LDL-cholesterol can clog arteries; the level should be low

◆ HDL-cholesterol is moving away from artery walls; the level should be high

◆ As the total cholesterol level rises, so does the risk of heart disease

◆ Most people in the UK have a raised cholesterol; the average is 5.9 mmol/l

◆ A total cholesterol of 5.0 mmol/l or less is recommended

◆ A cholesterol level of 4 mmol/l would be better still

Should we all be taking a drug, then?

After all, the majority of people in the UK have blood cholesterols above the recommended level – and even further above the Japanese average. Wouldn't it make sense to put everyone on a drug like pravastatin if it could cut down heart attacks by one-third?

OK, it costs a few hundred pounds a year to keep one person on pravastatin 40 mg daily (the dose used in WOSCOPS). And you'd have to treat something like 110 people for five years before you saved one life. But how do you value a human life?

Convinced? Personally, I think there is something quite obscene about the idea of drugging the population en masse to try to prevent a disease that results from poor diet and lifestyle. (But if you already have heart disease, there may be a very strong case for using pravastatin or a similar drug; this is discussed in Chapter 25.)

I would much rather reduce my risk of heart disease by enjoying the rich variety of a healthy diet than try to offset the damage of a poor, unbalanced diet with drugs. Wouldn't you? If so, read on.

Food

'Food is an important part of a balanced diet.'

Fran Lebowitz,
Metropolitan Life, 1978

"I'd rather die young than live on a diet of lettuce and boiled fish," you say. Who wouldn't? In any case, you would probably die prematurely from boredom and malnutrition on such a diet. We are designed to enjoy our food, so how can a boring diet be really healthy? And yet, so many health promotion messages are negative: "Don't eat this"; "You mustn't have that". You could be forgiven for thinking that if you enjoy it, it must be bad for you. Not so!

There is a great abundance and variety of enjoyable foods, which will help you to ward off ageing processes and maintain a healthy heart and circulation, so why leave room for unhelpful foods?

It is confusing when experts disagree with each other about the healthy diet and keep changing their minds. Now we are told to eat less salt. Next week it may be pepper!

Well I quite understand how newspaper headlines can give this impression. I am looking at one which says 'Sunday Roast is Healthier than a Salad'. There is nothing in the article to justify this eye-catching headline even if a Greek salad and garlic bread may contain more fat than some English dishes. And here's a newspaper report that claims that 'there is as much protection against heart disease in a piece of milk chocolate as in a glass of red wine'. How many readers settled down to a winter of red wine and chocolate in a new health drive? The advice seems to change daily.

'Journalism largely consists in saying "Lord Jones Dead" to people who never knew Lord Jones was alive.'

G. K. Chesterton,
The Wisdom of Father Brown, 1914

Chlamydia: beastly bug or red herring?

You may have seen newspaper reports suggesting that, at last, the real cause of heart disease has been found – infection with Chlamydia. Chlamydia belong to a group of microscopic organisms that can't really decide whether to be viruses or bacteria. Strains of *Chlamydia trachomatis* have earned the group a bad name by causing sexually transmitted diseases and eye infections.

For some years medical scientists have been looking at a possible link between another member of the family (*Chlamydia pneumoniae*) and heart disease. Also, a bacterium known to cause duodenal ulcers (*Helicobacter pylori*) has attracted some scientific limelight after Mendall and colleagues reported a connection with coronary disease in 1994. Such theories are quite difficult to sort out as half the population have Helicobacter infection anyway – usually with no symptoms.

It could well be that the mild inflammation resulting from years of infection with these bugs triggers increased risk factors for coronary heart disease. On the other hand, it could be that social conditions (since childhood) increase the risk of infection **and** of heart disease. A study by Wald and colleagues, published in the *British Medical Journal* in 1997, was designed to minimise the effect that social differences might have on the result; no link was found between Helicobacter infection and death from coronary heart disease.

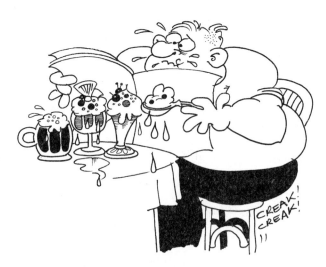

"I see they've found the bug that causes heart disease."

Back to fact

In fact, there is an overwhelming consensus about healthy eating, which is founded on firm evidence. In this book, we will be dealing with scientific evidence – not dreary dogma and not gimmicks. You will discover how to apply the evidence – how to make changes that will enrich your life and protect your heart.

No doubt you have heard that we should eat less fat, sugar and salt but more fibre. Put like that it sounds rather negative: cut down three tasty things and increase one boring one. It doesn't help if your image of fibre is a bowl of bran.

The reality of healthy eating is quite different. We can translate nutritional wisdom into everyday eating that is far more enjoyable and satisfying than the average British diet. First, we need to know more about what our food is made of.

The nutrients in our food can be divided into these important categories:

1. protein;
2. fat;
3. carbohydrate;
4. vitamins and minerals.

Protein

When it comes to dietary influence on coronary risk, fat and carbohydrate lie at the heart of the matter and they get chapters all of their own. What little we need to say about protein can be said right here.

Much of our body is made of protein and we need a regular supply in our food for the growth and repair of body tissues. The average UK diet contains more than enough.

Proteins are large molecules constructed from hundreds or thousands of small units called amino acids. Each amino acid consists of carbon, hydrogen, oxygen and nitrogen. When protein is digested in the intestine, it is broken down into amino acids again and these are absorbed into the bloodstream and used to make new proteins for the body's maintenance and construction programme.

Some of the amino acids are called 'essential' because the body is unable to make them; they must be supplied in the diet. Proteins that contain adequate quantities of all the essential amino acids are known as 'high biological value' (HBV) proteins. Those deficient in one or more essential amino acids are termed 'low biological value' (LBV) proteins.

Animal foods (meat, poultry, fish, dairy products, eggs) provide HBV protein while many plant foods contain LBV protein. Amino acids lacking in one plant will be present in another and, provided complementary foods are combined (such as pulses with grains), even a vegan need not go short of any amino acids.

◆ There is strong evidence for the importance of good food in preventing heart disease

◆ A good diet is *not* a boring diet

◆ The secret of success lies in the balance of nutrients

◆ To begin with, fat and carbohydrate must be balanced

Chapter 4

Fat

A fatuous phrase

If you need to lower your blood cholesterol level, the doctor advises a 'low-cholesterol diet', right? Wrong! Well, some doctors have been heard to use that fatuous phrase.

Many people imagine that the main change you should make if your cholesterol is too high is to eat less cholesterol. In fact, if it were possible merely to eat less cholesterol, it would achieve very little, but a 'cholesterol-lowering diet' is far more to the point. For a start, eating less saturated fat can make a big difference to the amount of cholesterol in your blood.

- ◆ Just eating less cholesterol makes little difference
- ◆ Eating less saturated fat lowers blood cholesterol
- ◆ The high fat content of UK diets increases heart disease and cancer
- ◆ Heart attacks are caused by atherosclerosis and thrombosis; saturated fats increase both

---

Get your fats straight

Fats in our food are made up of various 'fatty acids'. These fatty acids are divided into three main groups according to their chemical structure as shown in Table 2.

27

Table 2 Types of fatty acids and their sources

Saturated fatty acids (SFA, saturates)	The molecule has no room for any more hydrogen atoms. It is SATURATED with hydrogen	Lauric	Coconut oil, palm kernel oil
		Myristic	Coconut oil, dairy products
		Palmitic	Palm oil, dairy products, meats
		Stearic	Cocoa butter, meats
Mono-unsaturated fatty acids (MUFA, mono-unsaturates)	There is only ONE area of the molecule that is not saturated with hydrogen atoms	Oleic	Olive oil, rapeseed oil, meat, fish
Polyunsaturated fatty acids (PUFA, polyunsaturates)	There is MORE THAN ONE area of the molecule with room for extra hydrogen	Linoleic	Corn oil, sunflower oil, soya bean oil
		Linolenic	Linseed oil
		Eicosapentaenoic	Fish
		Docosahexaenoic	Fish

Now if all this detail about fat seems a bit heavy, don't worry. It's like that when you're dealing with fat; it does seem a bit heavy at first (but don't forget it actually floats on water). This is just necessary preparation before we lift off. The book gets easier to read as we go along – honestly.

Table 2 shows some fatty acids that you gulp down every day, without even a thought for their names. As you see, some of the names give you a clue as to where you'd find the fatty acid.

Animal, vegetable or mineral?

You will often hear that saturated fat comes from animals while the polyunsaturated and mono-unsaturated fats come from vegetable sources. I don't want to make life complicated, but this really is too simple. There are some very important exceptions. Palm oil and coconut oil contain a lot of saturated fatty acids (Table 3). So, when a food label lists 'vegetable oil' as an ingredient, beware! This could

Table 3 Fatty acid content of fats and oils

Oil/fat	Total fat (g/100 g)	Saturates (g/100 g)	Mono-unsaturates (g/100 g)	Polyunsaturates (g/100 g)
Oils				
Coconut oil	99.9	85.2	6.6	1.7
Corn oil	99.9	12.7	24.7	57.8
Olive oil	99.9	14.0	69.7	11.2
Palm oil	99.9	45.3	41.6	8.3
Peanut oil	99.9	18.8	47.8	28.5
Rapeseed oil (low erucic acid)	99.9	6.6	57.2	31.5
Safflower oil	99.9	10.2	12.6	72.1
Sesame oil	99.7	14.2	37.3	43.9
Soya oil	99.9	14.5	23.2	56.5
Sunflower seed oil	99.9	11.9	20.2	63.0
Spreading fats				
Butter	81.7	54.0	19.8	2.6
Low-fat spread	40.5	11.2	17.6	9.9
Margarine: Hard, animal and vegetable fat	81.6	30.4	36.5	10.8
Hard, vegetable fat only	81.6	35.9	33.0	9.4
Polyunsaturated	81.6	16.2	20.6	41.1
Olive/rapeseed oil reduced-fat spread	59.0	13.5	32.3	10.4
Very low-fat spread	25.0	6.5	13.5	3.5
Other fats				
Dripping, beef	99.0	54.8	36.7	2.5
Lard	99.0	40.8	43.8	9.6
Suet, shredded	86.7	48.0	32.1	2.1
Ghee (clarified butter)	99.8	66.0	24.1	3.4

Data from *McCance and Widdowson's The Composition of Foods*, 5th edition, Holland *et al.*, 1991, © Crown copyright. (with additional manufacturer's data)

The fatty acid content of oils depends on the variety and maturity of the seed as well as growing conditions. The fatty acids listed do not account for 100% of the weight of a fat; triglyceride fats have a glycerol component as well. You should also note that this table does not show trans fatty acids.

mean anything from highly desirable olive oil (70% mono-unsaturates) to unhelpful coconut oil (85% saturates). If it were olive oil, the label would probably say so. On the other hand, you may find that a bottle labelled 'vegetable oil' contains pure rapeseed oil – or a blend of soya, rapeseed and corn oils. You do need to know what you're getting.

However shaky your biology, you probably realise that fish are animals, not plants, but oily fish are a rich source of the special polyunsaturated fatty acids, eicosapentaenoic acid (EPA) and docosa-hexaenoic acid (DHA). They don't roll off the tongue but they can be a joy to eat and we'll learn more about them in Chapter 7.

More fat please. We're British

'If you want to eat well in England, eat three breakfasts.'

W. Somerset Maugham

Most people in the UK are eating far too much fat. If you don't want to be swallowed up in the epidemic of heart disease, your fat intake should be well below average.

In a typical UK diet, about 40% of the calories come from fat. The Department of Health's expert committee (COMA), reporting in 1994, recommended that this be reduced to 35%. The reduction was to be made by cutting down *saturated fat*. COMA reports in 1991 and 1994 set a target of 10% of calories for people's saturated fat intake (a significant reduction on the actual average of 16%).

Don't get confused here. You might be thinking, "I don't eat any-thing like 40% fat!" Having 40% of your calories as fat does **not** mean that 40% of the weight of your food is fat. Fat is 'energy-dense': a little fat gives a lot of energy. Much of the fat we eat is hidden in processed foods. Meals with no visible fat can push you above the 35% mark in no time. Needless to say, when fat is obvious (as in greasy sausages and chips, pork crackling or cream cakes) your fat intake can shoot beyond the 40% level – and a lot of that will be saturated fat.

Slashing saturated fat is the cornerstone of the cholesterol-lower-ing diet because the body lowers blood levels of the harmful choles-terol (LDL-cholesterol) when it receives less saturated fat.

It has become clear that the different saturated fatty acids in our food don't all have an equal effect when it comes to raising choles-terol. In fact, stearic acid doesn't seem to raise it at all.

Before you search your cookery books in vain for stew of stearic acid, remember the importance of thrombosis – clot production. Coronary arteries get clogged up because of two disastrous processes: atherosclerosis **and** thrombosis. Fatty deposits of atheroma stick to artery walls when the blood cholesterol concentration is too high. Well, what sets off thrombosis? You'll discover more answers to that later in the book but we now know that some saturated fatty acids make thrombosis much more likely. Even though stearic acid doesn't raise cholesterol, it does raise the risk of thrombosis.

In 1991, Professors Ulbricht and Southgate published a paper in the *Lancet*, drawing attention to the fact that some fatty acids increased atheroma while others triggered thrombosis. They proposed a league table of 'atherogenicity' and 'thrombogenicity'.

It seems that myristic acid and lauric acid are particularly 'atherogenic' because they push up LDL-cholesterol levels. In addition, myristic acid, like stearic acid, makes thrombosis more likely.

So, even though stearic acid doesn't raise cholesterol, steer clear of stearic and give myristic a miss!

How? That's a very good question. You won't find them in your recipe books or on a restaurant menu. Advice to avoid this or that fatty acid isn't much help, is it?

Some saturated fatty acids raise cholesterol levels while others are worse at causing thrombosis. And food contains a mixture of different fatty acids. So the only practical course is to cut down on all foods with a high saturated fatty acid content.

- ◆ A 'low-fat spread' containing 40% fat is still a very high-fat food
- ◆ A healthy diet does not mean lots of sunflower margarine or spread
- ◆ Too much polyunsaturated fat could be harmful; it lowers good as well as bad cholesterol

---

A fat lot of good

To meet legal requirements, something labelled 'butter' or 'margarine' will contain a standard amount of fat (about 81 g/100 g) but there are important differences in the types of fat used. A 'low-fat spread' containing 40% fat (40 g/100 g) is still a very high-fat food.

Many people have got the message that a healthy diet means eating sunflower margarine – or reduced-fat spread. Certainly, changing from butter to a low-fat spread high in polyunsaturates is a good idea. Replacing saturated fat with polyunsaturates helps to lower blood cholesterol. This does not mean, as some people seem to think, that polyunsaturated fat is so good for you that you should have as much as possible!

Increasing your intake of linoleic acid (that's the polyunsaturated fatty acid in sunflower, safflower, soya bean and corn oils) can help to lower the blood cholesterol level. Unfortunately, as well as bringing down the **total** blood cholesterol, large amounts of polyunsaturated fat also tend to reduce the helpful cholesterol (HDL-cholesterol). In addition, there is some concern that overdosing on polyunsaturates could be harmful in other ways, such as increasing the process of oxidation, which could put more fatty deposits in arteries. The real problem is that we do not know of any natural population that uses linoleic acid extensively, so we cannot be certain how safe it is to use it as a major source of energy. The 1991 Government guidelines recommended that polyunsaturated fatty acids should contribute 6% of the total calorie intake. Sparing use of a low-fat sunflower spread is no problem at all.

A lot of good fat

'. . . and you can enjoy the fat of the land.'
***

Genesis 45:18,
New International Version

Studies carried out in the 1950s and 1960s showed that cholesterol levels fell when saturated fat in the diet was replaced with mono-unsaturated fat (mainly oleic acid in olive or rapeseed oils). Simply adding oleic acid to the diet without reducing saturated fat did not lower cholesterol. It was concluded that mono-unsaturated fatty acids had a neutral effect on cholesterol levels.

Some more recent studies have shown active cholesterol reduction by mono-unsaturates equal to that of polyunsaturates. (These studies have generally used 'liquid formula' diets and there is a debate about how much the mono-unsaturates in natural diets can lower cholesterol.) However, when saturates in the diet are replaced by mono-unsaturates, the total blood cholesterol level falls without the damaging reduction in HDL- cholesterol caused by polyunsaturates. This may partly explain why the Mediterranean diet is associated with low rates of heart disease. In addition, olive oil and rapeseed oil (in small quantities) can help to protect against thrombosis. The 1991 COMA report recommended that we obtain 12% of our energy from mono-unsaturated fatty acids, but the 1994 report did not give a figure.

ACTION POINTS

◆ Beware 'vegetable oil'! It could contain lots of saturated fat

◆ Cut down on all foods with a high content of saturates

◆ Avoid hard margarines; they contain lots of trans fatty acids

◆ Avoid foods with 'hydrogenated vegetable oil' – especially when it's near the top of the ingredients list

What about 'trans fatty acids'?

I have already mentioned sunflower spread and there are also palatable spreads containing high levels of mono-unsaturates – no doubt excellent choices if you must spread fat on your food. In addition to the olive oil suggested by their name, these spreads are likely to be derived from rapeseed oil; in fact rapeseed oil is usually the main ingredient. But a word of caution: although lower in fat, in some ways a margarine (or reduced-fat spread) may not be as good for you as the oil from which it is made. Changing the oil from a liquid into a spread involves 'hydrogenation' – adding hydrogen atoms to some of those spare places on the fatty acid molecules. 'Hydrogenated vegetable oil' is a term you will often see on food labelling; you should regard it as similar to saturated fat and keep your intake to a minimum.

Another important point about this process of hydrogenation is that it results in some **trans fatty acids**. Now a trans fatty acid is a chemical variant of the more natural form of the fatty acid molecule.

The natural form of the molecule is called cis, but the trans version has part of its structure twisted round to produce a different shape (see page 34). Think of a trans molecule as someone with the lower half of his body twisted round until his bottom faces forwards. Obviously, he'd have to put on his underpants and trousers back to front (not so much transvestite as TRANS-pants-SITE).

You can see the problems that this unnatural arrangement might cause in the everyday life of a fatty acid, and a little metabolic mayhem would not be surprising. He couldn't sit next to cis to watch TV and would probably end up standing; trans fatty acids are straight but the natural, cis molecule is bent at the double bond.

The percentage of saturated and trans fatty acids in a hard margarine is likely to be much higher than in a soft margarine or spread. A margarine made from hardened vegetable fats might contain 15% trans fatty acids compared with only 0.7% in a low-fat sunflower spread.

There is mounting evidence that high levels of artificially produced trans fatty acids in the diet are harmful. Several studies have shown that when people eat more trans fatty acids, LDL-cholesterol goes up and HDL-cholesterol goes down – a very undesirable combination. To make matters worse, they increase the risk of thrombosis. In 1993, Willett and colleagues reported findings from the Nurses Health

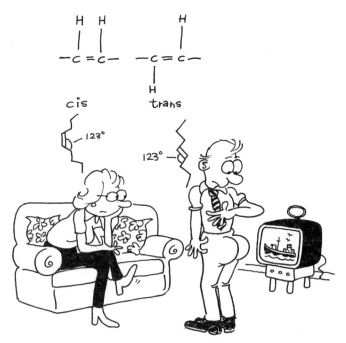

cis and trans isomers of an unsaturated fatty acid.

Study, which involved 85,000 women. The women who ate more trans fatty acids were more likely to have heart disease. Less than 2% of your calories should come from this type of fat, so watch those processed cakes and biscuits as well as margarines (Table 4).

Table 4 Recommendations of COMA report (1991)

Type of fatty acid	Contribution to total dietary energy
Saturated	10%
Mono-unsaturated	12%
Polyunsaturated	6%
Trans	less than 2%

What are 'essential fatty acids'?

Most people in the UK eat far too much fat but we all need some. A completely fat-free diet would be virtually impossible to achieve, but also very dangerous. Linoleic acid (from the omega-6 fat family) and alpha-linolenic acid (from the omega-3 family) are called 'essential' because the body cannot make them from other fatty acids. If you follow the guidelines in this book – and make sure your diet includes enough cereal grains (for omega-6 fats) and fish (for omega-3 fats) – you will have all the fatty acids you need. If you are a vegan, seeds, nuts and cooking oils are important sources; it is helpful to use olive oil, or rapeseed oil (rather than sunflower, safflower or corn oil) to reduce the proportion of linoleic acid in your fat intake. (Vegans sometimes get as much as 60% of their fat in the form of linoleic acid and at this level it can interfere with the body's ability to make the 'fish oil' docosahexaenoic acid, which is not included in the vegan diet.)

If it's 'good fat', can I have as much as I want?

The 1994 COMA report specifically considered diet and cardiovascular disease (diseases of the heart and circulation). It recommended replacement of fats rich in saturates with those rich in mono-unsaturates, as long as the total fat intake does not provide more than 35% of calories. The committee recommended increased consumption of fish, vegetables, fruit, potatoes and bread.

The **total** amount of fat in your diet (saturates, polyunsaturates, and mono-unsaturates) – and not just the **type** – makes a difference to your risk of heart disease (not to mention your weight). Dr Miller and colleagues have found that higher-fat diets increase the risk of blood clots by affecting the activity of an important clotting factor (factor VII). Indeed, it seems that even one very high-fat meal increases the risk of thrombosis – so it's not just a question of your average intake over the week.

For convenience, we often talk of eating less 'saturated fat', but do remember that all fats in our diet are a mixture of different fatty acids (see Table 3). What we need to do is to select foods that have a very low content of saturated fatty acids.

◆ Trans fatty acids raise harmful cholesterol, lower helpful cholesterol and increase the risk of thrombosis

◆ A balanced diet, including cereal grains, seeds, nuts and fish, contains the fatty acids you need – even without adding cooking oils or fat spreads

◆ If you are a vegan, use olive oil or rapeseed oil

◆ 'Friendly fat' is found in olive oil, rapeseed oil, some nuts, avocados and fish

◆ Eating *too much* fat, even if it isn't saturated, increases thrombosis risk

Fat chance of enjoying a healthy meal then?

How can I enjoy my food if I'm worrying about the percentage of saturated fat in it? Don't worry. Once you've learnt a few basic principles, you will find it easier and easier to select low-fat foods that provide the foundation of your low-fat diet. Be more relaxed about good sources of mono-unsaturated fatty acids (e.g. olive oil, rapeseed oil, hazelnuts, almonds, avocados) and include some oily fish (e.g. sardines, pilchards, mackerel, herring, salmon). This approach will provide the right balance of fats and soon becomes second nature.

To learn those principles, let's look at the major sources of fat in our food.

Dairy products

Milk

'Things are seldom what they seem,
Skim milk masquerades as cream.'

Sir W.S. Gilbert, *H.M.S. Pinafore*, 1878

Milk is an excellent source of important nutrients like protein, calcium and vitamins but it also makes a big contribution to the nation's saturated fat intake. Whole, fresh milk is about 4% fat, two-thirds of which is saturated. This may not sound very much but you must consider the quantity of a food you consume as well as the percentage of fat it contains. If you used milk like a condiment – just sprinkling a few drops on your dinner – the amount of fat would be insignificant but a pint a day is a different matter.

The answer is to use skimmed or semi-skimmed milk. I thoroughly recommend skimmed milk (but not for children under five). This provides all the protein and calcium of whole milk but virtually no fat at all. Yes, it does taste different, but most people soon get used to this if they give themselves a chance. If you really feel you cannot adapt to skimmed milk, semi-skimmed will give you half the fat of whole milk. (Remember: too many compromises will undermine your efforts to make an impact on heart disease risk.) Even then, I recommend skimmed milk for cooking (including sauces and custard) because the chances are that you won't notice the difference in taste.

Another great advantage of fully skimmed milk is that you can buy it in powder form. Provided you reconstitute it in advance (by mixing with water in a pint jug and leaving it in the refrigerator until it is cold) you would never know it hadn't come from a bottle. I hate the thought of making the milkman redundant, but it is a great convenience to stockpile skimmed milk powder when it is on special offer in the supermarket; you need never run out of milk and you don't have to remember to cancel the milk when you go on holiday.

ACTION POINT

◆ Use skimmed milk. It contains all the goodness of whole milk – without the fat

Cream

Cream is no help to you at all when it comes to eating a low-saturated fat diet (Table 5).

Table 5 Fat content of creams

Type of cream	Total fat content
Single	19%
Whipping	39%
Double	48%

Two-thirds of the fat in cream is saturated. It is best to exclude cream completely from your regular diet, then you can feel free to enjoy it on that special occasion. (Special occasions arise occasionally – not every weekend.)

Low-fat yoghurt (e.g. 1% fat) and very low-fat yoghurt (e.g. 0.1% fat) are good substitutes if you enjoy them, but they are not to everyone's taste. Greek yoghurt has a much creamier flavour but, being 7–9% fat, should be used sparingly. (Fat-free versions are now available but the creamy flavour is reduced accordingly.) Cows 'strained' Greek yoghurt is about 9% fat, whereas the 'set' variety is only 4% fat. Typically, a 'set' sheep yoghurt would be 7.5% fat.

Fromage frais (8% fat) and virtually fat-free fromage frais (0.1% fat) are acceptable substitutes for cream. I particularly recommend vanilla-flavoured virtually fat-free fromage frais. (Try saying this five times quickly. Good: now you're ready to ask for some when it doesn't appear on the supermarket shelf.) If you have this instead of cream with strawberries on a summer's day, you won't feel deprived at all. If nothing but cream will do, at least dispensing it from a spray can bulks out the fat with a bit of air.

Be wary of cream substitutes based on vegetable oil, as they may still contain a lot of saturated fat.

- ◆ Virtually fat-free fromage frais is a useful alternative to cream; 'synthetic cream' is not
- ◆ Cottage cheese is a low-fat food. Half-fat cheddar is still a fatty food

Cheese

'Poets have been mysteriously silent on the subject of cheese.'

G.K. Chesterton

Like cream, most cheeses have a high fat content, two-thirds of which is saturated (Table 6).

Table 6 Fat content of cheeses

Variety of cheese	Typical fat content
Brie	27%
Camembert	23%
Cheddar	34%
Cheddar – reduced fat	15%
Cottage cheese	4%
Cottage cheese – reduced fat	1.5%
Parmesan	33%
Pecorino	33%

Clearly, cottage cheese is an exception to the general rule and is a genuinely low-fat cheese (although two-thirds of the fat is still saturated). Be careful about 'lower fat' or 'reduced fat' cheeses because, while they will contain less fat than the traditional version, they are still likely to be high-fat foods and you need to read the nutritional information carefully.

Quark (typically 0.2% fat) is a soft white cheese and you can use it freely. I wouldn't want to eat it by the lump as if it were delicious boursin. You could spread it on bread instead of butter when making savoury sandwiches but it is especially useful when cooking a whole variety of recipes that call for cream cheese or even cream.

Parmesan and pecorino are useful cheeses because they have a high flavour-to-fat ratio. Small quantities grated into a dish will add a lot of flavour and not much fat.

So, don't stint on dairy products. Skimmed milk and a variety of products with a similar fat content (e.g. buttermilk, very low-fat yoghurt, virtually fat-free fromage frais, quark) are invaluable to the cook. They contain all the calcium and protein of full-fat products –

without the fat. When you discard the fat, some fat-soluble vitamins go with it, but skimmed milk powder is fortified with vitamins A and D.

ACTION POINTS

◆ Save cream for really special occasions

◆ Use: virtually fat-free fromage frais, very low-fat yoghurts, quark and buttermilk

---

Meat and meat products

This group of foods is a rich source of protein but also of fat – much of it saturated. British cuisine places too much emphasis on meat. A mound of flesh dominates the plate while one or two demoralised vegetables pay homage at the margin. Six ounces of meat or poultry a day is a sensible limit and, of course, it is quite possible to be a healthy vegetarian.

Red meat

'The fat was so white, and the lean was so ruddy.'

Oliver Goldsmith (1728–1774),
The Haunch of Venison, 4

If you want to include red meat in your diet, buy lean cuts and trim off all visible fat. Typically, roast shoulder of lamb would be over 25% fat, while roast lean topside of beef would be less than 5% fat (Table 7).

As well as trimming fat before cooking, it is often worth draining or skimming off fat during or after cooking. Minced meat can conceal a lot of fat. Buy the leanest mince you can get or, better still, select lean meat and ask the butcher to mince it. Even then, browning the mince in a non-stick pan, transferring it to a sieve, and drying it with paper kitchen towelling before proceeding with the recipe will get rid of a lot of redundant fat. Another approach is to refrigerate a finished dish and carefully remove all the hardened fat from the surface before re-heating.

So remember: SLIM, TRIM, and SKIM. Select SLIM meat; TRIM before cooking; SKIM after cooking.

Table 7 Fat content of meat and meat products

Meat	Total fat (g/100 g)	Saturates (g/100 g)	Mono-unsaturates (g/100 g)	Polyunsaturates (g/100 g)
Beef				
Brisket (boiled)	23.9	9.5	11.8	0.5
Rump steak (grilled)	12.1	5.2	5.8	0.5
Topside (roast)	12.0	4.1	6.4	0.7
Topside (roast) lean only	4.4	1.4	2.2	0.2
Lamb				
Breast (roast)	37.1	18.4	14.3	1.8
Leg (roast)	17.9	8.9	6.9	0.9
Leg (roast) lean only	8.1	3.9	3.0	0.4
Shoulder (roast)	26.3	13.1	10.2	1.3
Shoulder (roast) lean only	11.2	5.4	4.2	0.5
Pork				
Belly rashers (grilled)	34.8	12.9	14.1	5.2
Chop (grilled)	24.2	9.0	9.8	3.6
Leg (roast)	19.8	7.3	8.0	3.0
Leg (roast) lean only	6.9	2.4	2.7	1.0
Chicken				
Meat and skin (roast)	14.0	4.2	6.5	2.5
Meat only (roast)	5.4	1.6	2.5	1.0
Light meat (roast)	4.0	1.2	1.9	0.7
Dark meat (roast)	6.9	2.1	3.2	1.2
Duck				
Meat, fat and skin (roast)	29.0	7.9	15.7	3.5
Meat only (roast)	9.7	2.7	5.3	1.2
Turkey				
Meat and skin (roast)	6.5	2.1	2.7	1.3
Meat only (roast)	2.7	0.9	1.1	0.5
Light meat (roast)	1.4	0.4	0.6	0.3
Dark meat (roast)	4.1	1.3	1.7	0.8
Meat products				
Pork sausages (grilled)	24.6	9.5	11.0	2.7
Pork pie	27.0	10.2	12.5	2.7
Cornish pastie	20.4	8.9	8.7	2.2

Data from *McCance and Widdowson's The Composition of Foods*, 5th edition, Holland *et al.*, 1991, © Crown copyright.

Game

Game (for example venison, rabbit and pheasant) is generally less fatty than farm animals – the four-legged ones, anyway.

Poultry

> 'Long as there is chicken and gravy on your rice
> Ev'rything is nice.'
> ———————————
>
> Johnny Mercer,
> 'Lazybones', 1932

Properly prepared, chicken and turkey can make a delicious contribution to a low-fat diet. Remove the skin and any visible fat (otherwise the fat content may be trebled). For many recipes, it is convenient to buy skinless chicken breasts (e.g. 2.2% fat) or skinless turkey breasts (e.g. 1.1% fat). Thigh meat has a higher fat content (typically 3.5% for turkey thigh).

Extra lean turkey mince is an excellent, lower-fat alternative to minced beef in anything from burgers to bolognese.

You can even buy smoked turkey rashers which taste just like bacon but are only 1% fat. Do yourself some good with a cooked breakfast – turkey rashers, mushrooms and tomatoes cooked in a tiny amount of olive oil or rapeseed oil. But you do need to ration those rashers on account of their salt content.

Meat products

Beware unidentified frying objects. What's in a sausage? For a start, it's unlikely to be packed with lean meat when a bit of cheap fat makes the filling go so much further. In fact, sausages, salami, and samosas, pies, pâtés, and pasties are all disastrously loaded with fat. If you can't identify it, best not buy it.

Meat substitutes

Tofu, or soya bean curd, is widely used in Japanese cuisine. If you have never met it, you are probably rather wary but, once you have become acquainted, you will find it a very versatile alternative to meat or dairy products. Using soya protein in place of animal protein helps to lower the total blood cholesterol and LDL-cholesterol. Their large intake of soya, and various other vegetables and grains, may help to

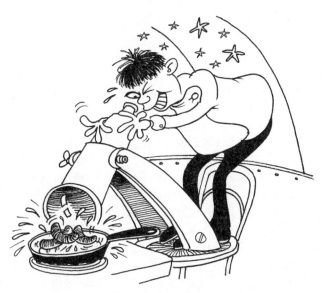

Beware unidentified frying objects.

explain why oriental men have such low rates of prostate cancer (until they change to Western diets).

Unlike most plant proteins, the protein from soya beans contains all the essential amino acids – making it a very good meat substitute from the nutritional point of view. Even if you dislike great lumps of soya masquerading as meat, you will probably find one or two packs of soya mince invaluable when you want to knock up a quick 'chilli con carne' – without the meat.

Quorn is a low-fat, high-protein meat substitute made from a fungus (like mushroom) and egg white. It has a chicken-like texture and will take on the flavour of any sauce in which it is cooked.

Of course, you can always compromise by using meat substitutes together with meat as a way of reducing the fat content of a dish.

ACTION POINTS

◆ Avoid processed meat products (such as sausages, salami, meat pies and pâté). They contain lots of saturated fat

◆ Quorn, tofu and soya mince can be used with meat to reduce the fat content of a dish

Fats and oils

Of all the fatty foods in our diet, this group is the fattiest. After all, any cooking oil will be 100% fat. The term 'oil' merely indicates that it is a liquid at room temperature. Adding large quantities of pure fat to your food will not help you to achieve a low-fat diet so these products should always be used as sparingly as possible.

Often, when a traditional recipe calls for added fat, you can leave the fat out altogether with very satisfactory results. For example, when making a white sauce you can simply use cornflour with skimmed milk instead of making a roux with butter and flour. Bland? Don't forget your white sauce is normally destined for greater things. It may be the basis of a brandy sauce to accompany your Christmas pudding (see Chapter 27). Believe me, by the time you've added some sugar and plenty of brandy (or white rum), you won't miss the fat at all.

On other occasions, a little fat makes all the difference – when roasting potatoes, for example. You could produce an ultra low-fat version by cooking in vegetable stock. I much prefer to toss the par-boiled potatoes in a little pre-heated olive oil or rapeseed oil and roast them in a very hot oven until crisp and golden. The result is exquisite and will do you nothing but good.

You will note that I do not suggest using a little lard! Choose an oil with a high content of mono-unsaturated fatty acids and a low content of saturates. Olive oil meets the criteria, being about 70% mono-unsaturates and 14% saturates. It is a good first choice because of its track record: Mediterranean countries, with olive oil at the heart of their cuisine, have low rates of heart disease.

Rapeseed oil is an excellent choice too. In fact, it has a lower saturate content than olive oil and is about 60% mono-unsaturates but it cannot claim the track record of olive oil.

You see, the wild rapeseed plant contains a lot of erucic acid – a mono-unsaturated fatty acid, but one which we have no experience of eating in large quantities. It would be an unwise experiment to start eating large amounts of erucic acid; it might be good for us – but it might not.

Commercial production of rapeseed oil had to await the selection of a variety with very low levels of erucic acid. Don't worry. The rapeseed oil on your supermarket shelf will be a low-erucic acid variety; the high mono-unsaturate content is all down to oleic acid – exactly the same fatty acid as in olive oil. So I have every confidence in rapeseed oil (and it certainly stands beside the olive oil in my kitchen) even though it cannot yet claim to have been tried and tested through the centuries like olive oil. Mind you, as well as oleic acid, rapeseed oil is a good source of alpha-linolenic acid, which is in the same family as fish oils. The Japanese on Kohama Island and the people of Crete eat diets rich in alpha-linolenic acid and have remarkably low rates of heart disease. Rapeseed oil has the advantage of being much cheaper than olive oil and it is also one of the main crops produced by British farmers.

It may be that the name puts people off rapeseed oil. It's very popular in the USA but they call it canola oil. After all, 'sunflower' conjures up positive images of a summer's day and 'olive' probably reminds you of a nice girl. A more cuddly name to replace 'rapeseed' might double its popularity overnight. Perhaps a manufacturer should run a competition to rename the oil: the promotion would be a heartening boost for British farming and for the beleaguered British heart.

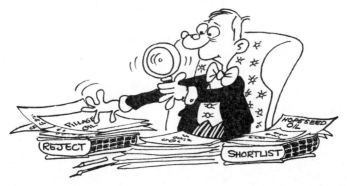

Perhaps we should have a competition to rename rapeseed oil.

Olive oil or rapeseed oil will meet most of your culinary requirements and it is not essential to buy any other oils or fats. If you want the flavour of olive oil (for example in salad dressing) extra virgin olive oil is useful. An oily salad dressing can give you an awful lot of fat, so, even if it is friendly fat, go easy. If you don't want an olive oil flavour (for example when making flapjack) select olive oil with a light flavour; the fatty acid content is similar but the taste is delicate. Of course, an alternative would be to use rapeseed oil. Other oils with a significant proportion of mono-unsaturated fatty acids are peanut oil (also called groundnut or arachis oil) and grapeseed oil.

Table 8 divides some common fats and oils into three groups. Those rich in mono-unsaturates are recommended and it is best to

Table 8 Fats and oils

High in mono-unsaturates	High in polyunsaturates	High in saturates
Olive oil	Sunflower oil	Palm oil
Rapeseed oil	Corn oil	Coconut oil
Peanut oil	Safflower oil	Butter
'Olive oil' spread	Soya oil	Lard
	Walnut oil	Dripping
	Sesame seed oil*	Suet
	Sunflower spread	Margarines

*Sesame seed oil contains a reasonable helping of mono-unsaturates (37%) as well as poly-unsaturates (44%).

Hard margarines are particularly to be avoided. Not only do they contain high levels of saturated fatty acids but also of trans fatty acids which may be even more damaging (see page 34).

avoid completely those with a high saturated fatty acid content. Sparing use of fats and oils containing a high proportion of poly-unsaturates is acceptable. DO NOT re-use oils after cooking; re-heating can oxidise polyunsaturated fats, making them more damaging to blood vessels.

ACTION POINTS

◆ When cooking oil is needed, use a little olive oil or rapeseed oil

◆ Don't re-use cooking oils

What about baking if olive oil and rapeseed oil are the only fats in your kitchen? Most recipes that call for a hard fat work perfectly well if you use oil instead. The general rule is to replace 4 oz (100 grams) of butter or margarine with 5 tablespoons (75 ml) of oil. Oil works extremely well in biscuits, cakes and bread. It is even possible to use oil in pastry and crumble but you may prefer a reduced-fat spread (high in mono-unsaturates) which is suitable for baking. You can mix oils; replacing some of the rapeseed oil in your flapjack with peanut oil will give it a more nutty flavour.

> **ACTION POINT**
>
> ◆ Adapting recipes: for every 4 oz (100 g) of butter or margarine use 5 tablespoons (75 ml) of rapeseed or olive oil.

So remember:

- the traditional fat in a recipe often can be left out altogether;
- if you need to use fat:

    – choose an oil rich in mono-unsaturates;

    – use as little as possible.

What about my bread and butter, then? If you cannot contemplate life without putting butter on your bread, you had better learn to spread it thinly. A scraping of reduced-fat spread (high in mono- or polyunsaturates) would be preferable, but most people could surprise themselves by discovering how happily they adapt to new habits. I love toast and marmalade. An intervening layer of fat is entirely superfluous. The French habit of eating unbuttered bread with a meal is a healthy one.

The new fat spreads – a spreading revolution?

If you were on Mars or in a monastery at the time, you may have missed the launch of the new fat spreads – Benecol and Flora pro.activ – specially formulated to lower blood cholesterol levels.

These spreads belong to a new group of products known as 'functional foods' – foods that are claimed to do more for you than merely supply tasty nourishment. We are likely to see many more functional foods in the future. (What would you think of a contraceptive cheese, or a sandwich spread that makes tax returns seem interesting?)

The new fat spreads have had prominent places in the media, but what role, if any, do they have in our fight against heart disease?

Benecol products contain plant stanols while Flora pro.activ is fortified with plant sterols. Sterols occur naturally in the cell membranes of plants and animals. (Cholesterol itself, which is found only in animals, is a sterol.) It has been known since the 1950s that

plant sterols can lower blood cholesterol levels. Stanols are produced by adding hydrogen to sterols and have a similar effect.

Sterols and stanols reduce the absorption of cholesterol from the
intestine. (We normally absorb about half the cholesterol in the
intestine; eating one of these products cuts that in half so we absorb
about a quarter.) This raises an obvious question: do they still work
if you are eating a low-cholesterol, low-fat diet?

A study by Denke was reported as showing that stanols weren't
effective in men on a low-fat diet. But it probably wasn't the low-fat
diet that reduced the effect of the stanols: it's much more likely that
the stanols didn't work properly because they were given in gela-
tine capsules. Sterols and stanols work better when delivered with
a fatty food so a spread is ideal. Indeed, two studies published in
the *American Journal of Clinical Nutrition* in 1999 showed that
stanols (dissolved in margarine) effectively lowered LDL-cholesterol in people eating low-fat, low-cholesterol diets.

You see, these products don't just reduce absorption of the cholesterol you eat. Some cholesterol that you make in your liver
passes into the intestine before being absorbed into the bloodstream. Sterols and stanols reduce absorption of this cholesterol
too, so it's not surprising that they lower blood cholesterol levels
even when there's very little cholesterol in the diet. (Actually the
body responds to this reduced absorption by making more cholesterol – but not enough to prevent a drop in blood cholesterol.)

To achieve a 10–15% reduction in LDL-cholesterol, you need to
eat 2 g of plant sterol or stanol a day; this amount is added to the
average daily portion of spread. Eating more than the recommended amount is unlikely to lower your cholesterol further.

Middle-age spread?

The average reduction in LDL-cholesterol produced by 2 g of sterol
or stanol a day depends on the ages of the people studied. The
average fall in LDL-cholesterol is 0.54 mmol/l in people aged
50–59, 0.43 mmol/l in those aged 40–49, and 0.33 mmol/l in those
aged 30–39. So if you divide the average age by 100, it tells you the
expected drop in LDL-cholesterol in mmol/l.

This is a very worthwhile reduction (especially when you consider how easily it's achieved) and amounts to a 25% cut in coronary risk. (Although the drop in cholesterol is smaller in a
35-year-old than in a 55-year-old, there is still a 25% risk reduction

because raised cholesterol is a relatively more important risk factor in the younger person. The difference between relative risk and absolute risk is explained in Chapter 24.)

Are these spreads safe? They seem to be and Flora pro.activ has been approved under the EU Novel Foods regulations. One concern is that sterols and stanols reduce absorption of the antioxidants beta-carotene and vitamin E, but this isn't a problem if you eat enough fruit and vegetables. On current evidence, these products wouldn't normally be recommended for pregnant women or for children under 5.

Of course, these spreads cost a lot more than standard fat spreads. That's because you need 2500 tons of vegetable oil to extract one ton of sterol. In middle age, you might be glad to spend about half the cost of a daily paper on staying alive, instead of saving up for a lavish funeral.

If you're in the habit of spreading fat on your bread, switching to Flora pro.activ or Benecol could be a wise move. But if, like me, you ditched that layer of fat long ago, what will you gain from adding 20 g of fat spread to your daily diet? Middle-age spread?

Nuts

'I am Charley's Aunt from Brazil, where the nuts come from.'

Brandon Thomas (1857–1914) *Charley's Aunt*

Nuts are nutritious. They are high-protein foods but they also have a very high fat content so this is a convenient place to deal with them. Nearly all the fat in coconut is saturated. You can see from Table 9 that, if you went nuts, a pile of brazils would give you a hefty dose of saturated fat as well.

Generally, though, nuts are quite helpful to your heart. Including some walnuts in a low-fat diet can lower blood cholesterol levels, according to a study published in the *New England Journal of Medicine* in 1993. Almonds too have been shown to have a cholesterol-lowering effect.

An investigation on over 30,000 Seventh-Day Adventists found that those who ate nuts frequently (more than four times a week) had about 50% fewer heart attacks than those who indulged infrequently (less than once a week).

Table 9 Fat content of common nuts

Type of nut	Total fat (g/100 g)	Saturates (g/100 g)	Mono-unsaturates (g/100 g)	Polyunsaturates (g/100 g)
Almonds	55.8	4.7	34.4	14.2
Brazil nuts	68.2	16.4	25.8	23.0
Cashew nuts (Roasted)	50.9	10.1	29.4	9.1
Chestnuts	2.7	0.5	1.0	1.1
Coconut (creamed block)	68.8	59.3	3.9	1.6
Hazelnuts	63.5	4.7	50.0	5.9
Macadamia nuts	77.6	11.2	60.8	1.6
Peanuts	46.1	8.2	21.1	14.3
Walnuts	68.5	5.6	12.4	47.5

Data from *McCance and Widdowson's The Composition of Foods*, 5th edition, Holland *et al.*, 1991, © Crown copyright.

You don't have to belong to a particular religious group to benefit from nuts. You could be a nurse. Findings of the Nurses' Health Study on over 86,000 women were published in the *British Medical Journal* in 1998. Women who ate nuts at least five times a week had a 35% lower risk of coronary heart disease than those who rarely ate nuts.

Mind you, sorting out the real cause of such observations is always a tough nut to crack. It could be that frequent nut eaters have generally healthier lifestyles; perhaps it's because they also eat more fruit and vegetables, smoke less, and take more exercise that they have less heart disease. Researchers have concluded that when all these 'confounding factors' are stripped away, the kernel of truth remains: nuts do offer some protection against heart disease. How?

In a nutshell, they contain more friendly fat than unfriendly – apart from coconut, that is. They supply the essential polyunsaturated fatty acid, alpha-linolenic acid (related to fish oil); walnuts are a particularly good source of this. Almonds and hazelnuts major on mono-unsaturates. Nuts also supply vitamin E, an important antioxidant.

So, it's worth shelling out on a few hazelnuts, almonds and walnuts; they make a healthy contribution to muesli and many other recipes. Remember that lots of calories come with the fat in nuts so, if keeping your weight down is a problem, nuts won't help you to crack it. Chestnuts are the exception that proves the rule: they contain very little fat. Enjoy roast chestnuts whenever you want but shy away from coconut.

◆ Apart from chestnuts, nuts are very high in fat

◆ Avoid coconut; it's loaded with saturated fat

◆ Other nuts give you more friendly (unsaturated) fats

◆ Eating a few walnuts, almonds or hazelnuts may help your heart

---

Snack foods

'My wife's on a strict fast again.
She won't eat a thing – except fast food.'

Anon.

We all have a little gap to fill between meals sometimes. That's where snack foods come in. If you choose the wrong ones, you'll overshoot your saturated fat allowance before you can say "Jack Sprat".

If you want lots of sugar with your fat, you'll get that in chocolate, pastries and commercial cakes and biscuits. Heavily salted fat is conveniently packaged as potato crisps, corn snacks etc.

Normal crisps are over 30% fat, while reduced fat versions may be about 25% fat – and, when one quarter of the total weight is fat, you cannot pretend it's a low-fat snack. Multigrain 'chips' containing less than 10% fat ('Jordan's naturally seasoned chips') are now available and, although still bristling with salt, they make an appealing option.

Unfortunately, factory-made cakes and biscuits frequently utilise hydrogenated vegetable oil and, as a result, contain significant quantities of trans fatty acids – which may be more damaging to your arteries than saturated fatty acids.

Fresh fruit is an ideal snack. Make sure it is either washed thoroughly or peeled. Many vegetables, like carrots, celery, mange-tout peas or sugarsnap peas, make great gap-fillers too.

Dried fruits (such as apricots, pears, prunes, raisins, dates and figs) are available – ready to eat – in convenient, resealable packs. Next time you get that irresistible urge, try a handful of nuts and raisins instead of a bar of chocolate – hardly a low-calorie snack, but most of the fat is friendly.

Of course you like to have cakes and biscuits sometimes and, if you make them yourself, you can enjoy them without worrying about saturated and trans fatty acids. It may sound strange but, in many cakes, prune purée can be used instead of fat, and the results are excellent (see Chapter 27). When fat is required, select rapeseed oil or lightly-flavoured olive oil.

◆ Making your own cakes and biscuits can avoid saturated and trans fatty acids

◆ When baking, you can often replace fat with prune purée

◆ Reduced-fat crisps still contain lots of fat (and salt)

◆ Suitable snacks include: fruit, dried fruit, carrot sticks, sugarsnap peas; Japanese rice crackers, mackerel pâté on pitta bread, home-cooked poppadums and popcorn; home-made sandwiches, cakes and biscuits

When you have friends round for drinks, you will no doubt offer them crisps and other traditional, high-fat snacks. Why not include some healthier options as well? Japanese rice crackers have a relatively low fat content. Poppadums cooked by immersion in hot oil are obviously very fatty but they are surprisingly acceptable when cooked dry on a paper towel in the microwave oven (e.g. 40–60 seconds on high power). I still prefer the genuine, high-fat article but, if you cook them yourself in rapeseed oil, as a very occasional treat, at least you know what fat you're getting. Popcorn is a variety of maize, a good wholesome grain, which is usually coated in butter or hydrogenated vegetable oil. Try popping it yourself in a covered saucepan with a very little rapeseed oil. Alternatively, if you are partial to popcorn, it's worth investing in one of the excellent machines that simply pops the corn with hot air, avoiding the need to add any fat at all.

Smoked mackerel pâté is easy to prepare, rich in desirable fish oils, and always popular (see Chapter 27). Toasted triangles of wholemeal pitta bread are a great accompaniment to this. A variety of low-fat dips can also be served with toasted pitta, wholemeal rye crispbreads, matzos, low-fat crackers or raw vegetables. Be careful to read nutritional information on savoury biscuits and crackers. You may be surprised at the quantity of fat in some of them.

If you enjoy smoked salmon, why not serve it on thinly-sliced wholemeal bread with plenty of lemon juice? There's no need to muffle the flavour with butter.

'TRAMP: Would you give me twenty-five pence
for a sandwich, lady?
LADY: I don't know – let me see the sandwich.'

Gyles Brandreth,
1000 Jokes: The Greatest Joke Book Ever Known, 1980

Sandwiches can be anything from banal to bizarre. What you put between two pieces of bread is limited more by your imagination than by anything else. And you can cater for every taste without including large amounts of saturated fat. Fresh salad and wholemeal bread are always a good start. Low-fat yoghurt, virtually fat-free fromage frais, quark or cottage cheese lend themselves to a great variety of low-fat dressings; tomato ketchup, lemon juice, Tabasco sauce, Worcestershire sauce, Hoisin sauce, Dijon mustard and curry paste are great for adding flavour. If you want to dress it with something 'off the peg', and I don't recommend your hat, you could try one of the commercial fat-free dressings (such as yoghurt and chive or Thousand Island style). Tinned fish and cooked chicken or turkey usually go down well.

With ingredients like these, there is no need for butter but consider Benecol or Flora pro.activ. A layer of grease will waterproof the bread. Mind you, there is nothing wrong with moist bread – as long as it's not soggy – unless you are trying to emulate British Rail. (BR earned a reputation for reliability in catering: if you ordered a sandwich, it always turned up – just round the edges.)

Mini sandwiches are ideal for parties, and you can always use shape cutters for extra fun.

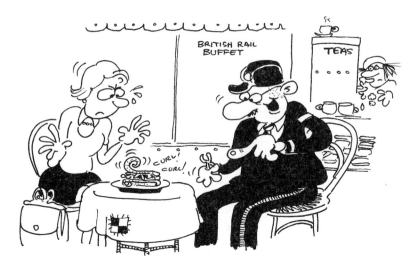

"I see your sandwich has turned up."

Fat substitutes

'Seeing is deceiving. It's eating that's believing.'

James Thurber, *Further Fables for Our Time*, 1956

The perfect fat substitute has all the feel and flavour of fat with none of the calories and is completely safe. This last point is always rather difficult to prove with a new substance, but food manufacturers know that there is a lot of money to be made from increasingly fat- and calorie-conscious consumers who won't want to change the habits of a lifetime when offered an alternative on a plate.

Polydextrose (by Pfizer) and Simplesse (by Nutrasweet) have acquired 'generally regarded as safe' (GRAS) status and are used in foods like margarine, mayonnaise, ice cream and confectionery. They cannot be used in any foods that will be heated and a margarine made with Simplesse is no good for cooking.

Procter and Gamble have developed Sucrose Polyesters (trade name 'Olestra') by combining fatty acids with a sugar backbone in a different configuration from any natural fat molecule. Olestra is stable when heated and can even be used as a cooking oil. It behaves just like a normal fat, except for one crucial point: it is not digested. It passes right through the body unscathed by digestive enzymes. So you have double the fun: all the fun of eating it, and all the fun of excreting it. Indeed, one of the concerns about Olestra has been that some people may experience the latter very rapidly after the former. Further development of Olestra has greatly reduced its laxative properties, but some concern remains that vital fat-soluble vitamins could go down the pan along with the unwanted calories.

Like artificial sweeteners, good, safe fat substitutes will have their uses. The commercial potential is huge and they will be hailed as the answer to obesity and heart disease. I doubt that they will ever fulfil this hope. They will never be a satisfactory substitute for developing good food habits and enjoying the rich variety of a balanced low-fat diet.

◆ Fat substitutes can be useful in low-fat processed foods

◆ There is no substitute for learning to appreciate a balanced diet of unprocessed foods

Chapter 5

Carbohydrate

As the name suggests, carbohydrates are made of carbon and the elements in water (hydrogen and oxygen). They are an important energy source, but the proportion of dietary calories consumed as carbohydrate varies greatly across the world. The population of a developing country might obtain 85% of its calories from carbohydrate, while the diet of an industrial country contains much more fat and may provide less than 45% of the energy as carbohydrate.

The carbohydrates in our food comprise sugars, starches and fibre.

Sugar

Sugars are SIMPLE CARBOHYDRATES. In the simplest sugars, the molecule consists of only one 'building block' and these are known as the monosaccharides – glucose, galactose and fructose. When two of these are joined together, a disaccharide sugar is formed. Sucrose is a combination of glucose and fructose. Other disaccharides are maltose and lactose.

Sugars in our food can be divided into 'intrinsic sugars' and 'extrinsic sugars'. Intrinsic sugars remain where nature put them – within the cell structure of the food; they are an intrinsic part of the food. An example would be the small amount of sugar that occurs naturally within a fresh bean. Extrinsic sugars, on the other hand, have been separated from this natural structure – like table sugar and the sugar added to a can of baked beans.

Fructose (fruit sugar) is found in fruit, and lactose (milk sugar) is found in milk, but sucrose (table sugar) is found **on** tables.

Starch

Starches are COMPLEX CARBOHYDRATES. They are polysaccharides because they consist of many sugar units joined together. The starch in our diet is made up of lots of glucose molecules linked to one another. We get most of our starch from cereal grains and potatoes, but it is also found in peas, beans and other vegetables.

Fibre

Fibre, which used to be called 'roughage', is also in the COMPLEX CARBOHYDRATE group. In fact, nutritionists prefer to talk about non-starch polysaccharides (NSP) these days, but I suspect you will feel more comfortable if I keep calling it 'fibre'. So I will.

In westernised diets, fibre has had to play Cinderella to all those glamorous nutrients. After all, we can't digest it; it's just the dross that's left behind after the intestine has extracted all the goodness from our food. But, like Cinderella, fibre turned out to be something special and, without it, even the most princely diet would be desperately deficient.

Indeed, the relative lack of fibre in our diet may go a long way towards explaining why many medical problems (including constipation, diverticular disease, acute appendicitis, bowel cancer and gallstones) are so common here but so rare in some parts of the world (e.g. rural Africa). In addition, diets containing plenty of high-fibre foods are associated with low rates of heart disease.

There are two main types of dietary fibre.

Insoluble fibre provides bulk, which helps you to feel satisfied without devouring too many calories. It is also important for normal bowel function and helps to prevent constipation. Simply adding insoluble fibre to the diet probably doesn't lower blood cholesterol but, in practice, when people eat more high-fibre foods, they get less of their energy from saturated fat and the cholesterol level falls. Vegetables (including the skins) and cereal husks provide insoluble fibre. Good sources are: wholemeal bread, wholegrain cereals, brown rice and jacket potatoes.

Soluble fibre does have a direct cholesterol-lowering action. That means that adding enough soluble fibre to the diet, without changing anything else, causes some drop in blood cholesterol levels.

We do not fully understand the mechanisms responsible for this cholesterol reduction. It may be partly that soluble fibre clings to bile acids in the large intestine and prevents their re-absorption back into the body. These bile acids contain cholesterol that has been made in the liver. In this way soluble fibre could encourage the excretion of cholesterol produced by the liver.

Even so, the big reductions in blood cholesterol are seen in people who eat plenty of high-fibre foods *instead* of foods containing a lot of saturated fat.

We obtain soluble fibre from fruit and vegetables generally, and especially from pulses (peas, beans, lentils, chickpeas), as well as from oats. Apples, pears and citrus fruits (such as oranges) are important sources of pectin – one form of soluble fibre. Experiments have shown that adding pectin to the diet lowers cholesterol, but you would generally have to eat a big pile of fruit every day (e.g. five pounds of apples) to match the quantities of pectin given in these experiments.

Too much of a good thing?

Very high carbohydrate diets, in which more than 60% of the calories come from carbohydrate, can raise blood triglyceride levels and lower HDL-cholesterol – the 'good cholesterol' (Chapter 3). The rise in triglycerides may be temporary, settling back to baseline after several months on such a diet, but the reduction in HDL-cholesterol continues. This would appear to be a very unwelcome effect. However, the people that eat these very high-carbohydrate diets also eat very little saturated fat; they have low levels of LDL-cholesterol – the 'bad' cholesterol – and low rates of heart disease.

So what should I eat?

Where carbohydrate is concerned, standard advice is simple: keep it complex.

It has been generally assumed that simple carbohydrates (sugars) are bad for you because they cause a rapid rise in blood sugar, while complex carbohydrate (starch) is good for you because it releases energy slowly.

It turns out that this view is far too simple. The very fibre of this dietary doctrine has been dealt a death blow by recent research into the glycaemic index of foods.

What's the glycaemic index?

The starch in our food is broken down by digestion and absorbed into the bloodstream as glucose. It doesn't matter whether the food is bread, rice, pasta, potato or something else: the starch it contains has to be converted to simple glucose before it can be absorbed. Some foods are easily broken down causing a rapid rise in blood glucose, while others take longer to digest so that glucose is released more slowly.

The glycaemic index (GI) of a food is a measure of the blood glucose response to eating a standard portion (50 g of carbohydrate). The rise in blood glucose produced by eating a portion of a particular food is measured in groups of volunteers and compared with their response to having 50 g of glucose in a drink.

Pure glucose is given a GI of 100; it's absorbed immediately, causing a rapid rise in blood glucose. A food producing only half this glucose response has a GI of 50. The more slowly glucose is released from the food, the lower the GI. Table 10 shows the GI numbers of some common foods.

Perhaps it always was naïve to think that sugar was of the devil, and wholemeal bread a virtuous food – when the starch in bread ends up as simple blood sugar. But the big surprise has been the finding that some starchy foods, such as bread, have a higher GI than table sugar! And wholemeal bread has virtually the same GI as white bread.

When blood glucose shoots up after eating high-GI foods, more insulin is released to reduce it again. Raised insulin levels make you feel hungry and can lead to fat storage. It is bad news for the heart and arteries if insulin levels are persistently raised, as they are in the 'insulin resistance syndrome' (see page 232).

More enlightened doctors have realised for some time that people with diabetes benefit from eating a low-GI diet. Conventional advice in recent years, however, has been to control blood glucose by cutting out sugary foods and eating plenty of low-fat, starchy foods, such as bread and potatoes. How much sense does this make when wholemeal bread and baked potatoes push up blood glucose faster than table sugar?

Not only that, but in the light of recent research it seems that those of us who don't have diabetes are better off on a low-GI diet as well. For a start, eating a higher proportion of low-GI foods helps to reduce fat storage and control body weight. It also seems to improve the balance of blood lipids, raising protective HDL-cholesterol and lowering triglycerides. There is now evidence that men and women who keep to a low-GI diet are less likely to develop diabetes and heart disease.

How do I follow a low-GI diet?

Have a look at Table 10 and simply replace foods that have a high number with ones that have a low GI. It is, of course, a continuous scale but foods are sometimes divided into three bands:

- low GI (less than 55)
- medium GI (55–70)
- high GI (over 70).

If you get into the habit of choosing the foods with low numbers, while cutting right down on those with a GI above 70, the overall GI of your diet will be low.

You will see that new potatoes have a lower GI than baked potatoes. Basmati rice has a lower GI than instant rice. Apples, pears and plums have lower GIs than tropical fruits such as melons and pineapples. In general, pastas and pulses (peas, beans and lentils) have lovely low GI numbers – although broad beans are a notable exception.

How can the glycaemic index help athletes?

The slow release of energy from low-GI foods can keep you going for longer than the quick rise in blood sugar that results from eating foods with high GI numbers. Endurance will be increased by eating a low-GI meal, such as pasta, 1 or 2 hours before embarking on strenuous activity that goes on for more than 90 minutes. So whether you plan to climb a mountain or go cross-country skiing, if you're going to be at it for at least 90 minutes, stoke up with long-range (low-GI) fuel about 90 minutes beforehand.

On the other hand, when athletes are training hard every day, they need to put energy (glycogen) back into their muscles quickly after each training session. Experiments have shown that foods with *high* GI numbers are better for this because they allow the body to make glycogen more rapidly.

Table 10 Glycaemic index of foods

Food	GI	Food	GI
Breakfast cereals		*Rice (continued)*	
All-Bran	42	White rice, low-amylose	88
Porridge	42	Instant rice (boiled 6 mins)	90
Special K	54	*Pasta*	
Muesli (variable)	56	Fettucini	32
Shredded Wheat	69	Vermicelli	35
Weetabix	70	Spaghetti, wholemeal	37
Cheerios	74	Spaghetti, white	41
Puffed Wheat	74	Macaroni	45
Rice Krispies	82	Noodles, instant	47
Cornflakes	84		
Bread		*Potatoes*	
Pumpernickel	41	Sweet potato	54
Mixed grain	40–50	New potato	62
Pitta	57	Mashed potato	70
Wholemeal	69	Instant potato	83
White	70	Baked potato	85
Baguette	95	*Pulses*	
Cereal Grains		Beans:	
Barley, whole or pearl	25	soya	18
Rye	34	kidney	27
Bulgar	48	butter	31
Barley, cracked	50	haricot	38
Buckwheat	54	blackeye	42
Couscous	65	baked	48
Millet	71	broad	79
Rice		Chickpeas	33
Brown rice	55	Lentils	26–30
Wild rice	57	Peas:	
Basmati rice	58	frozen (boiled)	48
White rice, high-amylose	58	dried (boiled)	22

Are low-GI foods always healthy?

No. Don't fall into the trap of thinking that all foods with a low GI are a good choice. Crisps have a GI of 54 – much lower than a baked potato; that's because the fat in crisps delays digestion. The GI only tells you about one thing – the effect on blood glucose. Low-GI foods – like crisps – can still be loaded with unhelpful fat and salt.

All-Bran has a lower GI than Shredded Wheat, but it also contains added salt while Shredded Wheat is nothing but whole-wheat. Although wholegrain foods aren't guaranteed to have a low GI, they are still preferable to overprocessed products which are spoilt by having important nutrients and fibre removed, and undesirable ingredients added. A good variety of whole grains each day can help to protect you against heart disease and cancer.

So don't just look at GI. Look at how much the food has been mucked about by the manufacturer and, in particular, how much fat and salt has been added.

◆ **The glycaemic index (GI) of a food tells you how fast it pushes up blood glucose and insulin levels**

◆ **A low-GI diet helps to control body weight and cuts the risk of diabetes and heart disease**

◆ **Some foods rich in complex carbohydrate have a higher GI than table sugar**

◆ **Pastas and pulses have lovely low GI numbers**

Less simple

Discoveries about the glycaemic index of different foods have revolutionary implications, but advice to have less simple carbohydrate (sugar) is still valid. When sugar is added to your food, it gives you calories without nourishment (so-called 'empty calories').

Don't worry about the intrinsic sugar in fruit and vegetables, but try to cut down the extrinsic sugar that is added to so many foods and drinks. The table sugar added to a bowl of cereal or to a cup of tea is obvious, but so much extrinsic sugar is hidden – in breakfast cereals, soft drinks, and many different processed foods, both sweet and savoury. Check food labels to spot the hidden sugar, remembering that ingredients are listed in order of quantity present (by weight). Sugar will probably be the first ingredient listed on a jar of jam. This simply means there is more sugar than anything else in the jam.

Sugar appears in many guises. Honey, molasses, sucrose, maltose, lactose, fructose, glucose, glucose syrup, dextrose, invert sugar and caramel are all variations on the same theme – sugar.

Sugar is bad for the teeth (especially when eaten frequently throughout the day) and may contribute to obesity. It often comes with fat in factory-made cakes, biscuits and other snacks.

Here are a few practical tips for cutting down unnecessary sugar:

- If you are still adding sugar to tea and coffee, why not join the millions who now find that drinks taste better without?

- Most of us would benefit from drinking more water. Carbonated drinks like cola and lemonade conceal an awful lot of extrinsic sugar, so the low-calorie varieties are better from that point of view. (A can of soft drink might contain seven teaspoons of sugar.)

- Artificial sweeteners have their place but, if you use them routinely instead of adjusting your palate (or your 'tooth'), you end up having sweeteners in addition to too much sugar.

- Many recipes, including those for jams and marmalades, can stand a big reduction in sugar. Reduced-sugar jams or pure fruit spreads are best kept in the fridge once opened.

- Dried fruits – such as dates, raisins, sultanas, apricots, figs and prunes – can be used to sweeten cakes and biscuits. The sugar is intrinsic and they are also high in fibre.

- Select low-sugar breakfast cereals (less than 10% sugar) and enhance them with chopped bananas and dried fruit.

- Get into the habit of finishing meals with fruit. Save traditional puddings for special occasions.

- Buy tinned fruit in natural juice, not syrup.

'JACKIE: **Pity there's no such thing as Sugar Replacement Therapy.**
VICTORIA: **There is. It's called chocolate.'**

Victoria Wood,
Mens Sana in Thingummy Doodah, 1990

More Complex

In the light of recent research, the simple recommendation to eat more complex carbohydrate is not wrong; it's just that choosing the best complex carbohydrates is a little less simple than it appeared. Starch, insoluble fibre and soluble fibre are often provided together, in varying proportions, by the same foods.

The extra information provided by GI numbers (see Table 10) can help you make the very best choices. You can see that a baguette will send your insulin levels soaring almost as much as pure glucose, while a mixed-grain loaf – especially one containing barley and rye – would be a particularly good option.

Regular **pulses** are good for your heart: peas, beans (including baked beans, kidney beans, soya beans, borlotti beans, butter beans) lentils and chickpeas are great sources of soluble fibre that can help lower cholesterol. Beans also provide quality protein reducing the need for meat; replacing animal protein in the diet with vegetable protein reduces both total and LDL-cholesterol. On top of all this, we now know that pulses (except broad beans) have lovely low GI numbers, so give them leading roles in your cuisine.

Starchy foods like bread, rice, pasta and potatoes can be helpful too, but go for those with lower GI numbers. Pasta is a clear winner (and this is why it's popular with athletes looking for a source of sustained energy). Spaghetti, macaroni, lasagne, noodles, tagliatelle, trottole and vermicelli are just some of its many forms. The important thing with foods in this group is to avoid cooking them or serving them with unnecessary fat.

'**Bread that must be sliced with an axe is bread that is too nourishing.'**

Fran Lebowitz, *Metropolitan Life*, 1978

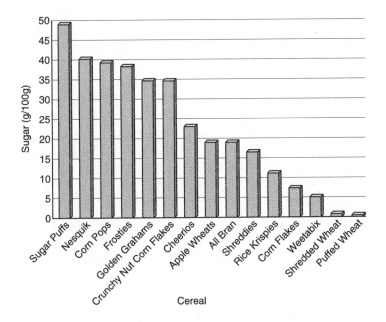

Figure 4 Sugar content of some common breakfast cereals.

Cereal grains give you starch and fibre (as well as protein). Many breakfast cereals contain a lot of added sugar. This is quite obvious if the product is advertised as honey- or sugar-coated, but with other cereals you will often find that sugar is still the second ingredient listed. Shredded Wheat (including 'Bitesize') and Puffed Wheat are remarkable for having only one ingredient – wheat – with no added sugar or salt. A bowl of Shredded Wheat and skimmed milk needs no extra sugar if topped with sliced bananas and raisins or other dried fruit. Soft fruits (like raspberries, strawberries and blackberries) and stewed fruits also make lovely accompaniments to breakfast cereals. If you feast frequently on very sugary cereals, consider mixing them with less sugary ones (see Figure 4). Mix your Sugar Puffs with a good helping of Puffed Wheat and you'll munch through much less sugar. Don't bother with this advice if you need to gain weight and you've already lost all your teeth.

> 'Breakfast cereals that come in the same colors as polyester leisure suits make oversleeping a virtue.'
>
> Fran Lebowitz, *Metropolitan Life*, 1978

ADAPTING TO CHANGE

We are creatures of habit. Don't forget that you've been eating
food for longer than you can remember. It's a habit. If you've been
having porridge with cream for 20 years, don't expect to be ecstatic
the first time you try it with skimmed milk. Don't chuck it away in
disgust and conclude that healthy eating's not for you. Give yourself
a chance. You've spent years getting used to a high-fat, high-salt
diet; you can learn to enjoy a low-fat, low-salt diet much quicker
than that. But don't give up on day one because it's not what
you're used to.

I'm not suggesting you should force yourself to eat porridge made
with water every day until you feel grateful! For a start, you can
make changes gradually. You could change from cream to skimmed
milk via whole milk and semi-skimmed milk – or any blend of
these – if you wanted. It may be that porridge is not for you at all.
A recipe that I enjoy may not appeal to you. Don't let that put
you off. There are countless other possibilities.

You are embarking on a voyage of discovery. Don't turn back at
your own front gate.

Oats and oat bran are useful sources of soluble fibre – not to mention
taste and texture. A bowl of porridge oats with skimmed milk or
water takes less than four minutes to cook in the microwave oven, and
there's no dirty saucepan! Top this with skimmed milk and just a little
golden syrup.

Why not make your own muesli with a mixture of cereal grains
and dried fruit? (See Chapter 27.) If you are buying ready-made
muesli, it's worth avoiding brands with a very high sugar content and
those with coconut.

'The critical period in matrimony is breakfast-time.'

A.P. Herbert, *Uncommon Law*, 1935

The average intake of fibre in Britain would need to be increased by
50% to reach the recommended level.

Of course, you can boost fibre intake by adding wheat bran to porridge or any other moist food, but overdoing this may reduce absorption of certain minerals, and not everybody's intestine takes kindly to having large quantities of wheat bran dumped in it. It is better generally to eat plenty of foods (pulses, fruit and vegetables, starchy foods and cereal grains) that have not had their natural fibre removed.

There is an important principle here: try to eat as much of your food as possible in its natural, whole, unprocessed form. A whole apple gives you starch, fibre, intrinsic sugar, vitamins, minerals and water. If it's a good apple, you may eat a second one, but you are unlikely to eat more than two in one go. Now, if you convert apples into apple juice, most of the sugar becomes extrinsic and you lose the fibre. You can gulp down the juice of a dozen apples without a second thought – all those calories without the fibre. I'm sure that new juicer will be a godsend on occasions, but perhaps it should go to the back of the cupboard.

ACTION POINTS

◆ Eat less sugar. Watch out for hidden sugar in processed foods

◆ Eat plenty of starchy foods – e.g. potatoes, pasta, rice, grains (including bread)

◆ Choose wholegrain cereals, bread, pasta and rice when possible

◆ Fruits and vegetables provide fibre and starch – eat plenty

◆ Large amounts of soluble fibre (from beans, oats and fruit) help to lower cholesterol

◆ Eat most of your food whole/unprocessed. Apples rather than apple juice

Chapter 6

Salt

'But Lot's wife looked back and she became a pillar of salt.'

Genesis 19:26, New International Version

We all need just a little salt (not a Lot). You are probably consuming at least six times as much common salt, or sodium chloride, as you need. Yes, even if you don't add any salt to your food, you will be eating several times the amount your body requires.

So what? The problem is that there is a link between eating excessive salt and having raised blood pressure – hypertension. If your blood pressure is high, you are more likely to have a stroke or heart attack.

◆ Our high-salt diet is linked with high blood pressure which leads to strokes and heart attacks

◆ On *very* low-salt diets, blood pressure doesn't rise with age

◆ Up to 85% of our salt comes from processed foods

◆ Reducing average UK salt intake by a third would dramatically cut strokes and heart attacks

◆ The palate adjusts to salt reduction, but do it gradually or food will taste bland

◆ Potassium helps to lower blood pressure; you get it from fruit and vegetables

The salt of the earth

Although salt is abundant on the surface of the earth, many folk around the world eat much less of it than we do.

In 1988 the *British Medical Journal* published the findings of the Intersalt study. This huge research project (on 10,079 men and women from 52 population samples in 32 different countries across the world) investigated the relationship between salt consumption and blood pressure. The researchers measured the quantity of sodium excreted in the urine over a 24-hour period as an indicator of salt intake.

The conclusions were inescapable. People with very low salt intakes had low blood pressures; high average salt consumption was linked with high average blood pressure.

And that wasn't all. We are so used to blood pressure rising as we get older that it is commonly considered a normal part of the ageing process. It isn't. The Intersalt study showed that it didn't happen in the groups of people with very low salt intakes. And the higher the average salt intake of a population, the more pronounced the age-related rise in pressure.

Inescapable conclusions? Yes, but, predictably, the Salt Institute (the salt producers' trade organisation) has made every attempt to escape them. The Institute criticised the statistical method that the Intersalt team had used to reveal the link between salt intake and the rise in blood pressure with advancing age. The Intersalt researchers responded with a complete re-analysis of their data – published in the *British Medical Journal* in 1996. In fact, *four* different methods of analysis all confirmed the link between bigger salt consumption and higher blood pressure in middle age.

The great salt scandal

You might think that a few grains of salt are neither here nor there but, of course, the salt producers are in business to shift mountains of salt from their mines to our meals. They have fought fiercely to undermine the evidence and obscure the facts. The Salt Institute pooh-poohed the statistical method of the Intersalt team, then ignored their new analyses that used methods suggested by the Institute itself, and rubbed salt into the wound by producing its own analysis of Intersalt data, riddled with statistical and biological flaws. The *British Medical Journal* was good enough to publish this; it shows the contortions of a group with a commercial interest. The Institute's analysis involved fictional figures such as the estimated blood pressure at birth (based on data about ages 20–59). This is nonsense! But it is symbolic of the salt producers' strategy. They take a grain of truth and make a mine of misinformation.

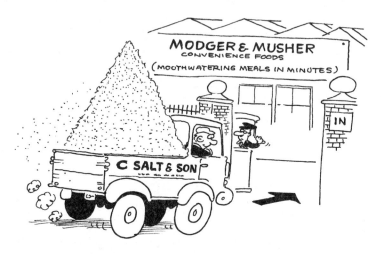

**In business to shift mountains of salt
from their mines to our meals.**

To be fair, the salt producers are not the only ones to have expressed doubts about the implications of Intersalt. Notably, Professor John Swales urged caution before applying the results of a population study to individual people. Mind you, further analysis of the Intersalt data has strengthened the evidence that, *within* populations, salt consumption of the individual is linked with blood pressure. Apart from Intersalt, there is a lot of other experimental evidence that the blood pressure of individuals is influenced by salt intake.

Evidence comes from several types of study.

- Clinical trials on people with raised blood pressure have shown a reduction in blood pressure when salt is restricted; in some cases this has avoided the need to take drugs to treat raised blood pressure .

- Migration studies on people who move from primitive rural areas to towns have shown that when salt intake goes up, so does blood pressure.

- Animal studies have confirmed that blood pressure can be pushed up and down by varying the salt content of the diet. (I know chimpanzees aren't people but they are certainly individuals.)

There's no doubt that some people are more sensitive than others to the effects of salt on blood pressure. And there is still a debate about the value of restricting salt intake in people with normal blood pressures. Indeed, you may even have been told by a doctor that you needn't bother about salt because your blood pressure's OK. But what will your blood pressure be like in five or ten years' time? The crucial point that is so often overlooked is that blood pressure tends to rise with age – except in communities with very low salt intakes. Anyway, although your blood pressure is 'OK' now, you would probably be better off if it were lower still. Besides, a high-salt diet may raise the risk of other problems such as osteoporosis (weak bones) and cancer of the stomach.

Although some independent scientific voices have posed proper questions about the significance of salt, many of the salt cynics turn out to be driven by the food industry. Adding salt is a cheap way of making processed foods palatable – to palates that have adapted to salt concentrations similar to that of sea water. Unfortunately, our physiology is not well adapted to marine life. To improve flavour by increasing the content of real food, such as fruit and vegetables, would be expensive. It is far cheaper to feed the consumer if you feed the controversy too.

Similar ploys have been used by other groups with commercial interests to protect. Within the food industry, makers of full-fat dairy products have fought their corner fiercely. Over the years, the tobacco industry has done its best to defend the cigarette on 'scientific' grounds in the face of mounting evidence to condemn it.

The evidence on salt is less mature than that on fat or tobacco – but it's seasoning. The food industry is enjoying a measure of success. Disguising salty evidence is a distasteful tactic but confusion abounds. Not only does the food industry believe much of its own propaganda, but many doctors are unsure about the real importance of salt. Although some people will be genetically more sensitive to salt than others, this is a big problem for the population as a whole.

In fact, the evidence suggests that merely reducing the average salt intake of our population by one-third would prevent more strokes and heart attacks than all the current treatment for high blood pressure!

In 1994 the British government's committee of experts recommended that the average daily salt intake of the population should be reduced from its present level of 9 g to 6 g. Note that we are talking about salt here – sodium chloride – and not sodium. Six grams of salt contains a little less than 2.4 g of sodium (see Table 11). The recommended reduction in salt of 3 g is roughly half a teaspoonful. It was recognised that this would not be achieved without reducing the salt content of processed foods. The government endorsed the committee's recommendations on other aspects of food policy, but not this. It turned out that the food industry had lobbied ferociously against action on salt. Seven years later, in 2001, the Department of Health officially backed the recommendation that the average salt consumption of adults should be reduced to 6g a day.

Frustrated by the lack of government action, a number of eminent medical scientists formed a group for Consensus Action on Salt and Hypertension (CASH). Their aim is to work with the food industry to reach a consensus on salt and blood pressure and then to find ways of reducing the amount of salt in food. Having called themselves CASH, perhaps it is as well that they no longer look to politicians for action: the name could prove unhelpful when lobbying MPs – MPs who are terrified of being linked with 'cash for questions' and probably with questions for CASH.

Won't salt restriction cramp my style?

You can get cramps due to salt depletion, can't you? Well, this can happen to people labouring in tropical conditions, but it need not concern you in our climate.

Eating foods (such as fruit, vegetables, meat and fish) in their 'natural' state gives you all the sodium you need. Unfortunately, eating processed foods adds large quantities of superfluous salt to your intake. Using a saltcellar adds insult to injury. (Which is more insulting to the cook: to add salt to a meal before even tasting it, or to taste it first and then add salt? I'm not sure.)

Table 11 Sodium content of foods

Food	Sodium content (mmol/100 g)	Sodium content (g/100 g)	Equivalent concentration of sodium chloride (g/100 g)
White bread	23.04	0.53	1.35
Brown bread	23.48	0.54	1.37
Wholemeal bread	23.91	0.55	1.40
Wholemeal flour	negligible	negligible	negligible
White flour	negligible	negligible	negligible
Self-raising flour	15.65	0.36	0.92
Cornflakes	48.26	1.11	2.82
Rice Krispies	54.78	1.26	3.21
Weetabix	11.74	0.27	0.69
Bran flakes	43.48	1.00	2.54
All Bran	39.13	0.90	2.29
Cream cracker	26.52	0.61	1.55
Rye crispbread	9.57	0.22	0.56
Digestive biscuit	26.09	0.60	1.53
Spaghetti (boiled)	negligible	negligible	negligible
Spaghetti (in tomato sauce)	18.30	0.42	1.07
Rice (boiled)	negligible	negligible	negligible
Potatoes (boiled)	0.30	0.01	0.02
Salted butter	32.61	0.75	1.91
Margarine	34.78	0.80	2.04
Cheddar cheese	29.13	0.67	1.70
Edam cheese	44.35	1.02	2.59
Processed cheese	57.39	1.32	3.36
Cottage cheese	16.52	0.38	0.97

Based on data from *McCance and Widdowson's The Composition of Foods*, 5th edition, Holland *et al.*, 1991, © Crown copyright.

Nutritional labels normally state the **sodium** concentration in grams per 100 grams (g/100 g).

Don't imagine that anything up to 6 grams of **sodium** a day is OK: that would be 15.3 grams of salt (sodium chloride)! It is actually impractical for you to keep a running total as so much sodium slips in silently.

There are 393 mg of sodium in every 1 g (1000 mg) of sodium chloride. So, to convert grams of sodium into grams of sodium chloride, you would divide by 0.393 (or simply multiply by 2.5).

To convert mg of sodium into mmols of sodium, you divide by 23 (the atomic weight of sodium).

Assault on the taste buds

If you stop adding salt in the kitchen and at the table, you'll be surprised at how quickly your palate adjusts. Cut down gradually and you will avoid the initial shock. Before long you will begin to appreciate natural food flavours, which once you would have overpowered with salt, and heavily salted food will taste unpleasant.

This is a change worth making. Unfortunately, though, most of the salt in the UK diet (65%–85% of it) comes from processed foods (Figure 5). It's already in the food before it reaches your kitchen. Salt, like fat, is a cheap ingredient and you'll get a good helping of both in sausages, pâtés, pies, crisps and a host of other manufactured savoury foods. I'm sure these fatty foods won't be top of your shopping list any more.

Here is a shocking fact: the biggest single source of salt in the British diet is factory-made bread! Fortunately, since the first edition of this book was published, it has become easier to find reduced-sodium loaves in the shops. Still, the best way to get the

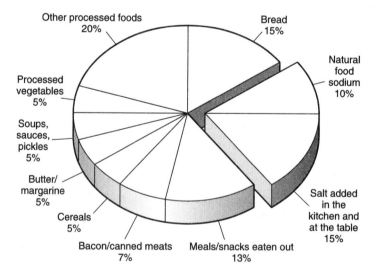

Figure 5 The contribution of various foods to the sodium intake of the population will be something like this. The picture will be quite different in some individual people. For example, bacon or canned soup will account for higher proportions in those who eat a lot of these foods. The natural sodium in food makes up no more than 10% of the intake; 15–25% is added during cooking or eating; 75% comes from food processing.

bread you really want is to make it yourself. Wait! Don't hold your hands up in horror. This has never been easier. With an automatic bread maker, just a few minutes of your time to throw in the ingredients is all it takes to have a fresh loaf whenever you want. And there's certainly no need to add the standard quantity of salt. Even though salt is said to 'stabilise the yeast', you can make lovely loaves with a lot less than the recipe suggests. Admittedly, if you are on the breadline, a machine like this seems expensive, but it can soon pay for itself if you eat a lot of bread.

Some savoury foods, such as crisps, are very obviously salty. But it probably wouldn't occur to you that the concentration of salt in those cornflakes or Rice Krispies is higher than in sea water (see Table 11). When the label tells you about sodium, YOU MUST MULTIPLY BY 2.5 to convert it to salt. Atlantic sea water contains about 1 g/100 g sodium (2.5 g/100 g sodium chloride).

Lots of good products are spoiled by their high salt content. Why buy a can of sweetcorn with added sugar and salt when there are excellent brands without? So check those labels for sodium content. Any supermarket worth its salt will offer reduced-sodium alternatives. You will find some tinned soups with 0.3 g/100 g sodium or less, and other varieties with three times that quantity. (Even the lower-salt brands will give you about a gram of sodium per can; a really low-salt home-made soup would be better.)

A tin of tuna in water (not brine) might contain only 0.1 g/100 g sodium, while a tin of anchovies in olive oil would have about 6 g/100 g – yes, sixty times the concentration. Of course, you may well eat the whole tin of tuna in one meal, but the thing to do with the anchovies is to scatter a few finely cut shreds on your pizza topping.

Apart from sodium chloride, common salt, various other compounds can bump up the sodium content of manufactured foods. The most notable example is monosodium glutamate, which is frequently used as a flavour enhancer.

Keeping your sodium intake down is a wise move. A small reduction in blood pressure could make all the difference – the difference between having a stroke or heart attack and not having one. Sadly, there will always be those who take this kind of advice with a pinch of salt. It's not just a question of lowering your blood pressure now: a reduced-sodium diet helps to prevent blood pressure rising with age.

Potassium, on the other hand, helps to lower blood pressure. We all get too much sodium but many of us could do with more potassium. Don't worry. You don't have to go round checking food labels for potassium content. This is another problem which is solved by eating enough fruit and vegetables.

What about salt substitutes?

It is far better to re-educate your taste buds than simply to load your saltcellar with a salt substitute, but on those occasions when you really feel a little salt makes all the difference, you could use a tiny amount of 'LoSalt' or 'Solo'; these are low-sodium products containing a mixture of potassium chloride and sodium chloride. You can use them in home-made bread. One container should last for ages. If it doesn't, you're using too much.

There are other salt substitutes consisting entirely of potassium salts. These are useful for people on very low sodium diets for specific medical reasons, but they are less palatable than products containing some sodium.

There's always pepper, I suppose

True. We still haven't discovered anything terrible about pepper. And freshly ground black pepper can do a lot for a meal. But seasoning doesn't end there. Reducing salt opens the way to an exciting exploration of herbs and spices. Get fresh herbs whenever you can. Why not grow some in your garden (or window box)? Don't forget garlic, mustard powder, lemon juice and vinegar (including wine vinegars and balsamic vinegar). It's no surprise that celery salt is mostly salt, but beware other ready-made seasonings: you may find salt is the main ingredient.

So, should I rid my larder of salt? No. It would be wise to be well stocked – or you'll regret it when the path freezes over.

ACTION POINTS

◆ Eat as much of your food as possible whole/unprocessed

◆ Don't add salt when cooking or eating

◆ If you feel added salt is essential, consider 'LoSalt' and 'Solo'

◆ When buying processed foods, go for lower-sodium products

◆ Season skilfully with: pepper, garlic, herbs, spices, mustard, lemon, wine, sherry, vermouth, vinegar, etc.

◆ Take care with ready-made flavourings such as stock cubes, soy sauce, etc.

◆ Season for a reason. Halt! That's salt!

Chapter 7

Fish

A fishy theory

It is often said that Inuit people, eating their traditional diet which was very rich in fish oils, had low rates of coronary heart disease. This may be true but there must be some doubt about the causes of death as they were not determined by post-mortem examination. As Professor Durrington has pointed out, we cannot be certain that some of the deaths put down to 'hypothermia' or 'drowning' were not, in fact, caused by heart attacks. So could the oily fish turn out to be a red herring?

Inuits aside, we do have good evidence of the beneficial effects of eating fish, including oily fish. In the Zutphen Study, the dietary habits of 852 Dutch men were examined and these men were followed up for 20 years. During this time, 78 men died from coronary heart disease, but the death rate from heart disease was more than 50% lower in the men who ate at least 30 g (1 oz) of fish a day than in those who did not eat fish. About one-third of the fish consumed was of the oily type.

The Japanese generally eat lots of fish and have low rates of heart disease. Japanese fishermen eat more fish than the general population and have even lower rates of heart disease.

A large study on men who had recently suffered a heart attack found that those advised to eat oily fish (at least two portions a week) were significantly less likely to die (during a follow-up period of two years) than those who were not given this advice.

- ◆ High fish diets are linked with low rates of heart disease
- ◆ Fish oils (EPA and DHA) reduce the risk of thrombosis and abnormal heart rhythms
- ◆ All fish are helpful to your heart – especially oily fish (e.g. sardines, mackerel, salmon)

What do you mean by oily fish?

This does not refer to tinned tuna in vegetable oil! Fish contain the special polyunsaturated fatty acids, eicosapentaenoic acid (EPA) and docosahexaenoic acid (DHA). These are also known as omega-3 fatty acids. You may remember that polyunsaturated fatty acids have more than one area of the molecule with room for extra hydrogen. Well, 'omega-3' simply means that the last position on the molecule that is not saturated with hydrogen is the third carbon atom from the end of the chain. This chemical structure makes these omega-3 fishy fatty acids behave quite differently from the omega-6 polyunsaturates like linoleic acid found in vegetable oils.

The quantity of EPA and DHA present in a fish depends particularly on the species of fish, but also on factors like the season and whether the fish is wild or farmed. Fish with high levels of these omega-3 fatty acids are often called 'oily fish'. They live in cold water. Common examples are mackerel, salmon, herring, sardines and pilchards. You will sometimes find tuna listed as an oily fish and, indeed, fresh tuna can be a good source of omega-3 fatty acids, but the tinned tuna you are likely to find in the supermarket will probably have a very low fat content (e.g. 0.5 g/100 g) – provided you don't buy it in vegetable oil!

The total fat content of oily fish is very variable (see Table 12) and only a small proportion of this is made up of omega-3 fatty acids, but in every case the saturated fatty acid content is low.

One way of ensuring a regular intake of fish oils is to take a concentrated supplement. The GISSI-Prevenzione trial published in the *Lancet* in 1999 recruited 11,324 people who had recently survived a heart attack. Adding 1 g/day of omega-3 fatty acids (one Omacor™ capsule daily) to the standard treatment reduced the overall death rate by an extra 20% and the risk of sudden death by 45%.

What's so special about these omega-3 fatty acids?

Consumption of fish oils has several significant effects on the circulation.

First, the blood doesn't clot as easily. Tiny cells in the blood called platelets have to stick together before a blood clot can form in the circulation. EPA gets into the platelets and makes them less 'sticky'. 'Coronary thrombosis', which means the formation of a blood clot in one of the coronary arteries supplying the heart, is another name for a heart attack. We saw in Chapter 4 that saturated fats can make thrombosis more likely, increasing the risk of a heart attack. Fish oils make thrombosis less likely.

Secondly, large amounts of fish oil can reduce the level of triglycerides in the blood. Permanently raised triglyceride levels do seem to increase the risk of heart disease. Fish oils do not normally make a significant difference to the blood cholesterol level.

There is some evidence that large doses of EPA and DHA can slightly reduce raised blood pressure. The effect on people with normal blood pressure seems less consistent. One study in older people found that fish oils were better at lowering blood pressure if salt intake was reduced as well.

More fish in the sea

Other sea fish (such as cod, haddock, bass, flatfish, red snapper, and dogfish) contain some EPA and DHA even if it's not enough for them to be classed as oily fish. And fish don't have to come from the sea to contain useful amounts of oil: trout and carp have enough to qualify as oily fish.

There's more to fish than omega-3 fatty acids. All fish from sprats to sharks will do you good (as long as it's **you** eating **them**). They make an excellent, low-saturated fat replacement for meat. As well as protein, they provide important vitamins, minerals and trace elements. Fish are good suppliers of various B vitamins (e.g. niacin, vitamin B_6, vitamin B_{12}) and oily fish contain vitamin D. They will top you up with iron and potassium; sea fish will give you iodine and the important antioxidant, selenium. Canned sardines and pilchards are excellent sources of calcium. And, of course, fish is delicious as well as nutritious.

Table 12a Fat content of white fish

	Total fat (g/100 g)	Saturates (g/100 g)	Mono-unsaturates (g/100 g)	Poly-unsaturates (g/100 g)
Bass, sea (raw)	2.5	0.4	0.6	0.6
Cod (raw)	0.7	0.1	0.1	0.3
Cod (steamed)	0.9	0.2	0.1	0.4
Cod (fried in sunflower oil)	15.4	1.8	3.1	9.7
Coley (raw)	1.0	0.1	0.3	0.3
Haddock (raw)	0.6	0.1	0.1	0.2
Halibut (raw)	1.9	0.3	0.6	0.4
Monkfish (raw)	0.4	0.1	0.1	0.1
Mullet, grey (raw)	4.0	1.1	0.9	0.5
Plaice (raw)	1.4	0.2	0.4	0.3
Rock salmon/Dogfish (raw)	9.7	1.4	2.6	2.7
Shark (raw)	1.1	0.2	0.2	0.4
Skate (raw)	0.4	Trace	0.1	0.2
Turbot (raw)	2.7	0.7	0.6	0.6
Whiting (raw)	0.7	0.1	0.2	0.2

I know some people say they don't like fish; they are missing so much and I do hope you're not one of them. If you are, perhaps I could ask you just to consider the possibility that you have been put off by some ill-chosen or badly presented fish. Smelly fish and slimy fillets are excellent bait for crab fishing, but they are not fit for your table, however well seasoned or cooked. Fish should be fresh – firm and bright-eyed (but not bushy-tailed). And overcooking is a common mistake.

Fish come in so many forms, and can be prepared in such a variety of ways, that most people can find something acceptable. If grilled plaice doesn't appeal, a tuna salad might be more to your liking. If you are put off by a whole trout staring you in the face, you may feel at ease with a fillet. Or perhaps you'd prefer your fish disguised in a casserole or pasta sauce. Most of us can appreciate any of these but, if you're not a fish lover, it's well worth finding one or two fish dishes you can enjoy. To start you

Stop that heart attack!

Table 12b Fat content of oily fish

	Total fat (g/100 g)	Saturates (g/100 g)	Mono- unsaturates (g/100 g)	Poly- unsaturates (g/100 g)
Herring (raw)	13.2	3.3	5.5	2.7
Kipper (raw)	17.7	2.8	9.3	3.9
Mackerel (raw)	16.1	3.3	7.9	3.3
Pilchards (canned in tomato sauce)	8.1	1.7	2.2	3.4
Salmon (raw)	11.0	1.9	4.4	3.1
Salmon, pink (canned in brine, flesh only)	6.6	1.3	2.4	1.9
Salmon, red (canned in brine, flesh only)	9.0	1.7	3.7	2.4
Sardines (raw)	9.2	2.7	2.5	2.7
Sardines (canned in oil, drained)	14.1	2.9	4.8	5.0
Swordfish (raw)	4.1	0.9	1.6	1.1
Trout, rainbow (raw)	5.2	1.1	1.8	1.7
Tuna (raw)	4.6	1.2	1.2	1.6
Tuna (canned in brine, drained)	0.6	0.2	0.1	0.2

NOTE: the fat content of fish varies with the season and the maturity of the fish. Oily fish caught in British waters (such as mackerel and herring) contain more fat in winter. Herring, for example, might contain 5 g/100 g in spring and 20 g/100 g in winter.
Data from *Fish and Fish products*, the 3rd supplement to *McCance and Widdowson's The Composition of Foods*, Holland, Brown and Buss, 1993, © Crown copyright.

ACTION POINTS

◆ Eat fish at least twice a week

◆ Avoid fish canned in 'vegetable oil'; choose those in olive oil or water

◆ If you're not a fish fan, disguise fish in casseroles, etc.

◆ Grill, bake or microwave; avoid deep-fried fish; shallow frying in a little rapeseed or olive oil is OK

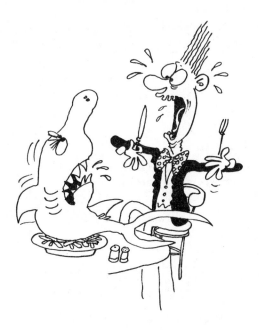

You may be more at ease with a fillet.

off, an outing to a first-class fish restaurant might be a good investment.

I'm not talking about fish and chips, of course. The problem with traditional fish and chips is that two excellent ingredients (fish and potato) have been drenched in fat. It wouldn't be so bad if you could be sure that a good quality oil, rich in mono-unsaturates or polyunsaturates, had been used. Even if it started that way, reheating may have caused oxidation, making the oil much less friendly to your arteries. For a healthier version of fish and chips, see Chapter 27. Oven chips have a much lower fat content (e.g. 5%) than those cooked in deep fat (e.g. 15%). Thin chips, such as french fries, are more fatty than fat chips.

All fins bright and beautiful . . .

The magnificent sight of a gleaming salmon or bass, dorsal fin erect, delights the fish enthusiast. All the better if he or she has hunted the creature in its habitat, cleaned it, prepared it and brought it to the table. What better way to procure fresh fish?

If you are the non-enthusiast, already squirming at my description, get your fishmonger to do as much of the preparation as possible. Gutting and filleting are not for you. Neatly packaged fillets, frozen or fresh (as long as they are), make a convenient option. Tinned fish is a good standby. Don't buy it in unspecified 'vegetable oil'. Sardines in olive oil, drained, are great with salad or on toast (see Chapter 27).

Despite all the salt in the sea, fish are naturally low in sodium but variable quantities of salt are added to tinned fish and it's as well to keep an eye on the sodium content.

How often?

When it comes to sex, it's pointless recommending a frequency. Some people are happy with twice a year; others prefer twice a day. As long as both parties are content, it's futile advising a change. Fish is different.

I recommend that you have fish at least twice a week. One of these meals should include oily fish (two or three portions of oily fish a week are recommended for those who have already had a heart attack). This is a minimum and, if you want to eat fish every day, so much the better.

Of course, oily fish contain a lot more calories than white fish. And there is some concern that the traces of toxic pollutants found in some oily fish could build up to significant levels if you overindulge – so you may prefer to keep oily fish down to once a week and eat other varieties the rest of the time. If you are looking for alternative sources of omega-3 fatty acids, see the box in Chapter 18 on *Fishing for alternatives*.

What about fish oil supplements?

Taking one Omacor capsule daily would give you the protection demonstrated in the GISSI-Prevenzione trial (see page 79) without excessive calories or the worry about pollution. Each capsule contains 460 mg EPA and 380 mg DHA, strictly purified to remove cholesterol, pesticides, heavy metals and other impurities. If you read the labels, you will notice that many other supplements contain much smaller amounts of EPA and DHA. Omacor is available on prescription for people who have had a heart attack

Table 13 Fat and cholesterol content of shellfish

	Total fat (g/100 g)	Saturates (g/100 g)	Mono-unsaturates (g/100 g)	Poly-unsaturates (g/100 g)	Cholesterol (mg/100 g)
Crustacea					
Crab (boiled)	5.5	0.7	1.5	1.6	72
Crayfish (raw)	0.8	0.1	0.2	0.3	105
Lobster (boiled)	1.6	0.2	0.3	0.6	110
Prawns (raw)	0.6	0.1	0.2	0.1	(195)*
Prawns (boiled)	0.9	0.2	0.2	0.2	(280)
Scampi, in bread-crumbs (fried in sunflower oil)	13.6	1.6	3.1	8.2	110
Shrimps (boiled)	2.4	0.4	0.5	0.8	130
Molluscs					
Clams, canned in brine (drained)	0.6	0.2	0.1	0.1	(67)
Cockles (boiled)	0.6	0.2	0.1	0.2	53
Cuttlefish (raw)	0.7	0.2	0.1	0.2	110
Mussels (boiled)	2.7	0.5	0.4	1.0	58
Octopus (raw)	1.3	0.3	0.2	0.5	48
Oysters (raw)	1.3	(0.2)	(0.2)	(0.4)	(57)
Scallops (steamed)	1.4	0.4	0.1	0.4	47
Squid (raw)	1.7	0.4	0.2	0.6	225
Whelks (boiled)	1.2	0.2	0.2	0.3	125
Winkles (boiled)	1.2	0.2	0.2	0.4	105

*Figures in brackets are estimated.
Data from *Fish and Fish products*, the 3rd supplement to *McCance and Widdowson's The Composition of Foods*, Holland, Brown and Buss, 1993, © Crown copyright.

(or those with very high triglyceride levels); you can also buy it from a pharmacist without a prescription.

Shellfish indulgence?

Shellfish are sometimes depicted as forbidden fruit for the cholesterol conscious on account of their reputation for being rich sources of cholesterol. In fact, if you have a passion for shellfish, there is no reason why it should not be indulged.

The term 'shellfish' covers crustaceans like crabs, lobsters, shrimps and prawns as well as molluscs such as clams, mussels, oysters, scallops, squid and octopus. All have a very low total and saturated fat content. In addition, they contain useful quantities of the omega-3 fatty acids EPA and DHA – generally comparable with the quantities in non-oily fish (Table 13).

The reputation for being loaded with cholesterol probably comes partly from old figures which, for technical reasons, were too high. Also, it may be that two or three higher-cholesterol members of the group have tarnished the reputation of others. There are always a few shellfish individuals that get others into trouble.

Shrimps, prawns and lobsters have high cholesterol levels (but I don't know how often they get heart attacks). Even so, there is the question of portion size, and you needn't worry about the number of prawns in a prawn cocktail (unless you've discovered a generous restaurant); I'd be more concerned about whether it was a low-saturated fat seafood sauce. A 4 oz (100 g) portion of squid might give you 250 mg of cholesterol (quite enough for the whole day). Octopus, on the other hand, will probably have less than a quarter of this cholesterol content, but these terms cover many different species and a great deal depends on the method of cooking.

- ◆ Shellfish (such as mussels, oysters, prawns, crabs) are low in fat
- ◆ Have shellfish if you want to
- ◆ Use low-fat seafood sauces
- ◆ Shrimps, prawns, lobsters and squid are low in fat but not in cholesterol: keep to moderate portion sizes

Chapter 8

Antioxidants

A few years ago, antioxidants were stuck in the pages of scientific journals, but now they have hit the big time. Everybody's talking about them. You can't even buy a simple moisturiser these days without being told you need one with antioxidants to mop up the free radicals in your skin.

What are free radicals?

This has nothing to do with the release of political prisoners. Free radicals are unstable molecules which are formed as by-products of the body's normal metabolism. If you were being rude about a free radical, you might say it was 'one electron short of a pair' (and, indeed, the chemical definition is: 'having one or more unpaired electrons'). They are, in chemical terms, highly active and, just like an unstable political activist, they are always trying to provoke a reaction – and they can cause a lot of damage in the process.

> 'A conservative is a man with two perfectly good legs
> who, however, has never learned to walk forwards . . .
> A reactionary is a somnambulist walking backwards . . .
> A radical is a man with both feet firmly planted – in the air.'
>
> Franklin D. Roosevelt,
> 'Fireside Chat', 1939

◆ Free radicals are unstable molecules that cause damage

◆ The damage done by free radicals leads to heart disease, ageing and cancer

◆ Smoking produces extra free radicals

◆ The antioxidant vitamins (A, C & E) mop up free radicals

◆ Antioxidants can block the free-radical attack that clogs arteries

◆ Too much polyunsaturated fat without antioxidants causes atherosclerosis

Oxidation

When chemists refer to 'oxidation' of a substance, they are talking about a chemical reaction in which electrons are removed from the substance. ('Reduction' is the opposite process in which electrons are added.) Now free radicals are short of electrons and they will seize any opportunity to steal them. This is what makes them unstable, provoking the reaction of oxidation whenever they can.

The oxidative damage that free radicals cause to the body's fats, proteins and DNA plays an important part in the development of heart disease, ageing processes and cancer.

Normal body chemistry produces some free radicals, but they are also generated by pollutants, including cigarette smoke.

'I simply can't believe nice communities release effluents.'
———————
William Hamilton,
William Hamilton's Anti-Social Register, cartoon, 1974

Where do antioxidants come in?

Antioxidants are substances that stop these free radicals from acting and prevent them from causing damaging chemical reactions. You can think of an antioxidant as a 'scavenger' that goes round 'gobbling up' harmful free radicals. The best known antioxidants are beta-carotene (which is related to vitamin A), vitamin C and vitamin E; they are often called the 'ACE vitamins'.

Apart from these vitamins, we get several other important antioxidants from our diet (see Table 14). The chemicals that give vegetables their colour are called carotenes and flavonoids. Selenium is a chemical element found in small quantities in certain foods.

Table 14 Antioxidants

Antioxidant	Common sources
Vitamin E	Vegetable oils, whole grains, nuts, dark green vegetables
Vitamin C	Fresh fruit and vegetables
Carotenes	Yellow/orange fruit and vegetables (e.g. carrots, apricots, peppers) and green vegetables (e.g. broccoli, spinach)
Flavonoids	Apples, onions, red wine, tea, skins of fruits and vegetables
Selenium	Brazil nuts, cashew nuts, walnuts, bread, cereals, poultry, sea fish

Selenium

Concern has been expressed recently about the falling levels of the antioxidant selenium in British and other European diets. This is largely because we import less wheat from North America nowadays. The British and European varieties used for making bread have a lower selenium content. Selenium is one of the antioxidants that helps to prevent atherosclerosis (furring and hardening of arteries) but also has important roles in thyroid balance and sperm production.

You could certainly correct any selenium deficiency by eating brazil nuts, which are a very rich source of selenium. Just three brazil nuts contain all the selenium you need for a day, and only about 1.6 g of saturated fat. Lots of other foods (such as cashew nuts, walnuts, sea fish and cereals) contain useful amounts of selenium, although not in the concentration supplied by brazil nuts. Of course, if you can't stop at three brazil nuts, the dose of saturated fat will start to mount up.

What's the benefit?

This raises a useful point: don't just get carried away with the antioxidant content of a food; consider whether it is helpful in other ways. I am reminded of that newspaper article claiming that chocolate protects against heart disease – a claim which was based on the fact that chocolate contains certain antioxidants. Regrettably, any beneficial effect of the antioxidants obtained from a chocolate binge, would be overshadowed by the large intake of saturated fat.

How can antioxidants protect against heart disease?

It is likely that antioxidants are involved in a range of biochemical processes that help to prevent heart disease. Probably one of the most important of these is protection of LDL (low density lipoprotein) from oxidation by free radicals. A simple illustration of the way in which free radical attack on LDL can lead to fatty deposits in arteries is given in Figure 6.

Fat in LDL particles is attacked by free radicals producing oxidised LDL. Along come macrophages, which are special scavenging white cells, to engulf the oxidised LDL. Once the macrophages are laden with cholesterol droplets they are known as foam cells. These foam cells can deposit fat on the artery lining causing 'fatty streaks' and eventually atherosclerosis.

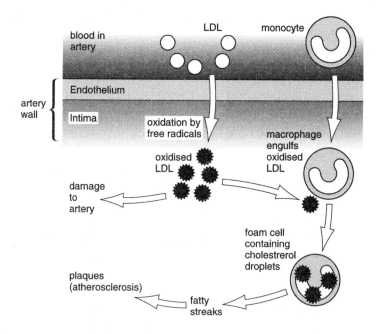

Figure 6 Free radical attack leads to fatty deposits in arteries.

Antioxidants block this chain of events by protecting the LDL from attack by free radicals. We have seen that polyunsaturated fatty acids in the diet can help to lower LDL-cholesterol – the 'bad' cholesterol – but they are not helpful unless there are enough antioxidants around. Too many polyunsaturates without enough antioxidants can increase this LDL oxidation by free radicals and lead to more atherosclerosis.

Vitamins C and E work together. As vitamin E gets used up in the battle against free radicals, vitamin C restores it and gets it fit to fight another day.

One of the damaging effects of smoking is to use up antioxidants, and smokers need more antioxidants than non-smokers. Unfortunately, you cannot reverse *all* the harmful effects of smoking by supplementing antioxidants.

◆ High levels of stored iron in the body could produce more free radicals

◆ Before the menopause, women have low iron levels and this could help protect arteries

◆ Men should avoid iron supplements unless a blood test shows they're needed

◆ Being a blood donor may lower a man's coronary risk by 15%

The irony in store

There is now some evidence that iron stored in the body can lead to the formation of free radicals; more free radicals could mean more atherosclerosis. Before the menopause, women usually store much less iron than men do because they lose iron every month with their periods. In fact, young women can easily become anaemic if there is not enough iron in the diet to replace this menstrual loss. It is very rare for women to develop coronary heart disease before the menopause (but, after the menopause, they start catching up with men; see Chapter 23). It is widely assumed that oestrogen is protecting them. Perhaps it is, but it's possible that lack of iron is another factor reducing the risk of heart disease in young women. (You have to be very bad at shaving to match a woman's menstrual blood loss; this could be a powerful argument for a man to become a blood donor – out of self-interest if nothing else.) It's quite reasonable for a young woman to supplement her diet with multivitamin tablets containing iron. Men may be better off taking preparations without iron.

What an irony if it transpires that being fortified with iron has brought some down, while others have been shielded by deficiency!

◆ High blood levels of homocysteine are linked with heart disease

◆ Homocysteine can trigger atherosclerosis and thrombosis

◆ Folic acid supplements can reduce homocysteine levels

◆ Tablets of 0.4 mg folic acid can be bought over the counter

◆ Green vegetables and blackeye beans are rich in folic acid

More about foam cells

I have explained to you how oxidised LDL is gobbled by macrophages resulting in foam cells, which cause atherosclerosis, and I can't leave the subject without mentioning homocysteine.

What's homocysteine?

Homocysteine is a breakdown product of a substance called methionine; methionine is an amino acid – a building block of protein. High blood levels of homocysteine occur for a short time after eating large amounts of animal protein, but persistently high levels have been found in many people with coronary heart disease. Excess homocysteine is converted into a substance called homocysteine thiolactone. This compound combines with LDL-cholesterol to form an abnormal structure, which is scavenged by macrophages (in just the same way as oxidised LDL) producing foam cells, fatty streaks and atherosclerosis. Not only that, but homocysteine triggers changes in the artery lining that can lead to thrombosis.

Just as the high average cholesterol levels in the UK raise the risk of heart disease, it looks as though we have a serious problem with homocysteine as well. Some people make too much homocysteine; the amount you produce is influenced by your diet and your genes. Researchers have shown that when some people are given a dose of methionine, they convert a lot of it to homocysteine, producing high blood levels. Alarmingly, it's likely that the majority of older people in the UK have homocysteine levels high enough to raise the risk of a stroke or heart attack. At the moment, you can't pop down to the doctor to have a homocysteine test like you can a cholesterol test; it is done in specialised clinics and for research purposes. You could pay for a test and now a testing kit is available to the public from Yorktest Laboratories.

Folic acid, vitamin B_6 and vitamin B_{12}

And the good news? Persistently raised homocysteine levels can be reduced to normal by dietary supplements of folic acid. Vitamin B_6 also helps to lower the concentration of homocysteine in the blood, especially after it has been raised by a dose of methionine.

Folic acid (also known as folate, folacin, and pteroylglutamic acid) is the B vitamin that women are advised to supplement (at a dose of 0.4 mg daily) before conceiving and in the first 12 weeks of pregnancy. This reduces the risk of neural tube defects (like spina bifida) in the developing embryo.

What dose of folic acid is needed to bring homocysteine levels down to normal? A lot of research is going on to test out different doses of folic acid (sometimes with vitamins B_6 and B_{12}). It is becoming clear that 0.4 mg of folic acid is normally very effective. Most people do not obtain this much folic acid from food. There is a big debate in government circles about whether extra folic acid should be added to foods such as bread. Of course, you don't have to wait for government action. You can buy 0.4 mg tablets of folic acid over the counter.

Green vegetables (especially Brussels sprouts, kale and spinach), blackeye beans, liver and fortified breakfast cereals are good sources of folic acid. Vitamin B_6 (pyridoxine) is found in green vegetables, breakfast cereals, fish, meat and poultry. You could get a supplement of vitamins B_6, B_{12} and folic acid from a multivitamin preparation but these often contain too little folic acid to treat raised homocysteine levels. The recommended maximum dose of vitamin B_6 to be taken as a supplement has recently been reduced to 10 mg.

A glance at the evidence on antioxidants

Leaving biochemical theory aside, what evidence is there that antioxidants protect against heart disease?

A lot of evidence has been gathered from animal work. For example, the arteries of rabbits or hens with high cholesterol levels will fur up quickly with fatty deposits, but this can be prevented by giving vitamin E to the animals.

Collecting good evidence about people is more complicated, but we are making progress. In the United States Nurses' Health Study involving 87,000 women, low intakes of vitamin E and beta-carotene were linked with an increased risk of coronary heart disease. Women with the highest antioxidant intakes had a 30–40% lower heart disease risk.

The death rates from heart disease in 16 European countries were compared and published in 1991. The six-fold difference between the countries' death rates was not adequately explained by differences in the established risk factors (such as smoking, high cholesterol and raised blood pressure). Vitamin E levels turned out to be more closely linked than any other factor to the rates of heart disease in the different communities.

Research on 1605 men from Eastern Finland published in 1997 found that men with vitamin C deficiency were more likely to have a heart attack.

Should I take supplements of antioxidants?

Studies of this sort support the view that a good intake of antioxidants – notably vitamins E and C – provides some protection against coronary heart disease. You may think that taking tablets or capsules containing antioxidant vitamins is a logical step, but we still have unanswered questions. Do we get all the antioxidants we need from a balanced diet or do supplements provide extra protection? Do supplements have any unwanted effects? Which antioxidants are most effective at preventing heart disease and in what doses?

We can get answers to these questions by carrying out 'controlled intervention trials', which compare large numbers of people who have been prescribed antioxidant supplements, with large numbers prescribed placebo (or 'dummy') capsules. Such studies have to be meticulously constructed to avoid misleading results and they take years to complete. Those published so far give some conflicting answers. Some important trials of vitamin E and C supplementation are in progress.

◆ Vitamin E stops atherosclerosis in animals with high cholesterols

◆ In people, low levels of vitamins C and E are linked with high rates of heart disease

◆ Fruits and vegetables are the main sources of antioxidant vitamins

◆ We aren't 100% certain that high-dose vitamin E supplements are safe

◆ Supplements are no substitute for a balanced diet

Supplements not substitutes

Whatever you do, don't fall into the trap of imagining that antioxidant, vitamin or mineral supplements can ever make up for a poor diet.

Much of this book is about the benefits of eating good food. It is a great mistake to think that, once we have identified the key nutrients, we can compress the value of a meal into a pill. There is strong evidence, from many investigations, for the importance of fruit and vegetables in the diet. A study by Timothy Key and colleagues published in 1996 followed over 10,000 health-conscious people for 17 years. Not surprisingly, the overall death rate for the group was lower than for the general population. Those who ate fresh fruit every day had even lower death rates – from all causes, as well as heart disease and stroke.

No doubt, the antioxidants in fruit and vegetables play a vital part in protecting us against heart disease, but we know that fibre and starch are important as well. If you extract 'pure nutrients' from whole food because you think that they are the most important, you may leave something even more important behind. Many observational studies have shown that eating foods high in beta-carotene is beneficial. Unfortunately, consistent benefit has not been shown in trials of beta-carotene supplements. Perhaps it was something else in beta-carotene-containing foods that was doing the good.

While evidence for the benefit and safety of antioxidant supplements is awaited, evidence for the value of fruit and vegetables in protecting against heart disease and cancer is overwhelming. You should eat at least five portions of fruit and vegetables every day. Nine would be better. A portion could be a piece of fruit or a serving of vegetables. When you don't have fresh vegetables, use frozen or tinned. They'll still do you good.

So what do I do about supplements? Well, although doctors and nutritional experts do not have enough information to recommend antioxidant supplements to the general population, we have to make a personal decision about whether to take them. Pending further evidence, I take 200 mg of vitamin E and 250 mg of vitamin C daily – as well as eating a good diet, of course.

200 mg of vitamin E is *20 times* the recommended daily allowance. While it is possible that extra protection is obtained from doses above the recommended level, we cannot be certain that such high doses are completely safe. There are plenty of people taking much higher doses of vitamin E than I take, but some of the evidence on megadoses of vitamin E gives cause for concern. The Heart Protection Study published in 2002 (see page 309) failed to show any additional benefit or risk when 600 mg of vitamin E and 250 mg of vitamin C were added to other treatment.

ACTION POINT

◆ Eat *at least* 5 portions of fruit and vegetables a day

Chapter 9

Garlic

It is, of course, an old wives' tale that garlic is good for you. It seems that this may be one of those occasions when old wives know best.

The medicinal powers of the garlic plant (*Allium sativum*) were proclaimed by the ancient Egyptians and by Hippocrates. Respiratory infections, boils, fungal infections and infestations with worms and other parasites are among the many conditions that have been treated with garlic over the ages. In recent times, science has provided some evidence that garlic can have remarkable effects on the cardiovascular system.

There must be something in it

Actually lots of different substances have been identified in garlic cloves, but the main ingredient that seems to be responsible for its medicinal properties is called allicin. Unfortunately, this is also the stuff that stinks. Attempts to extract a garlic essence with all the medicinal zest of fresh garlic and none of the odour have failed: you can't have the ping without the pong! Some odourless garlic preparations contain no active ingredients.

> 'I did not realize what it had done to my breath – one doesn't with garlic – until this afternoon when I stood waiting for somebody to open a door for me and suddenly noticed that the varnish on the door was bubbling.'
>
> Frank Muir,
> *You Can't Have Your Kayak and Heat It,* 1973

The quantity of allicin present in fresh garlic varies greatly and is influenced by agricultural conditions, as well as the origin of the garlic. When fresh garlic is stored at room temperature, the amount of allicin that can be obtained from it decreases substantially over a few weeks. However, when garlic powder preparations have been carefully dried and stored, they can retain up to 90% of available allicin over five years; those derived from the best Chinese garlic are good sources of allicin.

Allicin itself would be difficult to preserve as it is chemically unstable. Fresh whole garlic cloves contain the inactive, odourless amino acid called alliin. Crushing the garlic sets the enzyme allinase to work on alliin, releasing allicin and its familiar odour.

Of course, for most people, the aroma of garlic is a delight in the kitchen and at the dinner table – but not on the breath of your colleague the next morning. It is claimed that you can neutralise the odour of allicin by eating parsley. There may be something in this but I'm sure that there are many people blissfully believing that they are enjoying all the benefits of garlic without the social consequences; their friends don't like to tell them that they are living in a fantasy world – allicin Wonderland.

The best solution is for all of us to eat lots of garlic every day, so that we cannot detect it on anyone else's breath; then only the occasional alien will be offended. Of course, this is not such a fantastic

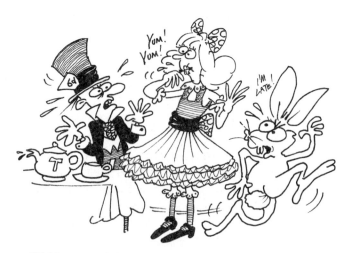

"I'd be a social outcast if it weren't for parsley."

idea. In some countries they have been doing it for centuries. It would be rather hard, I suppose, on that small minority of people who genuinely cannot tolerate garlic.

Kwai tablets contain garlic powder prepared by drying good quality Chinese garlic cloves. The special coating prevents the release of any allicin until the tablet reaches the digestive system. The tablets certainly are odour-free, but the people who take them may not be. In one large study, a garlic odour was reported (usually by the spouse) in 21% of those taking the tablets but also in 9% of the placebo group whose tablets contained no garlic!

Garlic and cholesterol

Various animal experiments, in which animals were fed diets that cause fatty deposits in arteries, have shown that garlic can protect the arteries against these changes. The studies have generally found a fall in the undesirable LDL-cholesterol together with a rise in the protective HDL-cholesterol in subjects treated with garlic.

In a large German study published in 1990, Dr Mader examined the effects of garlic in 261 people whose cholesterol and triglyceride readings were above the recommended levels. This was a randomised, double-blind, placebo-controlled trial: people were either given Kwai tablets or 'dummy' tablets, which looked the same, and neither the people nor researchers knew who was getting what until the code was cracked at the end. Reduction in cholesterol was significantly greater in those receiving garlic (12% at 16 weeks compared with 3% in the placebo group). Triglyceride levels dropped too (17% in the garlic group and only 2% in those receiving placebo tablets).

Garlic and thrombosis

If our blood didn't clot, we would bleed to death. On the other hand, if the blood clots too easily, thrombosis (the formation of a clot in the circulation) can cause a heart attack or stroke. The body is constantly keeping a balance between these extremes. Eating saturated fat increases the risk of thrombosis; several studies have shown that both garlic and onion can help protect against it.

The body's system for reversing the chain of events that leads to thrombosis is called 'fibrinolysis'. In one study there was a 70%

increase in fibrinolysis within a few hours of eating fried or raw garlic and this increase continued during a month of eating garlic. Onions contain a substance called cycloalliin (and you will notice the similarity to alliin in garlic). Cycloalliin significantly increased fibrinolysis 1½ hours after it was given to people who had suffered a heart attack.

Platelets (also known as thrombocytes) are the smallest blood cells but they are a vital part of the blood-clotting system. By sticking to each other or to the walls of a damaged artery they can help to bring bleeding under control. If platelets become too 'sticky', they can add to the plaques that cause narrowing of arteries and they can provoke thrombosis leading to a heart attack or stroke.

Various experiments in animals and humans have indicated that garlic can stop platelets clumping together too easily. This action of garlic is similar to the effect of aspirin; low-dose aspirin is prescribed for some people who are at increased risk of thrombosis (e.g. people who have had a heart attack or suffer from angina). We do not yet have enough information about the effect of garlic on platelet function to recommend it as an alternative to aspirin for people at high risk of thrombosis.

Garlic and blood pressure

Experiments on laboratory animals (such as rats, cats and dogs) have shown that garlic can reduce blood pressure. More relevant is the work done on humans. Auer and colleagues published a study in 1990 in which 800 mg a day of dried garlic powder (Kwai tablets) was given to people with raised blood pressure in a controlled trial. Very satisfactory reductions in blood pressure were observed in those taking garlic.

Survival in stink?

Maybe garlic does fight infection and protect against heart disease. You could propose that its widespread use around the world is explained by natural selection – that more garlic eaters have survived. Perhaps we too should become a nation of garlic eaters before we are wiped out by heart disease. I wouldn't go that far myself, but it is intriguing that this traditional, natural food flavouring could turn out to have so many beneficial effects.

The combination of actions on blood fats, cholesterol, blood pressure and thrombosis could make garlic a powerful protector against heart disease, but the evidence for this is incomplete.

Ideally we would have confirmation from carefully controlled trials that eating garlic results in fewer heart attacks. The trial design must ensure that the only difference between the groups under comparison is in their garlic consumption. As it is, a handful of experiments show that garlic reduces some important risk factors and we can point to groups of people that eat a lot of garlic and have low rates of heart disease (but also differ in other ways from groups of people with high rates).

If you enjoy garlic in your food, perhaps you will enjoy it all the more now. Unfortunately, it is likely that daily consumption of large quantities of good quality fresh garlic would be required to obtain maximum benefit, but nature has the last laugh and even tiny amounts can wreak havoc in your social life.

A practical way of eating the quantities of active garlic used in clinical trials is to take Kwai tablets, provided you are one of the eight out of ten who can do so without smelling of garlic, and you don't mind swallowing six to eight tablets a day. There is certainly not enough evidence for me to recommend this; more research is needed. It could never make up for an unhealthy diet or lifestyle, but at least you would have the assurance that you were simply taking a dried preparation of something that has been safety-tested on millions across the globe. It would also remove any pressure to add garlic to your food as if it were a medicine, leaving you free to delight in its flavour whenever it suits you and your diary.

GARLIC FACTS

- ◆ Lowers cholesterol and triglyceride levels
- ◆ Reduces platelet stickiness and the risk of thrombosis
- ◆ Lowers blood pressure
- ◆ The active ingredient, allicin, is the stuff that stinks
- ◆ Clinical trials used large amounts of allicin
- ◆ More research is needed
- ◆ Garlic is lovely. Enjoy it!

Chapter 10

Alcohol

'We drink one another's healths, and spoil our own.'

Jerome K. Jerome,
Idle Thoughts of an Idle Fellow, 1886

To your health!

Is that glass of wine a further step towards health and happiness or another nail in the coffin? It really depends whether it's the first drink of the evening or the fifth. A lot of research has been done on this subject and it is quite clear that light to moderate drinking can help to protect you against heart disease but heavier drinking will damage your health.

The J-shaped curve

A graph showing the link between death rate (from all causes) in an industrialised population and alcohol consumption is a J-shaped curve (Figure 7).

This means that the risk of death is higher for people who drink no alcohol at all than for those who drink a little. (Yes, I know 100% of us die eventually but when we talk about death rate or 'mortality' we are referring to the proportion of a population that dies in a specified period.) The lowest risk, the lowest part of the J, is at one to two units a day and the risk shoots up after four units a day.

This reduction in death rate among light and moderate drinkers results from reduced coronary heart disease (which is such a common

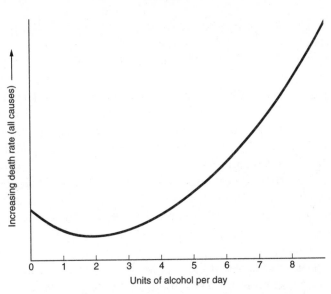

Figure 7 The J-shaped curve. This shows the link between alcohol consumption and death rate. The lowest risk, the lowest part of the J, is at one or two units a day.

killer that it has a big influence on total mortality figures). Heavier drinking increases the risk of having a stroke or developing liver cirrhosis, pancreatitis or certain cancers, or even damaging the heart muscle (cardiomyopathy) – not to mention road accidents or falling off a cliff.

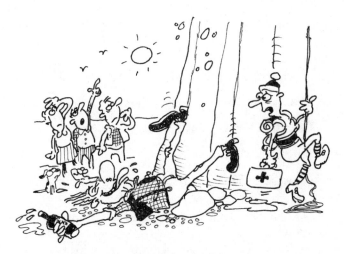

"At least he died with a healthy heart."

This J-shaped curve hides differences within the population. Alcohol is not politically correct. It is ageist and sexist.

Young adults (under 40) are more likely to die in an accident or as a result of violence than from a heart attack. The relationship between drinking and death rates in this age group is not a J-shaped curve. It's a straight line. The more you drink, the more likely you are to die. This is not surprising as alcohol is often involved in accidents and violent deaths. Older people are more likely to die from heart disease and less likely to die as a result of an accident or violence, so the protective effect of alcohol becomes significant. An interesting footnote for older people is that French researchers published an investigation in 1997, which concluded that older people who drink wine moderately are less prone to develop senile dementia and Alzheimer's disease than non-drinkers.

For women, the risk of heart disease rises after the menopause and the risk is higher for teetotallers than for light drinkers, but the recommended safe drinking limit is lower for women than men. This is not because the limits are set by a committee of men. In general, a woman's body contains less water than a man's and it takes less alcohol to reach a harmful concentration. There is some evidence that even modest consumption of alcohol can increase the risk of breast cancer.

What's the limit?

Adding up your alcohol intake is made easier by referring to units. One unit of alcohol is 8 g or 10 ml of ethanol and is based on standard pub measures.

The following drinks give you one unit of alcohol:

- 1 half pint of normal strength lager or beer;
- 1 small (125 ml) glass of wine;
- 1 measure (25 ml) spirits;
- 1 measure (50 ml) fortified wine e.g. sherry, Martini.

Remember, these are pub measures and home measures are usually doubles!

The latest official guidelines recommend that men should not drink more than three to four units a day and women should not go above two to three units a day. Drinking the maximum allowance every day is not recommended as this can damage health.

I have something very important to explain to you. These are the official limits because the really damaging effects of alcohol become apparent when people drink more than this. You'll be better off drinking less. You will get most of the protection that alcohol can give you against heart disease by drinking as little as one unit a day on five days of the week. For the under 50s, the risks of drinking up to the limit outweigh any benefits.

An important improvement in the revised guidelines was the emphasis on daily rather than weekly limits. Previously, the safe limits were said to be up to 21 units a week for a man and up to 14 units a week for a woman. So a man drinking 10 pints of beer a week would be meeting the guidelines, but if he drinks it all at the weekend it's a very unsafe pattern of drinking. Binge drinking is bad for you. Apart from the risk of accidents and the social problems that come with alcoholic intoxication, it pushes up the blood pressure and does not protect the heart like moderate drinking spread throughout the week. In fact, a bout of heavy drinking can bring on a heart attack even when the coronary arteries are normal!

◆ Light drinking helps protect against heart disease

◆ Heavier drinking damages health, risking strokes, cirrhosis and cancers

◆ In the under 40s, the benefits of alcohol are outweighed by the risks

◆ 1 unit of alcohol a day, 5 days a week is enough to help your heart

◆ Binge drinking is dangerous and can even cause heart attacks

How can alcohol protect against coronary heart disease?

It has often been pointed out that the higher rate of heart disease among non-drinkers does not prove that alcohol protects against heart disease. Perhaps this odd group of people who drink no alcohol at all is at higher risk because it includes those who have had to give up alcohol for health reasons. This is a very important point but researchers have now shown that the difference cannot be explained by ex-drinkers among the non-drinkers. After many studies on the subject, it is widely accepted that a modest alcohol consumption reduces the risk of coronary heart disease. But how?

An interesting case report published in 1984 by Breier and Lisch concerned a 69-year-old man with a condition known as familial hypercholesterolaemia. Sufferers from this inherited problem have very high cholesterol levels and, unless treatment is given to lower the cholesterol, arteries become clogged causing early heart disease. You may remember the actor Richard Beckinsale who died tragically young as a result of this condition. Well, the remarkable thing about the man studied was that he had reached the age of 69 without any evidence of narrowed arteries.

It seemed that, although he had a very high cholesterol level, his arteries were being protected by an unusually high concentration of HDL_2-cholesterol (a sub-fraction of the beneficial HDL-cholesterol). The other thing the doctors noticed was that this man drank 375 ml (three glasses) of red wine daily.

They decided to test whether the red wine was causing the high level of protective HDL_2-cholesterol. The man went through a cycle of drinking no alcohol for 21 days, followed by 21 days of drinking his usual three glasses of red wine a day. During the time without alcohol, the concentration of HDL_2 in his blood fell to about one quarter of the original level. After 21 days back on the red wine, the HDL_2 level had returned to its original value.

It is important to understand that this was a study on one particular man, and not everybody will have the same response. (Otherwise, we should adopt this dose of red wine as a standard treatment for familial hypercholesterolaemia for a start.) Nevertheless, several other studies have shown that drinking alcohol generally raises HDL-cholesterol levels. No doubt this is one of the ways in which alcohol can protect us against coronary heart disease. In fact, statistically, you could explain about half the extra heart disease occurring in non-drinkers in terms of lower HDL-cholesterol levels.

Raising HDL-cholesterol levels will help to stop arteries furring up over the years. Another very important way of reducing heart disease risk is to reduce the chance of a thrombosis – a blood clot in the circulation. Alcohol is known to make the blood platelets less active and to decrease fibrinogen levels; both of these actions will lower the risk of thrombosis.

Red wine contains antioxidants. The actual substances are polyphenols (notably flavonoids such as quercetin and epicatechin) but that shouldn't put you off your wine. On the contrary, their discovery is a cause for celebration because, like other antioxidants, they have been shown to reduce oxidation of LDL (see Chapter 8). So, theoretically at least, the antioxidants in red wine could help to stop fatty plaques forming in arteries. These antioxidants come from the grape skin and can also be found, in lower concentrations, in red (but not white) grape juice.

What's your poison?

Should you choose beer, wine or spirits to give your heart the best protection?

Much publicity has been given to 'the French paradox'. This has nothing to do with French paramedics treating heart attack victims. The point is that the French suffer fewer heart attacks than you would expect from the amount of saturated fat in their diet; it has been suggested that all the red wine they drink is protecting their hearts. The cynic might say that they die of alcoholic cirrhosis before they get a chance to have a heart attack. Certainly there are many factors apart from wine consumption that may contribute to this paradox (see page 140).

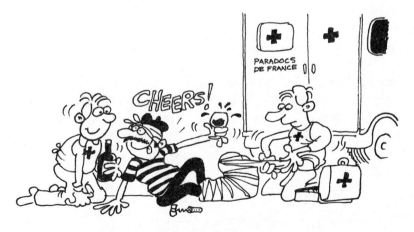

Nothing to do with French paramedics.

Over 60 studies have found lower rates of heart disease among light and moderate drinkers compared with non-drinkers. Some of these investigations have, indeed, concluded that wine offers better protection than other beverages but some studies have found in favour of spirits or beer. One of the problems is that one type of drink may be associated with a different drinking pattern from another type, according to the social customs of the community studied. If wine is normally consumed in moderation with meals, the effect will be very beneficial compared with binge drinking of spirits. A study on health professionals found spirits to be the most protective; spirits were the most commonly consumed type of drink and were generally taken in moderation throughout the week rather than in binges at the weekend.

Many studies on this subject were collected and analysed by Rimm and colleagues in 1996. They concluded that there was strong evidence linking all alcoholic drinks, when consumed in moderation, with a lower risk of heart disease, but not that one type of drink gives better protection than another.

It may be that the antioxidants in red wine offer additional benefits but, clearly, most of the protection against heart disease comes from the alcohol. On current evidence, then, despite what you may have heard about the health benefits of drinking red wine, it is pointless to take it like a medicine if you prefer to drink white. Personally, there is nothing I would rather drink with my evening meal than a glass of red wine, even if I am eating fish or poultry.

So, the important question is not so much "What's your poison?" as "How do you take it?" The beverage you choose is less critical than your pattern of drinking. This was borne out by an Australian study published in 1997 by McElduff and Dobson. They found the risk of having a heart attack was lowest in men who reported having one to four drinks a day – and in women who reported one or two drinks a day – on five or six days a week.

Should I start drinking?

If you do not drink any alcohol, you may be thinking by now that you should start. I would rather encourage you to concentrate on

◆ Alcohol can increase HDL-cholesterol and reduce thrombosis
  risk

◆ The pattern of drinking is more important than the type of
  drink:

  – 10 glasses of red wine on Friday night increases risk

  – ½ pint beer 5 times a week helps the heart

◆ Antioxidants in red wine may give added protection but this is
  not proven

◆ When society increases average alcohol intake, the number of
  heavy drinkers rises

all the other strategies in this book for reducing your risk of heart disease than to start drinking. And, if you are a young person, don't forget that the health hazards of drinking alcohol may outweigh the benefits. Obviously, nobody should mix drinking with driving.

Doctors have a problem when it comes to advising people about the benefits of light drinking. I don't mean that old saying about an alcoholic being defined as someone who drinks more than his doctor. Though it is true that heavy drinkers tend to underestimate how much they are drinking. Indeed, Dylan Thomas apparently said "An alcoholic is someone you don't like who drinks as much as you do". True alcoholics, of course, are one group of people who should not attempt light drinking. The only path for them is to avoid alcohol completely. No, the problem doctors have when advising about the benefits of light drinking is that there will always be those who say to themselves, "If a little will do me good, then a lot will do me more good." I hope you understand by now that nothing could be further from the truth. It is also a sad fact that the percentage of heavy drinkers in any group of people is related to the average alcohol consumption of that group. Encouraging more people to drink, however well-intentioned, is likely to result in more people drinking heavily. Our objective to convert the majority of people into light drinkers seems impossible to achieve.

Drinking to your heart's content

Alcohol is one of God's good gifts. It is there to be enjoyed but, tragically, is often abused. Savouring a glass of wine, five days a week is quite enough to help your heart; you can get most of the health benefit from a glass every other day.

Cheers!

ACTION POINT

◆ Enjoy up to 1 or 2 units of alcohol a day – not more!

Chapter 11

Coffee or tea?

'Look here, Steward, if this is coffee, I want tea; but if this is
tea, then I wish for coffee.'

Punch (1841–1992) vol. 123, 1902

You can often divide a roomful of people into coffee- and tea-
drinkers. Some people are coffee potty, while others are total-tea-
ers. Is there any evidence that our choice of beverage influences
our risk of getting heart disease?

Both coffee and tea contain caffeine, of course. Caffeine can stimu-
late the heart, provoking palpitations, and the brain, causing insomnia. It is also a diuretic: drinking a cup of strong coffee stimulates more
urine production than drinking the same volume of water. Caffeine
addicts will know the withdrawal headaches that occur if they abstain
for a time. For all this, there is no consistent evidence that caffeine is
linked with coronary heart disease and I see no reason for moderate
coffee- or tea-drinkers to be concerned about their caffeine intake (as
long as they are not suffering palpitations or insomnia).

The mystery ingredient

For years it has been suspected that drinking a lot of coffee might contribute to the development of heart disease. It has been established by
several research teams that drinking Scandinavian boiled coffee
causes a rise in blood cholesterol levels. If it isn't the caffeine in this
boiled coffee that raises cholesterol, what is it? It was discovered that

the mystery ingredient is removed by passing the coffee through filter paper; filtered coffee doesn't increase blood cholesterol.

We now know that two lipids, or fatty substances, called cafestol and kahweol are to blame. They seem to be unique to the coffee bean.

◆ Coffee beans contain lipids that raise LDL-cholesterol

◆ 6 cups of cafetière coffee a day could raise cholesterol by 10%

◆ Filtered coffee (paper filter) does not raise cholesterol

But we don't boil our coffee like the Scandinavians

It has long been known that the Scandinavians' coffee-boiling habit is disastrous for cholesterol levels, but, if cafestol and kahweol are present in the coffee bean, what about the types of coffee that we normally drink?

A Dutch group of researchers, Urgert and colleagues, published an interesting study in the *British Medical Journal* in November 1996. In this randomised controlled trial, half the subjects drank five to six cups (0.9 litres) a day of strong cafetière coffee and the other half drank the same amount of strong filtered coffee. The two types of coffee contained the same amount of caffeine. They kept this up for six months and repeated blood samples were taken before, during and after the six-month period.

Cafetière coffee raised the total cholesterol level by 6–10%. Worse still, most of that rise was due to increased LDL-cholesterol (the damaging one), which went up by 9–14%. These changes continued for the six months of coffee drinking. Every one percentage rise in total cholesterol results in a two percentage rise in risk of coronary heart disease. So, drinking five to six cups of cafetière coffee a day produced a 12–20% rise in coronary risk!

There was also a 26% rise in triglyceride levels in the cafetière drinkers but this had settled to 7% by the end of the six months. In addition, the researchers found that cafetière coffee raised the level of a liver enzyme (alanine aminotransferase) but there was no evidence of liver damage and the significance of this is uncertain.

Clearly, then, cafetière coffee can push up cholesterol levels just like boiled Scandinavian coffee but filtration removes the problem. A word of warning: the researchers used paper filters and you could not expect filtration through a metallic mesh to have the same effect.

What about other types of coffee?

Turkish coffee, although served in small cups, is very concentrated stuff. (I think it must have been the origin of that old joke. You know. Man: "Waiter, waiter, this coffee tastes like mud." Waiter: "It was only ground this morning, sir.") It contains similar quantities of cafestol and kahweol per cup to cafetière and boiled coffee.

Italian espresso coffee is also served in small cups and is a less concentrated source of cafestol and kahweol. It is estimated that about 25 cups of espresso would be equivalent to five or six of cafetière in this regard.

Instant and percolated coffee have low concentrations of the problem substances and their effect on cholesterol will be minimal.

Having filtered the evidence, what does it all boil down to? Remember: these alarming effects were produced by five or six cups of cafetière a day. If you are a frequent coffee drinker, you would be better off with instant, percolated or (paper) filtered. If cafetière coffee is an occasional indulgence, there is no need to lose any sleep over it (but you may do if you have it late at night).

ACTION POINTS
◆ Choose filtered/percolated or instant coffee
◆ Avoid regular consumption of strong cafetière coffee

What about tea?

'English cuisine is generally so threadbare that for years there has been a gentlemen's agreement in the civilized world to allow the Brits pre-eminence in the matter of tea – which, after all, comes down to little more than the ability to boil water.'

Wilfrid Sheed,
'Taking Pride in Prejudice', *GQ*, 1984

The good old English cuppa (of Asian tea) appears to be completely innocent as far as coronary heart disease is concerned. In fact, because tea contains flavonoid antioxidants, it may offer some protection against heart disease but, at the moment, no one can say how significant this is.

Isn't herbal tea more healthy?

Well, what is normal tea if it isn't a herbal tea made from the dried leaves of the shrub, Camellia sinensis? Of course, there is a wide variety of other plant extracts sold under the label 'herbal tea' and sometimes people imagine that they must be better for you than traditional tea. Indeed, some people think that anything 'herbal' or 'natural' must be quite safe and will probably do you a power of good. They overlook the fact that some of our most toxic drugs and poisons are simply plant extracts.

I'm not suggesting that any of the herbal teas in your local health food store are toxic. Some of them contain very familiar ingredients and offer a good caffeine-free alternative to tea. None of them will have been tried and tested and researched on anything like the scale of our traditional cuppa.

Hard to beat

Talking of making tea, isn't it a nuisance when the kettle element scales up in hard water areas? Before you rush to soften your drinking water, you may like to reflect on the fact that studies have repeatedly shown lower death rates from cardiovascular disease in hard water areas. The mortality difference is small, and you certainly shouldn't worry about it if you happen to live in a soft water area, but it has been a consistent finding. A water hardness level of 170 mg/l of calcium carbonate is fine and there is no apparent advantage in having it any harder than that.

'Eric: I always take my wife morning tea in my pyjamas.
But is she grateful? No – she says she'd rather have
it in a cup.'

Eric Morecambe and Ernie Wise,
The Morecambe and Wise Joke Book, 1979

◆ Tea appears safe and its antioxidants might even help your heart

◆ 'Herbal' teas are probably OK but have not been researched like tea and coffee

◆ Hard water areas have lower rates of heart disease; the difference is small

Having your fill

Chapter 12

Getting your balance

'When Marilyn Monroe was married to Arthur Miller, his
mother always made matzo ball soup. After the tenth time,
Marilyn said, "Gee Arthur, these matzo balls are pretty nice,
but isn't there any other part of the matzo you can eat?"'

Ann Barr and Paul Levy,
The Foodie Handbook, 1984

Variety is vital. How can we be sure our choice of foods is giving us
all the nutrients we need and in the right balance?

To make a detailed analysis of your diet, a dietitian would use food
composition tables or a computer to calculate your intake of various
nutrients. Don't even attempt this. There is quite enough to contend
with in the supermarket without taking a laptop computer.

A simple, practical method of making sure we keep the right
balance is to use food groups. Table 15 (page 118) shows the five
main food groups:

- Cereals and starchy foods;

- Fruit and vegetables;

- Milk and dairy products;

- Meat and high-protein foods;

- Fatty and sugary foods.

Every day you should eat a variety of different foods from each
of the first four groups.

The fifth group is foods containing lots of fat, lots of sugar or both. You don't need to select any items from this group for a healthy, balanced diet; if you do, keep the quantity right down. Yes, some of these foods (such as the cooking oils) are sources of essential fatty acids, but you can get these in adequate quantities from foods in the other four groups. This is not a completely comprehensive list of foods; the examples given will enable you to put other foods in the correct category (Figure 8).

Fruit and vegetables

Bread, other cereals and potatoes

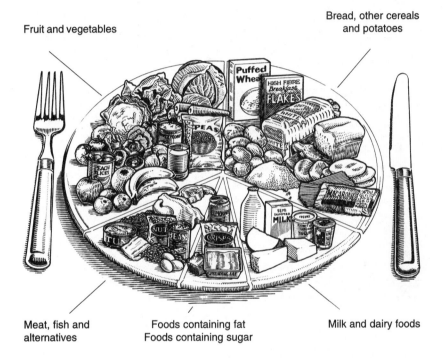

Meat, fish and alternatives

Foods containing fat
Foods containing sugar

Milk and dairy foods

Figure 8 The balance of good health. © 1996 HEA (now Health Development Agency).

Most of your food should come from the first two groups – the starchy foods and the fruit and vegetable group. Have several different portions from the starch group each day, where a portion is a bowl of cereal, or bread with a meal, or a serving of rice, pasta or potato. Include some higher fibre options such as wholemeal bread or brown rice. You needn't worry about having too much fruit and vegetable; most people in the UK are having too little. Eat **at least** five portions a day. A portion could be a piece of fruit, or a bowl of fruit salad, or a serving of vegetables.

Table 15 The five main food groups

---

1. Cereals and starchy foods

Bread, including wholemeal, mixed grain, granary loaves, white bread, French bread, pitta bread, rolls, baps

Crumpets, crispbreads, matzos

Breakfast cereals, muesli

Oats (including porridge), barley, rye, wheat, bulgar wheat, buckwheat, millet, maize, polenta, semolina, couscous, tapioca

Rice, including brown rice and wild rice

Pasta: spaghetti, lasagna, tagliatelle, macaroni, noodles etc.

Potatoes, including sweet potato, cassava, yam, taro

---

2. Fruit and vegetables

Salad vegetables, including lettuce, cucumber, tomatoes, peppers etc.

All vegetables (not potatoes) – fresh, frozen or canned

All fruit – fresh, frozen or canned (in fruit juice)

Dried fruit e.g. prunes, figs, apricots, raisins, sultanas

Unsweetened fruit juice

---

3. Milk and dairy products

Milk, skimmed recommended for most adults

Cheese: most have a high fat content
Cottage cheese, quark, and a little Parmesan/pecorino recommended

Yoghurt, especially very low-fat varieties

Fromage frais, particularly virtually fat-free

Buttermilk

---

4. Meat and high-protein foods

Meat: beef, pork, lamb (lean cuts, remove fat), lean bacon (or smoked turkey rashers), ham, rabbit, venison

Meat products: reduced-fat sausages/burgers (still not very low-fat)

Poultry: chicken, turkey

Fish: white fish – cod, haddock, plaice, sole etc.
Oily fish – mackerel, herring, sardines, pilchards, salmon
Shellfish – scallops, oysters, cockles etc.

Nuts: hazelnuts, almonds, walnuts, peanuts

Seeds: sunflower, sesame

Eggs

4. Meat and high-protein foods (continued)

Pulses: lentils, chickpeas, beans (e.g. baked beans, kidney beans, broad beans, mung beans, blackeye beans, pinto beans, soya beans), peas, split peas

Dahl, hummus, tofu, textured vegetable protein (TVP)

Quorn

5. Fatty/sugary foods

Fatty foods (some also have high sugar content):

Fat spreads, margarine, butter

Olive oil, rapeseed oil, corn oil, sunflower oil, safflower oil, soya oil, sesame seed oil, grapeseed oil, walnut oil, groundnut (peanut) oil, palm oil, coconut oil, 'vegetable oil'

Suet, lard, dripping

Oil-based dressings, fatty sauces, mayonnaise

Cream, ice cream

Cakes, biscuits, puddings, pastries, crisps

Chocolate, chocolate spread, toffee/butterscotch sauces

Coconut bars

Sugary foods (some also have high fat content):

Sweets

Sweet snacks

Sweetened drinks, squashes

Sugar, jams

Milk and dairy products are a very important source of calcium. They provide protein too. If you stick to skimmed milk and very low-fat dairy products, you can use them freely. Aim for three servings a day from this group. Examples of a serving would be the milk taken in tea throughout the day, or a carton of yoghurt, or quark added to a pasta dish.

Most Britons are eating more protein than they need and much of it comes with a good helping of saturated fat in meat products. Two servings a day from the protein group is enough. Use pulses and fish in abundance; use red meat sparingly. Pulses, of course, as well as providing protein, give you starch and soluble fibre.

Variety is the key. Five apples do not count as five portions.

ACTION POINTS

◆ Eat loads of cereal/starchy foods such as bread, rice, pasta, potato

◆ Eat *at least* 5 portions of fruit and vegetables a day

◆ Use skimmed milk, low-fat yoghurt, fromage frais, buttermilk, quark

◆ Have lots of pulses (peas, beans, lentils, chickpeas)

◆ Use fish, lean poultry (skinned), egg white (not yolk), tofu, TVP, Quorn

◆ Avoid meat products (sausages, burgers, pies, etc.) and fatty red meat

◆ Fill most of your menu with the first two food groups and beware the fifth

---

On balance

The food group principle can help people of all ages to achieve a balanced diet. Obviously, portion sizes and energy requirements vary from individual to individual. Some people have food allergies, or intolerances, or special dietary needs requiring professional advice, but everyone should get the best balance that they can.

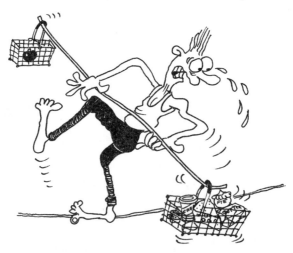

Getting your balance needn't be so difficult.

When you're getting on

It's a bit irrelevant at 80, isn't it? Not at all. Eating well and exercising are extremely important at any age. After the age of 65, there is a sharp rise in the rates of stroke and heart disease. You cannot avoid death – although you may postpone it – but this is particularly about life. It's about living it to the full, in the best health possible. "I will never be an old man. To me, old age is always fifteen years older than I am," is what Bernard Baruch had to say about it. On the other hand, as Bob Hope said, "You know you're getting old when the candles cost more than the cake."

By all means enjoy your birthday cake but, as you get older, please don't neglect vegetables, fruit and fish.

This book says more about eating than about not eating. If you are frail and have a poor appetite, it is all the more important that you get the right balance of nutrients. Misguided dietary restriction must be avoided; energy intake is crucial. You may need advice from your doctor or a dietitian.

When you're expecting

If you are pregnant, and here I am no longer addressing older readers, balanced nutrition based on the first four food groups is very important for you. There is no special pregnancy diet but there are a few important precautions.

To reduce the risk of a neural tube defect in the baby (such as spina bifida), you should take a folic acid supplement (0.4 mg daily); this should have been started before pregnancy, from the time of stopping contraception, and should be continued for the first 12 weeks of pregnancy. If you are less than 12 weeks pregnant and not taking folic acid, simply start now. The supplement should be taken in addition to eating foods containing folic acid (e.g. Brussels sprouts, spinach, cooked blackeye beans and fortified cereals).

Liver should be avoided during pregnancy as the high levels of vitamin A could harm your baby.

Toxoplasmosis is one of those infections which is not normally serious but in pregnancy it can be catastrophic. You can catch it from undercooked meat (and from handling cat litter).

Listeriosis (caused by the bacterium *Listeria monocytogenes*) is another infection to avoid in pregnancy. It can cause miscarriage, stillbirth or an ill baby. Some foods can be heavily contaminated with Listeria, which thrives at fridge temperatures but is killed by cooking. Foods to avoid are: soft cheeses like Camembert, Brie, goats' and ewes' milk cheeses; pâté and non-canned meat products like sausage rolls and pies; ready-made salads and coleslaw. Cottage cheese is fine.

Of course, pregnancy brings bizarre changes in appetite for some women. Cravings for certain foods (or even non-foods like clay or matchboxes) and aversion to others can temporarily threaten the balance of nutrition. All the more reason to get nutritionally fit well before getting pregnant.

◆ Balance is important at all ages

◆ Fish and fruit are often neglected

◆ In pregnancy, avoid toxoplasma, listeria and liver; take folic acid in the first three months

The balanced shopper

Help! The supermarket closes in half an hour and you have a family of four to feed. Don't panic. You've done it before. You know the layout of the supermarket. You collect a trolley and set off. Ah, the shopping list – it must be by the kitchen sink. How could you forget it? Are you finally going off your trolley? You dash up and down the aisles, hoping you'll remember what you need when you see it. Ugh! You're certainly going off this trolley; one wheel keeps making for the check-out and you're nowhere near finished. Oh, what are those? They look interesting. No time to check prices, let alone food labels. Sling them in the trolley. Was that your tummy rumbling? Those cakes would fill the gap.

All right. It's a good description of someone else – not you. That's good. Because, if you go to the supermarket hungry, hurried and harassed, there's no hope of the family eating a good and balanced diet for the rest of the week. What you put in that trolley ends up in their bodies (OK, not the toilet rolls, but the food). You cannot escape that consequence, but you can easily lose sight of it.

Healthy shopping means healthy eating. And vice versa.

Plan the shop, eat first, give yourself time, and take a list. The shopping list should be based on the first four food groups

(Table 15) because, if you have an unbalanced larder, you'll have an unbalanced diet.

At the end of the shop, you should be able to see at a glance that you have a balanced trolley – mainly full of fruit and vegetables, cereal and starchy foods, pulses and fish. No doubt you will also have a range of very low-fat dairy products and perhaps some skinless chicken or turkey breast or some game. Yes, you may have a little red meat or higher fat cheese, but these should be difficult to spot – swamped by other foods.

You have only to glance at the trolleys of some shoppers to see why heart disease is claiming people by the thousand – trolleys laden with fatty meat pies and sausages, fatty red meat and full-fat cheeses, whole milk, fat spreads, and manufactured cakes and biscuits. Two or three small bags containing fruits or vegetables have a tiny space at one end.

I realise that you may not buy all your food from a supermarket. Perhaps, for example, you get your fruits and vegetables from a market and your fish from a fishmonger. If you favour organic fruits and vegetables, it's well worth finding out if there is a local, weekly delivery service. This is a good way of ensuring that you never run out of fresh produce, provided you order enough. It's usually a matter of pot luck which particular items turn up each week and you may need to buy more with your weekly shop.

Why not make a shopping checklist based on Table 15? Of course, there are additional food items that are sometimes needed such as herbs, spices and seasonings.

Give yourself time to read food labels. Take a magnifying glass if you need one. In due course you will need less and less time to do this as you become familiar with more products.

As a general rule, reject processed foods with more than four grams of fat per 100 grams – especially when most of the fat is in the form of saturates. Remember to avoid unspecified 'vegetable oil' and hydrogenated vegetable oil unless the quantities are tiny. Don't worry: even if you don't add fat to your food, you can get all the fatty acids you need from the first four food groups. Certainly, if you use a little olive oil or rapeseed oil in your cuisine, and keep up a good intake of oily fish, there is no fear of lacking any fatty acids or fat-soluble vitamins; you simply have more control over the quantity and type of fat that you are eating.

Some items will be labelled as having no added salt or sugar. Anything approaching one gram of sodium per 100 grams is an awful lot when you are trying to limit your salt intake. Check how much of the total carbohydrate content is in the form of sugars. Table 16 gives you some help on food labelling.

Table 16 Guide to food labelling

A lot	A little
10 g sugars	2 g sugars
20 g fat	3 g fat
5 g saturates	1 g saturates
3 g fibre	0.5 g fibre
0.5 g sodium	0.1 g sodium

Source: Adapted from *Eating for Your Heart*, published by the British Heart Foundation, March 1999, with permission.

For many meals and foods you eat in large amounts, look at the amount per serving. For snacks and foods you eat in small amounts, look at the 'per 100 g' information. Work out from the table whether there is a lot or a little of each nutrient in the food. Remember – the most important nutrient to look for is FAT.

ACTION POINTS

◆ Make a shopping list from the 4 important food groups

◆ Don't go shopping on an empty stomach

◆ Take a magnifying glass if you need one to read food labels

◆ Reject processed foods with:

– More than 4 g fat/100 g (especially saturates)

– 'vegetable oil'/hydrogenated vegetable oil

– high sodium content (e.g. 0.9 g/100 g)

◆ Before you go to the check-out, make sure you have a balanced trolley

What about the bank balance?

'There are several ways in which to apportion the family income, all of them unsatisfactory.'

Robert Benchley

I'd love to eat a healthy diet, but how can I afford it? Food is expensive. This is a real problem for some people. Poverty has been defined as the need to spend more than 30% of available income on food. Certain foods mentioned in this book will be beyond the reach of some readers or could be an occasional luxury for others, but a healthier diet need not be a more expensive one.

Here are a few tips on eating well but keeping down the cost. For a start, eating more foods from the high-starch group (like bread, potatoes, pasta and rice), and less meat, is good for your heart and your budget.

There is a wide variety to choose from in the way of peas, beans and lentils, which are good sources of protein and cost less than meat. If you use them with foods from the cereal group, all your essential amino acids are provided. It's very convenient to buy them in tins, ready-cooked. Add them to casseroles, or any meat dish, and you'll need far less meat.

Buy foods on special offer. Cash flow permitting, stock up on canned foods or skimmed milk powder when the offer is good (as long as you know the brand, so there's no risk of being disappointed).

A freezer allows bulk-buying of many other foods when the price is low. Salmon steaks would be an extravagant luxury for many people but the price varies enormously. If you can afford it, stock the freezer (or freezer compartment of your fridge) when they are half-price.

Fruit and vegetable prices fluctuate with changes in season and agricultural conditions. Buy whatever is cheap at the time. You will often find much better prices on a market stall than in the supermarket. But beware: it's no economy if it goes bad before you can eat it. Be choosy. Get to know the good market stalls, and avoid the bad ones. Even better, grow your own fruits and vegetables. If you don't have a garden, consider an allotment. Sharing with another family can make this easier.

The same is true of shopping expeditions; if you don't have a car, sharing the cost of transport to a supermarket may be more economical than relying on local shops.

And finally, if worry about your budget is driving you to spend lots of money on cigarettes, you should read Chapter 22.

TIPS TO SAVE MONEY AND STAY HEALTHY:

◆ Eat more starchy foods and pulses, but less meat

◆ Buy foods on special offer

◆ For fruit and vegetables, use a good market stall and buy cheap

◆ Grow your own produce; consider a shared allotment

Chapter 13

Eating in – eating out

Eating in

> 'Kissing don't last: cookery do!'
>
> ---
>
> George Meredith (1828–1909)

Well done! A successful shopping trip has stocked your cupboards, fridge and freezer. A large basket of fruit; a full rack of vegetables; a shelf of cereal grains, rice and pasta; a fridge replete with fish, chicken breasts, low-fat dairy products and salad vegetables; and a full rack of spices: this sounds like a very good start. Of course, the fresh herbs, onion and garlic, and the sun-dried tomatoes (dry-packed) will help things along. And you can never have too many cans of pulses, tomatoes, pimentos and sweetcorn. The frozen peas, beans and spinach are an excellent standby.

So you're all ready to cook. Here are a few hints on doing it the healthy way.

For a start, like any job, food preparation is a lot easier with the right tools. A good set of knives is a sound investment (and with blunt ones you'll make a meal of it – eventually). You need at least two chopping boards so a separate one can be used for raw meat. Those made of soft white plastic are excellent: they won't blunt your knife and they can be washed with piping hot water or in a dishwasher. A food processor speeds up many recipes and, again, thorough cleaning is made easier if you have the luxury of a dishwasher.

The importance of scrupulous hygiene cannot be overstated. Like all family doctors, I frequently attend people with gastroenteritis, and many of these cases are avoidable. Raw meat must be treated like poison. Anything – whether a hand, a worktop or a cloth – that comes into contact with it must be properly cleaned before contamination is spread to something that will be eaten uncooked. Meat must be stored at the bottom of the fridge so that no drips can land on other food. Check the fridge temperature; it should be 4°C. Uncooked meat, even if pre-packed, should be placed immediately into a separate bag at the time of purchase to avoid contaminating other products. Assume all poultry has salmonella; if properly handled and cooked, this is no threat. If you are unfortunate enough to purchase a piece of beef contaminated with *E. coli 0157*, nothing short of the best kitchen practice will save you from disaster as so few organisms are required to cause catastrophic infection. Thorough cooking will kill bacteria in the meat, but woe betide you if the tiniest drop of uncooked meat juice ends up on your salad. (This is a good argument against buying cooked meats from someone who handles raw meat as well.)

Wash all fruits and vegetables carefully. A soft brush, such as a washing-up brush, is useful for fruit but a hard brush is good for root vegetables. Then there's no need to remove those potato skins: whether boiling, baking or roasting, they add to the flavour and nourishment.

ACTION POINTS

◆ Keep shelves stocked with fruits, vegetables, grains, pasta, pulses, etc.

◆ Use good knives and chopping boards

◆ Handle raw meat like poison

◆ Store meat at the bottom of the fridge

◆ Check that your fridge temperature is 4°C

◆ Wash fruit and vegetables carefully with a brush

You may have heard that you should chuck out the frying pan. I wouldn't – unless it's of poor quality. You'll need a good, heavy-bottomed pan, not so much to fry as to sauté – that is, to toss in the minimum of oil (sauter means 'to leap' in French). Or try sautéing in vegetable stock, perhaps with added wine or sherry, for a lower-fat dish. If using oil to fry or sauté, the oil must be hot enough to crisp the food quickly otherwise much more fat is taken up. You can now purchase an olive oil spray (one calorie per spray) which makes it easier to add tiny amounts of oil.

Another good way to move food quickly in a small amount of hot oil is to stir-fry in a wok. The trick is to have all the ingredients prepared and cut to similar sizes before starting and, working quickly, to add them to the hot oil – ending with those that need least time to cook.

Steaming is also an oriental method of cooking and a bamboo steamer that fits over a wok is not expensive. It's a particularly good way of cooking vegetables but can be used for rice, fish, or even chicken breasts.

If you boil vegetables, keep it short and shallow: use a short cooking time and shallow, boiling water. Put the lid on the pan, cook over high heat and serve immediately. How many children have been put off vegetables by limp and colourless specimens? Overcooking spoils nutrients. You can always use the water for stock.

◆ A heavy-bottomed pan is good for sautéing in very little oil and for 'dry-frying'

◆ To stir-fry, cut ingredients to similar sizes; move them quickly in the minimum amount of hot oil until cooked

◆ The microwave oven is ideal for vegetables, jacket potatoes and fish

◆ Vegetables are good steamed or boiled quickly in shallow water

---

A microwave oven is great for vegetables. They can be cooked in a covered serving dish and you generally need only a tablespoon or two of water – just enough to wet the bottom really. Not only is this a very convenient method, but it's also good at preserving the colour and texture of vegetables.

The microwave oven is ideal for cooking fish such as whole trout or salmon steaks. And jacket potatoes can be turned out in a fraction of the time needed in a conventional oven. It's a good idea to wrap them in foil after cooking, to keep them hot until you are ready to serve.

No kitchen is complete without a grill. Unlike frying, grilling allows fat to run away from the food. Oily fish do well under the grill; great care is needed to avoid overcooking white fish. Make sure meat is cooked right through: a fierce heat will burn the outside before the inside is cooked. A good marinade adds flavour and helps to stop the meat drying out. A charcoal barbecue is ideal for grilling – as long as you cook over hot charcoal and not in fierce flames. You don't have to opt for the traditional beefburgers and sausages; chicken kebabs and fish go down very well.

Even if you are a microwave enthusiast, you will probably do

EGGS IN PERSPECTIVE

Many recipes call for eggs. Egg white is just protein (albumen) and water. But the yolk contains a fair amount of fat and a lot of cholesterol. An egg yolk contains about 6.5 g of fat and almost 2 g of this is saturated. (Don't forget that nutritional information gives quantities per 100 g and one egg weighs about 60 g.) The amount of cholesterol in one egg yolk is spectacular – about 230 mg. We've seen that, when it comes to controlling blood cholesterol, the fat in food is more important than the amount of cholesterol. Even so, if you are struggling to get your blood cholesterol down, one egg yolk gives you quite enough cholesterol for the whole day.

A common recommendation is to have no more than three egg yolks a week. Personally, I choose to leave egg yolk out of most recipes. You can simply use two egg whites for every whole egg demanded by the recipe. An alternative is to use an 'egg replacer' (sold by health food shops). This is a powder containing no animal products; it's particularly useful for vegans and those with an allergy to eggs. In baked recipes, people aren't going to notice that you've used egg replacer instead of eggs, but you wouldn't use it to replace a fried egg, of course!

But do keep eggs in perspective. They won't bite (until well after they've hatched) and there's no need to be afraid of them (unless you suffer from egg allergy). Eating a couple of boiled eggs will give you a massive dose of cholesterol, but the amount of cholesterol in a small slice of a big cake made with three eggs is insignificant.

much of your roasting and baking in the main oven. Traditional recipes can often be made much healthier with a little modification.

The Sunday roast need not be steeped in saturated fat. Remember, the rule with meat is: SLIM, TRIM and SKIM (see page 40). Roast potatoes and parsnips are excellent if prepared by tossing the parboiled vegetables in a tiny amount of hot olive oil or rapeseed oil. Drain off the meat fat before making gravy.

When baking, remember that hard fats can often be replaced with rapeseed oil or lightly-flavoured olive oil (see page 46) or with prune purée (see page 341). Many recipes call for eggs. Because the egg yolk has a high fat and cholesterol content, the normal recommendation is to have no more than three eggs a week. Columbus eggs supply omega-3 fat but are still full of cholesterol. To avoid egg yolk, you can simply use two egg whites for every whole egg demanded by the recipe. It is often convenient to use dried egg white, which can be bought as a powder in sachets (made by Supercook). Alternatively, 'egg replacer' can be purchased in health food shops.

Make sauces with skimmed milk and cornflour. Forget the roux. It'll taste just as good without the added fat. You can always add extra skimmed milk powder to make it more 'creamy'.

Whatever you're cooking, consider doubling the quantity and freezing some. Ready-made meals in the freezer can save you from resorting to fatty takeaways when you haven't got time to cook.

ACTION POINTS

◆ Grill instead of frying

◆ Roast vegetables in a tiny amount of hot olive or rapeseed oil

◆ Replace hard fats with rapeseed or lightly-flavoured olive oil

◆ Use prune purée instead of fat for cakes/puddings

◆ Replace 1 egg with 2 egg whites, or use 'egg replacer'

◆ For sauces, use skimmed milk with cornflour instead of a roux; or use quark with skimmed milk for savoury sauces

◆ Cook and freeze big batches to avoid takeaways and convenience foods

Eating in – South Asian style

"The art of cooking is simple and needs to be so."

Das Sreedharan,
The New Tastes of India

If you are South Asian (having roots in India, Bangladesh, Pakistan or Sri Lanka), the information in *Stop that heart attack!* is especially relevant to you. The statistics for heart disease in South Asians are shocking. In the UK, the rate of premature death (i.e. before the age of 75) from heart disease is about 50% higher for South Asians than for white people. This epidemic affects both men and women, and risk factors for heart disease can even be found in South Asian children.

The explanation for this has a great deal to do with the 'metabolic syndrome' (see page 232), which is so common in South Asians. And the answer to it is to take enough exercise (see Chapter 19) and eat a protective diet; an unhealthy diet, full of fat and sugar, merely 'feeds' the metabolic syndrome and accelerates the decline into diabetes and heart disease.

Some simple changes to traditional methods of cooking can make all the difference. Here are a few tips:

- Don't use ghee, coconut oil, coconut cream or butter for cooking.

- Choose olive oil or rapeseed oil and measure it instead of pouring it directly into the pan; one tablespoon of oil is usually enough to make curry for 4 to 6 people, although it will seem too little if you're in the habit of using more; you'll soon adjust.

- Avoid deep frying. Foods such as chips, bajhias, sev, chevra/chevda, and samosas take up huge quantities of fat. Items like samosas can simply be brushed with a little oil and baked or grilled.

- Don't re-use cooking oils as some of the unsaturated fats become saturated.

- There is no need to add oil or ghee to chapati dough.

- Some dishes such as keema and dhal can be made very successfully without any added fat/oil.

- Avoid adding butter to cooked dhals and vegetables.

- Use a little water to replace some of the oil when cooking subjhis with more absorbent vegetables like methi (fenugreek), brinjals (aubergines) and karela (a bitter gourd).

- Choose lean meat and trim off all visible fat. If you use red meat such as beef, pork, lamb and mutton, keep to small portions.

- Use lots of high-fibre foods such as fruit, vegetables, dhals, chickpeas, beans (e.g. soya, red kidney and blackeye beans) and oatbran. Select wholegrain versions of chapati, bread and rice.

- Avoid full-fat dairy products and use very low-fat yoghurt, skimmed milk and cottage cheese. You can produce home-made yoghurt from skimmed milk. Remember that reduced-fat cheeses may still be very high-fat foods.

- Gradually reduce added salt, allowing all members of the family to adjust their palates. If you think a little salt is essential, use LoSalt or Solo.

- Avoid sweets such as jalebi and halva which are full of fat and sugar. A plate of chopped fresh fruit makes a refreshing end to a meal!

◆ **High rates of heart disease among South Asians living in the West are linked with the metabolic syndrome**

◆ **Regular exercise and simple changes in cooking methods can help to protect against diabetes and heart disease**

◆ **Cutting down fat (especially saturated), sugar and salt can make a huge difference to health without spoiling your food**

Eating out

'The best number for a dinner party is two –
myself and a damn good head waiter.'

Nubar Gulbenkian, quoted in the *Observer*, 1965

For most of us, eating out with friends is a great social pleasure.
With good food and good company you can't go wrong. But
restaurant food is loaded with fat, isn't it? How can you eat out
without damaging your coronary arteries? Watching your friends
tuck into steak and chips while you pick at your lettuce and
cucumber is not such a pleasure.

Certainly some restaurants have very little to offer the health-
conscious customer. Traditional French establishments use lots of
butter and cream; burger bars serving nothing but grease and chips
are no help either. Study the menu before selecting your restaurant.
There are plenty that offer enough variety to meet your needs.

While awaiting your meal, eat bread, if it is offered, but without the
butter or spread.

You will want to choose a starter such as melon or other fruit or
fruit juice. Seafood is fine if it isn't swimming in a high-fat sauce
(although if it is swimming at least you know it's fresh). Perhaps
you could have the sauce served separately and use it very sparingly. A deep-fried appetiser will get you off to a fatty start.

For the main course you could select grilled fish, chicken or turkey.
These can be absolutely delicious if they've been skilfully seasoned,
marinated and char-grilled. Beware any dishes covered with sauce
because sauces in restaurants usually have a very high fat content
– even though it's quite possible to make lovely low-fat sauces.

At a carvery you might choose lean turkey breast. Have plenty
of vegetables but avoid those smothered in butter or cheese sauce.
Go easy on the gravy.

It's a mistake to assume that vegetarian dishes are necessarily
low in fat. They could even be made with palm oil or coconut oil,
which would bump up the saturated fatty acid content.

Of course, you can always ask about the ingredients of a dish.
Don't be shy. You're paying. If the waiter or waitress doesn't know,
ask to see the manager or the chef. There's no reason why you
shouldn't request simple changes such as having your potatoes

sautéed in olive oil instead of butter. If the staff can't cope with such requests, it doesn't say much for the restaurant.

Boiled new potatoes or jacket potato would be wise choices in preference to sautéed potatoes, roast potatoes or chips. You won't want to top your jacket potato with sour cream or butter, but you could ask for some pickle instead.

You can never be quite sure what's in a creamy salad dressing; at least with vinegar and a little olive oil you know what you're getting.

The sweet trolley usually confronts you with cheesecakes, gateaux, pastries and lashings of cream. Wise options may be limited to fresh fruit, fruit salad or sorbet.

No doubt many different parts of the world are represented by the restaurants in your local town.

Although the native cuisine of some Mediterranean and oriental countries is ideal, you cannot rely on the Anglicised version being equally healthy. Again, you should ask how a dish has been prepared and which oil has been used.

From the orient, Chinese restaurants are the most familiar but Japanese and Thai restaurants are also worth exploring. Dishes that are stir-fried in a small amount of hot oil don't take up too much fat; deep-fried items, such as spring rolls, will generally take up more. Enjoy the variety of vegetables and have plenty of plain rice. Chicken and seafood are good choices; lamb and pork will be higher in fat. Unfortunately, Peking Duck is a very high-fat dish.

There's nothing quite like a curry. Sadly, much Indian cuisine involves the use of ghee (clarified butter) which has a very high saturated fat content. We have a local Indian restaurant that guarantees to use rapeseed oil – or to leave the oil out altogether if you prefer. In general, dishes without a sauce will be lower in fat. For example, chicken tikka would be less fatty than chicken tikka masala. At least the sauce in chicken jalfrezi is based on tomatoes and it should be a reasonable choice. Have plenty of boiled rice. It's better to fill up on naan bread than to have lots of high-fat dishes, but remember that naan bread contains about six times as much fat as ordinary brown or white bread. Enjoy side dishes such as raita (cucumber, yoghurt and spices).

Restaurants of a Mediterranean tradition, such as Greek and Spanish, usually have something acceptable on the menu, whether it's chicken kebab or grilled fish. Beware the pasta sauces in Italian restaurants: they are usually loaded with fat. Some pizza houses have excellent salad bars these days – enticing rows of wholesome ingredients. If you've paid for unlimited visits, you'll sample most of them. If it's one visit only, the bowl is too small. The secret here is to part-fill the bowl and then arrange cucumber slices vertically around the rim, secured with a ring of rice. The extra height greatly increases the capacity of the bowl. Watch the croutons (which are deep fried), salads in mayonnaise (e.g. coleslaw, vegetable salad) and oily dressings. Some outlets do serve fat-free or yoghurt-based dressings.

Eating out gives you far less control over your diet than eating in. If this is something you only do occasionally, the most important rule is this: relax and enjoy it!

ACTION POINTS

When eating out:

◆ Avoid restaurants with unsuitable menus

◆ Eat bread without butter or spread

◆ Select fruit, fruit juice or seafood (not covered in sauce) for starters

◆ Order grilled fish, chicken or turkey (without skin)

◆ Avoid sauces (or have them served separately and use very little)

◆ Choose boiled or jacket potatoes; or specify sauté in olive oil

◆ Request a low-fat topping for jacket potatoes (e.g. pickle) and avoid butter/sour cream

◆ Ask about salt and fat used; request olive oil rather than butter

Chapter 14

Foreign food

Nobody wants a heart attack, but eating a typical British diet is a good way to go about having one. It wasn't always so. The vast increase in heart disease throughout the UK over the past century has gone hand in hand with a huge change in our diet. Responding to this, a Welsh researcher conducted an odd experiment, which was discussed in the *British Medical Journal* in 1979.

He reconstructed a typical Welsh labourer's diet, as recorded in 1863, consisting mainly of potatoes, oatmeal and wholemeal bread. There was also a little cheese and milk but this diet was far lower in fat and higher in carbohydrate than a diet based on the Department of Health's current recommendations. The researchers didn't eat this diet themselves. They converted it into pellets, which they fed to a group of rats. An identical group of rats was fed pellets made from a contemporary Welsh diet. Rats on the 1863 diet lived far longer than rats on the modern diet.

I know you're not a rat. And I'm sure you are not attracted to the diet of a nineteenth-century Welsh labourer. However, there is a great deal for us to learn from interesting, contemporary diets around the world that are not linked with coronary heart disease. Nations with Northern European traditions have high cholesterols and high rates of heart disease, while people of Southern Europe, rural Africa and the Orient have low cholesterols and low rates of heart disease. Many of the low-risk people are eating delicious diets.

The Japanese diet

'You do not sew with a fork, and I see no reason why you
should eat with knitting needles.'

Miss Piggy

The Japanese have the lowest average cholesterol level and the lowest rates of heart disease in the developed world. Perhaps this is a
genetic characteristic of Japanese people. Not so. The Japanese who
settled in San Francisco adopted the American diet. As their saturated fat intake rose to mirror that of the Californians, so did their blood
cholesterol levels and rates of heart disease. On the other hand, the
Japanese who moved only as far as Hawaii took on a diet that was
somewhere between the Japanese and American diets with an inter-
mediate saturated fat intake. They developed more heart disease than
the Japanese who had stayed in Japan, but not as much as the Amer-
icans. Perhaps the Japanese would agree with Fred Allen's alleged
remark: "California is a great place – if you happen to be an orange".
    Japanese cuisine features:

- plenty of cereals (especially rice);
- fresh fruit and vegetables (which are not overcooked);
- lots of fish;
- soya beans including tofu (soya bean curd);
- very little red meat or saturated fat.

No doubt all these features play a part in reducing Japanese
rates of heart disease. Evidence for the role of soya protein in lowering cholesterol and protecting arteries has been building up in
recent years. The interesting thing is that this diet protects them
from heart disease even though smoking and raised blood pressure are common in Japan. The one thing that stands out as being
unsatisfactory in the Japanese diet is its high salt content. Since
making a big reduction in their sodium intake, the Japanese have
seen the prevalence of raised blood pressure decline dramatically
and the figures for heart disease have become even lower!
    Sadly, many young Japanese are now picking up some Western
eating habits and we may see rising levels of heart disease as they
reach middle age.

The least we can do is to return the compliment and pick up some oriental eating habits.

The Mediterranean diet

'In Rome people spend most of their time having lunch. And they do it very well – Rome is unquestionably the lunch capital of the world.'

Fran Lebowitz, *Metropolitan Life*, 1978

The people of Mediterranean countries such as Italy and Greece suffer much less heart disease than Northern Europeans. This may well have something to do with the olive oil that plays such an important part in their cuisine. Olive oil is a rich source of the mono-unsaturated fatty acid, oleic acid. We know that using olive oil instead of more saturated fats helps to lower the harmful LDL-cholesterol without reducing the level of protective HDL-cholesterol. Olive oil also provides antioxidants.

But it must be remembered that there are lots of other good things about the diet of Mediterranean countries apart from olive oil. Compared with a typical British diet, there is much greater emphasis on fruit and vegetables; evidence for their vital role in maintaining health has mounted. Seafood is given due prominence and use of garlic is the norm.

The Lyon Diet Heart Study was published in the *Lancet* in 1994. (This is the correct spelling and it was nothing to do with eating, or being eaten by, big cats.) It was a controlled trial involving people who had already had one heart attack.

The control group was given routine advice about a 'prudent diet', while the experimental group was put on a Mediterranean diet that was rich in oleic acid and alpha-linolenic acid (related to fish oils). They were advised to eat more bread, fruit, root vegetables, green vegetables and fish, but less meat – beef, lamb and pork being replaced by poultry. A special margarine based on rapeseed oil was supplied free to those in the experimental group and their families. They were allowed to use olive oil or rapeseed oil, but no other fats, for cooking and dressing salads. A moderate amount of wine was permitted with meals.

In just 27 months, there was a marked reduction in heart attacks among those on the Mediterranean diet.

'The French Paradox'

'France is the largest country in Europe, a great boon for
drunks, who need room to fall ...'

Alan Coren, *The Sanity Inspector*, 1974

The French appear to get off lightly. They put the pâté and
profiteroles on our menus but seem to have low rates of heart disease themselves. This disparity between their saturated fat intake
and their statistics for coronary deaths is known as 'the French Paradox'. (See also Chapter 10.)

Red wine has largely been given the credit for this. Certainly the
French drink a lot of it – too much, in fact. No doubt it reduces their
level of coronary heart disease but they pay for this with higher
rates of liver cirrhosis, cancer of the mouth and gullet, suicide and
violent death.

Apart from alcohol, there are other factors in the French diet
that would be expected to lower the risk of heart disease, including
the generous use of fruit, vegetables, onions and garlic and the tradition of eating plenty of unbuttered bread with meals. Also,
France is a big place and in parts the diet is more Mediterranean
with less saturated fat and more olive oil.

Bon appetit!

- ◆ Oriental, Southern European, and rural African diets are linked with low rates of heart disease
- ◆ The Japanese diet is high in cereals (rice), vegetables, soya and fish but low in red meat and saturated fat
- ◆ Mediterranean cuisine includes fruit and vegetables, bread/pasta, fish, olive oil, garlic, wine
- ◆ Rapeseed oil and nuts (e.g. walnuts) supply alpha-linolenic acid which is related to fish oil and helps to protect against heart disease
- ◆ There's more to the French Paradox than red wine

Chapter 15

Feeding children

'Maybe you know why a child can reject a hot dog with
mustard served on a soft bun at home, yet eat six of them
two hours later at fifty cents each.'

Erma Bombeck,
If Life is a Bowl of Cherries – What am I doing in the Pits? 1978

We all want our children to get off to a good start but how much of
the dietary advice in this book is relevant to young children? This
chapter explains easy ways to introduce healthy eating to children, so
that they learn to make heart-safe choices.

Feeding children can be a source of anxiety and frustration. If
you never have to do it, you may want to skip this chapter.

An early start

Some research has been done which discovered a link between the
size of a baby at birth, and death of the adult from heart disease or
stroke in later life. Professor Barker and his team followed the fortunes of 1586 men who were born in a Sheffield maternity hospital
between 1907 and 1924. They found that the bigger the baby (birth
weight, head circumference and weight/length^3) the lower the
death rate.

The weight of an infant at the age of one year is an even better
guide to his risk of coronary heart disease in adult life. Professor
Barker's team published findings on about 8000 men who were
born before 1931 in Hertfordshire. The results were striking. The

death rate from coronary heart disease was three times higher among those who had weighed only 17 pounds at one year than among those who had weighed 28 pounds. A similar trend has been found for women but such studies on women are harder to complete as so many have changed their name by marriage.

So it's never too early to start considering the child's adult health (before conception is ideal) but misguided attempts to impose a healthy diet on young children can be very damaging. Think of all the mothers who have fretted about their babies, and perhaps even tried to restrict their calorie intake, because their weight was well above average; it turns out that the big babies are the ones with a lower risk of heart disease.

◆ It's never too early to bother about healthy eating

◆ Nutrition, even before birth, can affect heart health in adult life

◆ Breast milk is the ideal food in the first few months

◆ Baby cereal fortified with iron is helpful from 4 months

◆ Giving fruit with a meal helps absorption of iron

Feeding an infant – the first two years

Infants are growing rapidly. They are not miniature adults. Unlike older children and adults, they need to take in about 50% of their energy as fat. Breast milk is the ideal food in the first few months of life. Either breast milk or infant formula should be continued during the first year but neither can supply all the nutritional needs of a baby in the second six months of life. Weaning foods add important nutrients and introduce a wide variety of tastes and textures. Food is fun (but it doesn't always seem that way when you find it behind a radiator several months later).

The commonest nutritional problem in infancy (in the developed world) is iron deficiency anaemia, which affects about 12% of one- and two-year-old children. It is even commoner in some Asian groups. We know that anaemia in early childhood can interfere with mental development so it is very important to avoid it. Although breast milk does not have a high iron content, the iron that is present is easily absorbed and utilised by the infant; it is helpful to introduce a baby cereal fortified with iron from about four months of age. Cow's milk is a poor source of iron and is unsuitable as a drink in the first year. Indeed, cow's milk, tea and wholemeal cereal foods can reduce the absorption of iron from food. The iron in red meat and offal such as liver is in a form (called 'haem iron') which is better absorbed than iron from plant sources. Vitamin C increases iron absorption, so giving fruit with a meal will help. Infant formula milks and certain foods (such as cereals and white bread) are fortified with iron.

Don't overdo the wholemeal and high-fibre foods at this age. Applying adult guidelines to infants is the origin of so-called 'muesli belt malnutrition'. Bulking out a meal with plenty of high-fibre foods is very helpful for adults, but infants have small stomachs and big energy requirements. They need a higher proportion of energy-dense foods or they can feel full before taking in enough calories.

Reduced-fat milk and low-fat dairy products are not suitable for children under two years.

Salt intake should be restricted, just as in adults, by choosing low-salt foods and by avoiding the addition of salt during food preparation.

The main reason why nuts are not recommended at this age is that they can cause choking. There is also concern that nut allergies, which can be life-threatening, are on the increase. It is possible that avoiding exposure to nut products during the first three years reduces the risk of developing this sensitivity.

Vitamin drops (such as those containing vitamins A, D, and C, which may be available from your health visitor) are a good idea from 6 months to 5 years. They are not a substitute for a balanced and varied diet.

ACTION POINTS

◆ Breast feed for as long as you can, but start solids by six months

◆ Don't give cow's milk as a drink in the first year

◆ Don't give low-fat dairy products to the under 2s

◆ Choose from the 4 important food groups to get the best balance you can

From two to five years

Changing from an infant into a schoolchild isn't easy: it presents a host of developmental challenges; it has its ups and its downs – not only emotionally, but also nutritionally. It is futile to try to impose any rigid dietary dogma on the pre-school child, and adult guidelines are still inappropriate at this age.

Semi-skimmed milk can be introduced as a drink from the age of two years. I didn't do this with my children and, on current evidence, I can't see a lot of point in most cases. One argument for semi-skimmed milk is that it is a step towards the grown-up diet of the schoolchild for, one way or another, this adaptation should be made by the age of five.

She hardly eats a thing!

'How to eat like a child.
Spinach: divide into little piles. Rearrange again into new piles.
After five or six maneuvers, sit back and say you are full.'

Delia Ephron, *New York Times*, 1983

You are bound to be anxious when your child appears to be starving or, at least, heading for severe nutritional deficiency. This is an extremely common anxiety in parents of pre-school children. Even the child who normally tucks in will lose his appetite for a few days with a bad cold. Toddlers rapidly sense their parents' concern and food becomes a powerful weapon in the battle for independence.

In the great majority of cases, plotting the height and weight on a chart confirms a completely normal growth pattern. Parents are sometimes puzzled that their child's negligible intake is enough to sustain normal growth. An interesting experiment was published by Birch and colleagues in the *New England Journal of Medicine* in 1991. They presented 15 pre-school children with a range of familiar foods and the children were allowed to have whatever they liked for a meal or snack. Their calorie intake varied greatly from meal to meal but the daily intake of each child remained fairly constant. The message is: healthy children don't starve themselves; they regulate intake to meet their nutritional needs.

A toddler is quick to realise that it doesn't much matter about eating at mealtimes if an anxious mother is only too glad to supply milk, biscuits or crisps to 'get something into him' (or her) at any other time of day. On the other hand, if a child discovers that no amount of lying on the floor and screaming will procure any nourishment until the appointed hour, mealtimes will soon be taken more seriously. Either way, the child will meet his or her nutritional needs.

This does not mean that, if you establish regular mealtimes, your child will always clear the plate! A child's requirements vary and you might have overloaded the plate. There will be passing food fads. The important thing is to relax in the knowledge that your child's appetite is a good guide to his needs. When you're hungry, eating is fun. It's important not to turn it into a deadly task. Once you are relaxed enough to show no concern about the unfinished meal, children work out that it's their loss, and not yours, if they don't eat when food is available.

Nor does establishing a routine imply three square meals a day. It is a very good thing for the family to sit down together for main meals whenever possible but small children have small stomachs and may need snacks. Crisps and biscuits are not the only possible snacks: some children enjoy sugarsnap peas or raw carrot or bread sticks.

While toddlers are very good at getting what they need as long as food is available, it is possible for parents to jeopardize their child's nutrition by restricting foods that are considered to be unhealthy or too fatty.

Aim to give your child something from each of the first four main food groups:

- Cereals and starchy foods: bread, breakfast cereals, rice, pasta, potatoes;

- Fruit and vegetables: fresh, frozen or canned are all excellent. Dried fruits (e.g. raisins);

- Milk and dairy products: milk, yoghurt, cheese;

- 'Meat' or high-protein group: meat, fish, poultry, pulses (peas, beans, lentils), eggs.

Chips, baked beans and banana custard (made with real banana) might not have been your first choice but you've covered the four important food groups. A few ideas for children's meals can be found in Chapter 27.

Young children don't demand a starter, a savoury course and a sweet. Small pieces of fruit, such as satsuma (seedless), banana, apple, pear or kiwi fruit, often slip down better nestling between pieces of meat, cheese or bread.

Children are often put off by the texture of food as much as the taste. Stewed fruit or vegetable purée (which can be added to other foods) will often go down better than lumps, and flaked fish can be smuggled in mashed potato.

You want your child to meet a wide range of tastes and textures but a new food is best introduced, just a little at first, alongside an old friend. Be prepared for rejection and conceal your disappointment; try again after a decent interval (several weeks).

When children are involved in choosing and preparing food, they are more likely to want to eat it. Another useful tip is to find out which of your child's playmates have good appetites, especially for foods your child rejects, and invite them round for meals. Example can be inspiring. Be less hospitable to the fussy ones.

Remember: food fads, awkwardness and manipulative behaviour are very common in pre-school children whereas failure to thrive is not. Of course, if there is any doubt about your child's growth or development you should discuss it with your health visitor or doctor.

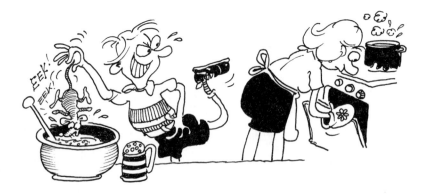

**When children are involved in the preparation
of food, they are more likely to eat it.**

- ◆ When food is available, healthy children make sure they get enough
- ◆ Food is fun! Don't turn eating into a deadly task
- ◆ Raw vegetables such as sugarsnap peas and carrot sticks make good snacks
- ◆ When children help to choose/prepare food, they're more likely to eat it

From five years

When a child reaches five, a diet based on the Department of Health's recommended averages for the general population is suitable – 35% of the calories coming from fat and 10% of them from saturated fat.

Ideally, a family with children of school age will sit at the table together, sharing a menu based on these guidelines. The recommended diet is significantly lower in fat than the current UK average diet. Achieving it will mean selecting some of the lower-fat options detailed in this book. A good variety of foods should be taken from each of the four main food groups, being sure to include enough fruit and vegetables as well as plenty of cereal and starchy foods.

From the age of five, fully skimmed milk can be used, not only in food but also as a drink. Of course, if you simply switch from whole milk one day to fully skimmed the next, we can predict the reaction. When the time came for our daughters to make the change, we started adding skimmed milk to their whole milk (out of their view, of course) – gradually increasing the proportion of skimmed milk. They were soon drinking fully skimmed milk quite happily.

For many adults, especially those at high risk of coronary heart disease, I would recommend a more radical diet than one based on the Government's targets for population averages (see Chapter 16). For children, who need plenty of energy for growth and to fuel the energetic lifestyle that should be encouraged, this moderate diet is sensible. It's still worth pointing out that the rapeseed oil in home-made flapjack is just as good at giving a child energy as the hydrogenated vegetable oil in a chocolate bar.

Why start so young?

If coronary heart disease is an adult problem, why bother about it in childhood?

Well, leaving aside the fact that eating well brings a whole range of health benefits apart from protecting the heart, it must be remembered that the foundations of coronary heart disease are laid in childhood.

Professor Barker's work suggests that nutritional factors in the womb and in infancy can influence adult heart disease. Other work has shown that risk factors for heart disease, such as raised cholesterol, can often be tracked from around two years of age into adult life. About 90% of the young adults with a cholesterol level of 6.2 mmol/l or above could probably be identified in childhood – either by the presence of obesity or by a raised cholesterol level (although the range is different in childhood).

Not only this, but the process of artery-clogging can actually begin in childhood! The formation of fatty plaques of atheroma in arteries begins with fatty streaks on the inside of the artery walls. Fatty streaks occur in tiny children. These streaks do not always go on to form plaques and in some cases they will be temporary. In some children, real artery-clogging plaques of atheroma appear around the time of puberty.

Isn't it worth stopping this process before it becomes established in the young adult?

Education, too, must be considered. Why should you suddenly start eating well at the age of 21 if you have never learnt how? You wouldn't leave piano playing or speaking French until then. You might be surprised at the healthy choices children can make when given the right opportunities from an early age.

◆ Adult guidelines (including fully skimmed milk) apply from age 5

◆ Children need energy-dense foods, but rapeseed oil is better than hydrogenated vegetable oil

◆ Clogging up of arteries starts in childhood!

Chapter 16

Moderation in all things?

'Moderation is a fatal thing. Nothing succeeds like excess.'

Oscar Wilde, *A Woman of No Importance*, 1893

Many books and articles on the subject of healthy eating will tell you that moderation is the key. At the same time, medical journals have frequently published articles lamenting the fact that giving people dietary advice has had very little impact on their raised cholesterol levels. I can tell you from my years of clinical experience that moderation is indeed the key – the key to failure in many cases.

Charts similar to that shown in Table 17 are often given out by practice nurses and doctors when they are advising people how to change their diets to lower cholesterol levels. You may have been given one yourself. These charts can be very useful. They tell you which things you can eat and drink regularly and which things to avoid altogether. The middle column shows which things you can eat and drink in moderation. Moderation is the downfall of many.

I recall a patient of mine called John. John was disappointed that after changing his diet for three months his cholesterol level had hardly altered. I asked him to keep a record of everything he ate and drank for one week. There was the roast lamb with roast potatoes and gravy, but he explained that he would only have roast lunch once a week, on a Sunday. His wife prepared this in the traditional way, using lard for the potatoes and meat fat for the gravy, but it was

149

Table 17 Extract from a chart used by some advisers

Eat regularly	Eat in moderation	Avoid
Dairy Foods		
Skimmed milk, low-fat yoghurt, skimmed milk soft cheese, cottage cheese, low-fat fromage frais	Semi-skimmed milk, medium-fat cheeses (e.g. Brie, Edam), reduced-fat cheeses, cheese spreads	Whole milk, cream, full-fat yoghurt, full-fat cheese (e.g. cheddar, Stilton), imitation cream
Meat		
Chicken, turkey (skinless), veal, rabbit, game, meat substitutes (e.g. Quorn, soya)	Beef, pork, lamb, ham, gammon (visible fat removed), very lean minced meat, duck (skinless), grilled lean bacon, liver, kidney, low-fat pâté	Sausages, pâté, salami, streaky bacon, corned beef, luncheon meats, burgers, meat pies, sausage rolls, goose

only once a week. Then there was the fish and chips (from the local shop) but that was only once a week, on a Wednesday, after his late shift. And by the time we had added up all the exceptions to his otherwise healthy diet, there wasn't a lot of room left for really helpful foods.

If you eat enough different foods that are moderately bad for you in moderation, there won't be much space on your menu for foods that are really good for you. Such a diet has very little impact on cholesterol levels or the risk of heart disease.

Some years ago, my own cholesterol level was over 7 mmol/l. I changed my diet and my cholesterol has been 5 mmol/l or below ever since; it's come down from a high reading to well below the population average (see Chapter 18). My 30% drop in cholesterol level amounts to a reduction in the risk of coronary heart disease by at least 60%! (A 2% reduction in risk for every 1% drop in cholesterol is a conservative estimate; in many cases, a risk reduction of 3% would be nearer the mark.)

I have found it is far easier simply to exclude unhelpful foods from my routine diet than to try eating them in moderation. Cheese is an example: I don't think about it because I'm too busy eating

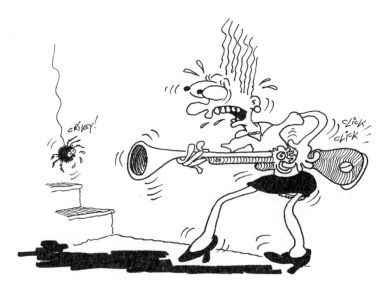

Nothing succeeds like excess

other things instead. And have you tried eating chocolate in moderation? Once you've started, it's difficult to stop. But if I went to a dinner party, which is something I do only occasionally, I would have no compunction about tucking into a piece of Camembert and some chocolate mints; it wouldn't matter at all because my routine diet is sound. After all, if you make a rule, you need the odd exception to prove it. Now if your social life is far more exciting than mine, and you're always off to dinner parties, you would need to take a different view.

Do you remember that advertisement for an anti-dandruff shampoo? Someone says to the shampoo user "I didn't know you had dandruff". The reply, of course, is "I don't". And when someone, seeing that I am careful about my diet, says to me, "I didn't know you had a cholesterol problem", my reply, of course, is "I don't".

Perhaps you have been told that your cholesterol is normal and you are thinking that all this discussion about eating a better diet doesn't concern you. It may be that you haven't had your cholesterol measured yet; when you do, Chapter 18 will help you to interpret the result. One of the most unhelpful things that health professionals can do is to give people the impression that because their cholesterol level is 'normal' they needn't bother about their diet! That's nonsense. If you've come away with this idea, your visit to the 'health promotion clinic' may have increased your risk instead of reducing it.

The average cholesterol level in our population is too high and lots of people have heart attacks with average and even below average cholesterols.

◆ Advice about diet often fails to lower cholesterol

◆ Moderation is the downfall of many

◆ Excluding unhelpful foods from your routine diet is easier than trying to eat them in moderation

◆ If your cholesterol is 'normal', healthy eating is still essential

---

If you think about earlier chapters in this book, you will realise that a good diet protects your heart and arteries in lots of ways that have nothing to do with lowering cholesterol. Reducing sodium intake helps to control blood pressure; cutting down saturated fat reduces thrombosis risk; fish oils make platelets less 'sticky'; and antioxidants in fruit and vegetables help to prevent fatty deposits forming in arteries. You need all this protection even if your cholesterol reading was 'normal'.

At the other end of the scale, there are people who have an inherited disorder of cholesterol metabolism resulting in a very raised cholesterol that cannot be brought down to normal by diet. They may need drug treatment, but, even if drugs control their cholesterol, a healthy diet is still vital to protect their heart and arteries in other ways.

Apart from avoiding heart disease, the diet recommended in this book reduces the risk of cancer as well.

What about the idea that giving people dietary advice doesn't make much difference to their cholesterol levels? It's often true. And why? In most cases it's because only moderate changes have been made to a basically unhealthy diet. The quality of dietary advice is often poor. People come away from it confused and poorly motivated. To give effective dietary education is very time-consuming. Doctors and nurses may conclude that their patient's raised cholesterol is 'metabolically resistant' – in other words, that it will not respond to a change in diet – when the real problem is that the diet hasn't changed enough. Certainly, as I have said, there are cases of metabolic resistance, but these are less common than the resistance of people to dietary change.

How do I know this? Studies carried out in metabolic wards or laboratories – where changes in diet are carefully controlled – show that big reductions in cholesterol levels can normally be achieved if the diet is altered enough.

Can this be achieved outside the laboratory? Yes. The Lifestyle Heart Trial published in the *Lancet* in 1990 was a properly constructed controlled trial on 48 people with coronary heart disease. The narrowing of their coronary arteries was carefully measured by a special investigation known as coronary angiography. Each person was then randomly allocated to either the experimental group or the control group. The 28 people in the experimental group were given a lifestyle programme that involved: a very low-fat vegetarian diet; help with giving up smoking; stress management and moderate exercise. The 20 people in the control group were given routine care. Those in the experimental group changed their diet so much that, after one year, their fat intake had dropped from 31.5% of total calories to just 6.8%. There was no significant change in the diet of the control group. Cholesterol levels fell significantly in the experimental group, but not in the control group.

After one year on the programme, all the people had their coronary arteries re-examined by angiography. The results were striking. In the control group receiving routine care, the coronary arteries had become narrower – the heart disease had progressed. This progression of heart disease had been prevented in the experimental group. Not only that, their coronary arteries were actually wider than they had been at the start of the experiment – their heart disease had gone into reverse!

And let's debunk the myth, once and for all, that a really healthy low-fat diet is boring, limited and unappetising. It may be radically different from the average British diet, but it can be more varied and interesting. Many people are stuck in a rut with their diet and don't know how to get out of it. They haven't begun to explore the range of cereal grains, pastas, fruits and vegetables, low-fat dairy products, pulses and fish available to them. Tastes vary but the choice is so wide that everyone can be satisfied without compromising the quality of the diet.

If you are attached to traditional British cuisine, most recipes can be adapted to use more desirable oils and low-fat cooking methods. My patient, John, could have continued his Sunday roast and his fish and chips with impunity if they had been prepared in the right way (see Chapter 27). Those who are fortunate enough not to have any problem keeping their weight down can be less stingy with the olive oil or rapeseed oil (or even sunflower, safflower, soya or sesame seed oils). Don't overdo it; high-fat diets influence clotting factors, increasing the risk of thrombosis.

The information in this book will allow you to discover for yourself that recipes containing very little fat can be every bit as delicious and satisfying as fatty ones. You may have already been advised by your doctor or practice nurse to adopt a low-fat diet and found it difficult to make the change. It would be impossible for a health professional to convey to you all the information contained in these pages. In this way the book can complement the efforts of your health advisers.

'The trouble with facts is that there are so many of them.'

Samuel McChord Crothers, *The Gentle Reader*

What's the point in changing my diet and lifestyle, you may ask, when I don't know whether my risk of getting heart disease is high or not? Perhaps I will live to 99 and die of cancer with a healthy heart. True, and Chapter 24 will help you to assess your risk. Whether the risk appears to be high or low, anyone living in a country where heart disease is epidemic would do well to reduce his or her risk. In any case the lifestyle that protects against heart disease also protects against cancer.

Now I have something very important to explain to you. We saw in Chapter 4 that the 1994 COMA report recommended that no more than 35% of calories should come from fat. The Government's expert committee was not making recommendations for the individual but for the population average. This is frequently misunderstood.

What's more, the committee set this target for the population – to reduce its fat intake from an average 40% of calories to 35% – because it was realistic and **not** because they believed it would result in the lowest possible risk.

In fact, I can reveal to you that some experts would have preferred a target of 20%! You may find that hard to believe, but it's true. That's not to say that 20% of calories coming from fat is ideal; the ideal figure is probably about 15%. The 1994 committee recognised that '... levels less than 10% have been achieved in some circumstances with evidence of benefit'.

The fact is that the committee's moderate target of 35% was a political compromise. It was reckoned that people weren't ready to make a bigger change. Even more to the point: the food industry just wouldn't stomach it.

That's the startling truth behind the recommendations of the 1994 COMA report. And yet, I come across health professionals who have picked up the idea that changing to a diet with less than 30% of calories from fat may be dangerous!

If your cholesterol has been measured and found to be high, you may need to make a much bigger change than this to bring it down to the ideal level.

If you have never had your cholesterol checked, consider arranging this through your doctor as part of an overall risk assessment (see Chapter 18).

Someone with a very low risk of heart disease would be well advised to maintain a healthy diet and lifestyle but can afford to relax: no drastic changes are needed. For those at high risk, moderation may be fatal.

Mind you, many people who are at high risk – especially those who have already developed heart disease – and yet fail to bring down their cholesterol by changing their diet, will, quite rightly, be offered drugs to control their cholesterol level. There is good evidence now that this can improve survival. The tragedy is that many of these people (though certainly not all of them) could avoid the need for lifelong treatment with cholesterol-lowering drugs if only they would change their diet substantially. But no. They scratch the surface. They make moderate adjustments. Their intake of saturated fat remains far higher – and their consumption of fruit, vegetables, starch, fibre and fish far lower – than that of many populations around the world that are not plagued by heart disease.

I can hear the voices of my critics saying that it's quite unreasonable and unrealistic of me to expect people to make radical changes to their diet. But it's not. Many have done it. I'm not actually asking you to adopt the diet of a Japanese fisherman. His tastes and preferences may be quite different from yours. With enough information, you, like many others, can discover that radically improving your diet need not mean deprivation; the great variety of helpful foods means you can satisfy all your needs without jeopardising your health. And with the right know-how, many of your family's favourite recipes can be adapted to slash the saturated fat but not the flavour. That's the purpose of this book: to give you the information and the know-how.

Current nutritional wisdom holds that there is no such thing as a 'good food' or a 'bad food' or a 'healthy food' or an 'unhealthy food' but there are good and bad diets because it's all a question of balance. OK, but I put it to you that foods with a high content of saturated or trans fatty acids are certainly very unhelpful to someone who is trying to reduce his heart disease risk – however unfashionable it may be to label them as 'unhealthy'.

- ◆ Big changes in diet and lifestyle can reverse heart disease!
- ◆ A radically different diet could be more interesting than the one you're eating now
- ◆ Modifying traditional recipes can make them much 'healthier'
- ◆ The COMA report recommended averages for the population
- ◆ Some people need to make much bigger changes than COMA advised

---

But we all need some fat, don't we?

Yes, some fat is essential – but not saturated fat. None of the saturated fatty acids is essential; we can make them for ourselves. Even if they were essential, you wouldn't have to worry: you can't avoid them altogether. Even olive oil is about 14% saturates. My advice is to avoid as much saturated fat as you can.

Surely there are dangers in making radical dietary changes?

Yes, just as there are dangers in continuing an unhealthy diet, making inappropriate changes can be damaging. I have argued that for those at high risk of heart disease on poor diets moderate changes are inadequate, but, although moderation is no answer, balance is essential. Never forget the five food groups (see Chapter 12). The radical change required means redressing the balance; it means enjoying enough of the helpful foods as well as avoiding unhelpful ones.

Isn't there a danger of wasting away on a very low-fat diet? No. Remember, I am talking about a balanced diet in which fewer calories come from fat, and more from carbohydrate. I would never recommend starvation; that can turn anyone into a skeleton. Most people in the UK – including those who are not overweight – would benefit from eating much less fat. We now know that this is unlikely to cause too much weight loss. Weight usually settles at a satisfactory level; it's as if the body has a 'set point' for weight.

It is just possible that you are losing more weight than you want to on a very low-fat diet, especially if you are young, slim and active. (Others wish they had your problem.) As well as monstrous portions of starchy foods (like bread, rice, pasta and potatoes) and enough low-fat, high-protein foods (such as turkey breast, skimmed milk and pulses) perhaps you should eat a little more fat. I'm not suggesting a high-fat diet as that would raise the risk of thrombosis, but there's no reason to stay on a **very** low-fat diet if you can't maintain your weight. Have a few almonds, hazelnuts and walnuts; use avocados if you enjoy them; dress your salads with olive oil; feast on oily fish from sardines to salmon; treat yourself to home-baked cakes and biscuits made with rapeseed oil. Enjoy it while you can: no doubt your weight will rise as you get older.

Is there a risk of vitamin deficiency on a low-fat diet? If you avoid high-fat and high-sugar foods, you have to get your energy from other foods – foods that will give you a good supply of vitamins and minerals. Fat contains the fat-soluble vitamins (A, D, E and K). Vitamin K is made in your intestine, and you won't miss out on vitamins A, D and E on the kind of diet I'm recommending which includes some nuts, oils and oily fish.

If you adopt a very low-fat diet to control your weight, make sure you include plenty of skimmed milk powder fortified with vitamins A and D. And the last thing you want to do if you are trying to reduce your risk of heart disease is to go short of the vital antioxidant, vitamin E; a supplement may be a good idea, although we cannot be certain that high doses are safe (see page

96). Don't take megadoses of vitamins A and D, as too much can make you ill, but by all means take a multivitamin containing the recommended daily allowances.

When we talk about changing dietary habits, a very real danger for some people is the development of unhealthy attitudes to food or even eating disorders such as bulimia and anorexia nervosa. No doubt the diet and fashion industries do a great deal to foster these unhealthy attitudes; it is certainly not my intention to do the same.

It is my hope that the information in this book will set you free – free to enjoy good food without harbouring feelings of guilt or worries about your health. Food should be delicious and satisfying, but the notion that it won't be unless it's loaded with saturated fat or hydrogenated vegetable oil is absurd. Food is all the more enjoyable if you know it's doing you good instead of fearing that it's doing you in.

If you are British, your risk of getting heart disease is vastly greater than it would be if you were Japanese. The difference comes down to lifestyle – mainly diet. You could make some minor changes and marginally reduce your risk. After all, you might get away with it. On the other hand, you could cut your risk dramatically to Japanese proportions. The choice is yours.

- ◆ Proper balance means eating enough helpful foods as well as avoiding unhelpful ones
- ◆ If you are losing too much weight on a very low-fat diet, include more oily fish, nuts, rapeseed/olive oil (as well as starchy foods)
- ◆ On a very low-fat diet, don't forget vitamins A, D and E
- ◆ You could cut your risk a little, or a lot. The choice is yours

Chapter 17

Losing weight

'I've been on a constant diet for the last two decades.
I've lost a total of 789 pounds. By all accounts,
I should be hanging from a charm bracelet.'

Erma Bombeck

◆ A growing number of people in the UK weigh far too much

◆ Your ideal weight depends on height. BMI should be 20–25

◆ If your BMI is in the right range, you may still have too much flab

◆ Being very overweight increases the risk of heart disease, diabetes, high blood pressure, stroke, gallstones and arthritis

◆ Losing weight could bring your blood pressure and cholesterol under control

Mass hysteria?

Everybody's at it. The diet industry is booming. Millions of pounds are spent on books telling you foolproof ways to lose weight and on miraculous remedies like 'fat-burning pills'. And yet, the nation is getting fatter! OK, there are the tragic anorexic exceptions but, if you travel on the tube in the rush hour, you won't need any statistics on body mass index to convince you that we are expanding.

What is body mass index?

You know the one about the man whose doctor told him he wasn't too heavy – just too short. Your ideal weight range, of course, depends on your height, so doctors use the body mass index (BMI). It's a simple way to check whether you're overweight. To calculate your BMI, you take your weight in kilograms and divide it by your height in metres squared:

$$BMI = \frac{\text{Weight in kilograms}}{(\text{height in metres})^2}$$

If your BMI is 20–24.9, congratulations. This is the 'normal' or desirable range. In fact, the World Health Organisation now accepts anything down to 18.5 as normal. Of course, it is important to measure your height accurately – not wearing platform shoes. And bathroom scales are notoriously inaccurate: sometimes they are so accommodating that you can get any reading you like by leaning in the right direction.

A BMI of 25–30 means you are 'overweight'. When doctors say someone is 'obese', it's not a vague term of abuse: it's simply defined as having a BMI over 30. A BMI over 40 would make you 'very obese'. Figure 9 shows you the acceptable weight range for your height.

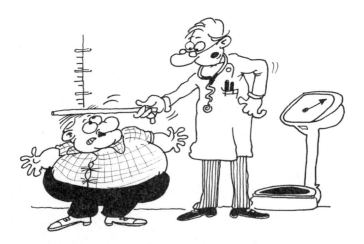

"Your weight is fine; it's your height that's the problem."

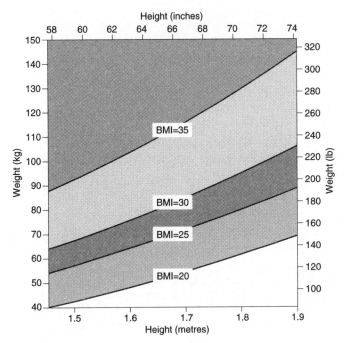

Use the chart or do this calculation to find out your BMI: divide your weight in kilograms by the square of your height in metres.

Your BMI score:
below 20: underweight
20–25: ideal
25–30: overweight
30+: seriously overweight – you need to see your doctor

Figure 9 What you should weigh. The BMI weight/height diagram.

Those who have built up very big muscles by weight training may be in the 'overweight' range although they are not fat. On the other hand, many people in the normal weight zone could do with more muscle and less fat.

A weighty problem

A growing proportion of the UK population is obese (BMI over 30). In 1980 about 8% of the adults were obese and by 1994 the proportion had almost doubled to reach 15%. And it's still rising! This is alarming – especially if you manufacture lifts. Obesity is the extreme end of the spectrum; many more people are overweight. Mortality shoots up as the BMI rises above 30; the risk of heart disease is increased fivefold, and of diabetes twentyfold. Many other medical problems – such as high blood pressure, stroke, gallstones, respiratory disease, arthritis and hernias – occur more commonly in people who are overweight or obese. It could be twenty years before an obese person runs into medical problems and, for this reason, the effects of obesity have sometimes been underestimated in the past.

If you have raised blood pressure or cholesterol, losing excess weight is vital. In some cases this will solve the problem and avoid the need for drugs.

◆ Eating more fat and being inactive are the main changes that have resulted in more people getting fat

◆ In general, fat people do not have slow metabolism

◆ Occasionally, weight gain results from lack of thyroid hormone

◆ Fat around the tummy (and a high waist–hip ratio) is dangerous

◆ Drinking excessively or smoking can increase abdominal fat

Why are we getting fatter?

Here's a simple fact: if you take in more energy (calories) than you use up, the spare energy will be stored. The body's main energy store is fat. So if you don't use up all the calories you eat, you must get heavier. And if you burn more calories than you take in, you get lighter. This is inescapable. Energy cannot be created or destroyed. That's the first law of thermodynamics.

So what's changed? Why have Western societies got fatter during this century? There have been two notable changes. Firstly, we get more of our calories from fat these days. Secondly, we are using fewer calories; we're much less active. Technology sees to that. We travel door-to-door by car and floor-to-floor by escalator. We are even spared the effort of opening doors. Adjusting the TV by remote control still means lifting a finger; perhaps future sets will respond to our thoughts.

The metabolic myth

Many overweight people complain that they have a slow metabolism: "If I so much as look at a lettuce leaf, I put on a pound." The popular idea that fat people have low metabolic rates is completely false. The bigger the body, the more energy it uses just to stay alive. In other words, the bigger you are, the higher your resting metabolic rate. Not only that, but as soon as you start moving your body, you use up more energy than someone who has a smaller body to move.

That doesn't mean that two people of the same weight will necessarily have the same metabolic rates. One of the most important things to understand is that muscle uses more energy than fat. If you stay the same weight but increase your lean body mass (that is to say, you increase your muscle and reduce your fat) your metabolic rate will rise. So when you lose weight, you must make sure you lose fat – not muscle – or you'll find it impossible to keep the weight off.

If you have been fighting a losing battle with your weight, I hope this book will change all that. Just occasionally, it turns out that the metabolic rate has been slowed down by inadequate production of thyroid hormone. Your doctor will be happy to check whether you have this problem. If you have, it's simply corrected by taking a daily thyroid supplement.

Fats and figures

Are you an apple or a pear? Our figure is largely determined by the distribution of fat on our body. The typical female figure is 'pear-shaped' – excess fat being stored on the hips and thighs. An obese man typically stores most of his fat on the abdomen – so-called central obesity – making him 'apple-shaped'. Despite these stereotypes, women often develop excess abdominal fat, especially after the menopause.

Being apple-shaped is a much greater health hazard than being pear-shaped. Central obesity is strongly linked with coronary heart disease; it also increases the risk of premature death, high blood pressure, stroke, diabetes and gallstones.

Another way of looking at the problem is to calculate the waist–hip ratio (that is, the waist measurement divided by the hip measurement). A ratio greater than 1 in a man, or 0.8 in a woman, would indicate an increased risk of coronary heart disease. For example, a man measuring 40 inches round the waist and 32 inches round the hips would have a ratio of 40/32 = 1.25, putting him at increased risk.

Recently, doctors have been using the simple waist measurement to pick out people at risk. For a woman, a 32-inch waist means some increased risk, and a 35-inch waist is serious. The equivalent values for a man are 37 inches and 40 inches. Professor Michael Lean has presented several papers on this. (With a name like that, he would, wouldn't he?) Writing in the *Lancet* in 1998, Professor Lean and colleagues argued that waist measurement could pinpoint people at risk as effectively as BMI.

Drinking excessive amounts of alcohol and smoking can increase the tendency to store fat on the abdomen. If you can pinch an inch or more of flab at the waistline, it's time to do something about it.

ACTION POINTS

◆ Don't 'go on a diet'; change to a healthy way of life

◆ Set realistic goals; aim for a weight loss of 1–2 lb/week (0.5–1 kg)

◆ Don't weigh yourself more than once a week

◆ Cut right down on fat. Eat plenty of high-fibre, starchy foods

◆ Don't go hungry. Eat regular meals

◆ Finish meals with fruit and carry a suitable snack (e.g. banana)

◆ As you get older, get smaller plates

◆ Cut down alcohol. It contains 7 cal/g

Dieting can damage your health

So, you've decided to take yourself in hand and lose that flab. What should you do? Go on a diet, right? Wrong! Think about it. Haven't you been here before? How many times have you been on a diet, lost weight and put it back on again? Yo-yo dieting is bad for you.

Whenever you 'go on a diet' that involves an unnatural pattern of eating – whether it's having meal replacement bars or eating nothing but yoghurt and grapefruit – you will lose weight initially as long as your calorie intake is less than your energy expenditure, but you cannot continue this unnatural behaviour for very long. Your diet comes to an end. Inevitably, the weight returns. And it's worse than that: if your diet has reduced your metabolic rate, the pounds will pile on even faster. All you have lost is your self-esteem.

Crazy diets are big business. Millions are drawn in by the promise of rapid weight loss, only to have their hopes dashed when the scales go back to their old ways.

Any diet involving a sudden reduction of calorie intake is likely to produce a substantial weight loss, typically about five pounds, in the first week. But don't get too excited. That's not five pounds of fat. It's mainly the water that goes as the body draws on energy stored as glycogen (a carbohydrate). You won't continue to lose weight at that rate (and you certainly shouldn't try as it would be very bad for you).

Very low calorie diets (VLCDs), in which meals are replaced by a broth, milkshake or snack bar of essential nutrients, certainly produce weight loss in the short-term. Unfortunately, as well as losing fat, you can lose good lean muscle tissue on these diets. That's a disaster. You want more muscle, not less. And don't forget that muscle burns more calories than fat does; when you start eating proper food again, it will be that much harder to control your weight. Very low calorie diets may have a place under close medical supervision in the management of very obese people – where weight loss is a matter of life and death.

The Atkins diet, a 1970's craze condemned by the American Medical Association, has enjoyed a resurgence of publicity and popularity. If you cut out carbohydrates and replace them with fat and protein, you go into 'ketosis' – the body's starvation mode. You may experience nausea and fatigue (not to mention the bad breath). Short-term weight loss is quite possible, but those who stay on a diet like this are inviting kidney problems, cancer and heart disease.

If you are really keen to try the Atkins diet, I strongly recommend that you modify it. You could cut out bread and potatoes, but keep up your fruit and vegetables. By all means increase your consumption of protein from **lean** sources such as grilled chicken, turkey and fish. Make sure your poultry is skinless and if you want to have more red meat, it must be very lean. Many people following the Atkins diet are consuming vast quantities of saturated fat, and the long-term effects of that could be catastrophic.

The cabbage soup diet may come with a warning that you shouldn't continue the diet for more than a week, but you don't really need to be told: ferocious flatulence will soon blast you back to reality. Restricting yourself to one or two foods is nutritional nonsense. Any weight loss is the result of calorie reduction, which could just as well be achieved on a balanced diet.

What about drugs?

If you are struggling to lose weight, the idea of taking a drug to suppress your appetite may be appealing. Unfortunately, these drugs have never been really helpful and have now been linked with serious side effects such as damage to heart valves. Steer clear of diet clinics that dish out drugs (including thyroid hormone) for cash.

Xenical (orlistat) was launched in 1998 and can be prescribed for obese people who first lose at least 2.5 kg (5½ lb) over 4 weeks by changing their diet. It interferes with fat digestion so that 30% of the fat you eat passes through the bowel without being absorbed. It's certainly not a wonder drug and those who try to continue a high fat diet on orlistat soon find themselves dashing to the toilet.

So how should I lose weight?

Nothing to lose?
The first question is whether you need to lose any weight. Figure 9 shows you if you are in the acceptable weight range for your height. If you are, you may still have excess fat, especially around the abdomen. Your task is to reduce the flab and increase the muscle while staying in the desirable weight range – to tone up. If you follow the advice on diet and exercise in this book, you will do just that.

I use the word 'diet' extensively in this book. It's a good word, but it's a word that's been hijacked by the diet industry. I use it, of course, to refer to a normal pattern of eating and drinking, a way of life. This has nothing to do with the abnormal behaviour of

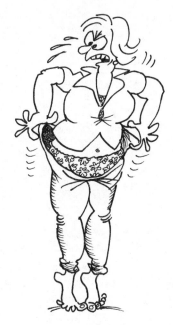

**"This diet's useless. I've been at it all day
and I still can't get into these jeans!"**

'going on a diet'. If you adopt the balanced diet explained in this book, you will control your weight **permanently** as well as reducing your risk of heart disease and cancer.

If your weight is **below** the normal range for your height, you certainly don't need to lose weight. Gaining weight may just be a matter of eating more food; but make sure you keep the balance right (see Chapter 12). You should see your doctor if you are very underweight. This is particularly important if you have lost weight recently. If you are afraid of putting on weight, even though the chart shows you are underweight, it may be that you are developing an eating disorder; the sooner you seek help, the better.

Setting goals

We all like quick results. We get instant tea and instant credit; why not instant weight loss? This desire for rapid results explains the commercial success of diet gimmicks. It also explains why diets fail.

If your goal is to lose half a stone before your holiday in two weeks, you can do it. If you imagine that the weight will stay off,

◆ Fat contains 9 cal/g; sugar, starch and protein contain only 4 cal/g

◆ You can be free from calorie counting

◆ Don't be enslaved by fat-counting charts – a gimmick

◆ Fat calories are more likely to be stored than carbohydrate

◆ Fat can give you lots of calories without switching off your appetite

◆ 'Friendly' fats like rapeseed oil are just as fattening as 'unfriendly' ones like lard

you'll be disappointed. After a series of diets producing rapid weight reduction, and followed by rapid weight gain, you become despondent. You're setting the wrong goals.

But let's be realistic. If you're overweight, you don't really want to lose a few pounds for a few weeks, and then put them back on again. You want a permanent solution to the problem. So don't go on a diet.

Let's suppose for a moment that your weight has been around 12 stone for a long time but you should be 10 stone. This means that the way you are eating and drinking at the moment is feeding a 12 stone person. If you go on a diet until you reach 10 stone, and then go back to your normal habits, your weight will return to 12 stone. If you adopt the lifestyle of a 10-stone person, you can stay at 10 stone – for good.

Once you discover that a properly balanced low-fat diet can be exciting, varied and delicious, you won't want to go back to your old ways! If you follow the plan in this book, you will feel much better about yourself and enjoy a new vitality.

Setting realistic goals is essential. Figure 9 will show you how much weight you need to lose to get into the ideal range. But don't be in a hurry. If you lose one to two pounds (half to one kg) a week (or up to half a stone, or 3 kg, a month), you can reach your target weight and stay there. Sudden, severe weight loss is likely to reduce muscle as well as fat, making things harder in the long run.

Don't weigh yourself more than once a week. It's pointless to pat yourself on the back or to get despondent because of day-to-day fluctuations that have more to do with fluid balance than anything else. In fact, monthly weighing makes more sense.

Reduce fat intake

This is the single most important step in the weight-loss plan. Fat is the most concentrated source of calories that can pass your lips. Every gram of fat delivers nine calories (or strictly kilocalories) of energy. That's more than twice as much as carbohydrate (sugar and starch) or protein. Both carbohydrate and protein provide only four calories per gram.

Forget calorie counting. A calorie counter and calculator will do about as much for your appreciation of food as a ruler and stopwatch will do for your love life. There's more to food than calories.

If you make a huge reduction in the amount of fat you eat, you are bound to lose weight. Getting your balance right (see page 117) means you can forget about calories; they will look after themselves.

Of course, if you serve your pulses or pasta with a big dollop of fat, the bathroom scales will react accordingly. Remember, you can eat twice as much protein or carbohydrate as you can fat (by weight) for the same number of calories.

And that's not all. Some people have the simplistic notion that if you eat fat it goes straight to your belly or your bottom because flab is made of fat whereas carbohydrate and protein, not being fat, can't add to the flab. This is simplistic indeed and nutritionists have pooh-poohed the idea. After all, we've known for a long time that the body can convert carbohydrate and protein into fat. But wait. There is now scientific evidence to support this naïve theory. Experiments have shown that it is, in fact, very unusual for the sugar and starch we eat to end up as fat.

An interesting experiment on 'volunteers' detained in Vermont State Prison, by Sims and colleagues as long ago as 1973, shed some light on this. The men were given diets containing the same number of calories but different amounts of fat. Those on high-fat diets put on weight much more easily than those on high-carbohydrate diets (even though the calorie intake was the same, remember). In fact, the men on high-carbohydrate diets had to eat at least 50% more calories than those on high-fat diets to maintain the same weight gain.

It may be politically correct to consider all calories equal, but the body doesn't appear to treat them that way. It seems that fat calories really are more likely to get under your skin – and that's the bottom line.

Perhaps this is the key to understanding another vital observation: fatty foods are not satisfying. It has often been said (possibly by rather fat people) that we need plenty of fat in our food to make it really satisfying and keep hunger pangs at bay, but serious scientific work has turned this assumption on its head.

It turns out that fat is not very good at suppressing our appetite. Protein and carbohydrate give a stronger signal to the body that we've had enough. Studies in obese women showed that they took in more calories during a high-fat lunch than during a high-carbohydrate lunch. Not only that, after a high-fat lunch, they continued to take in more calories during the following 24 hours!

It's as if the body says, "I recognise this: it's fat. Better store it for a future famine. Must keep eating until we get something we can use now. Oh, what's this? Carbohydrate – that'll do. We can get on and turn that into energy right away."

You know what it's like to go on a diet and, mustering great will-power, nibble your way through a really 'slimming' meal. Within half an hour you're looking for something else to eat and the diet goes to pot. The body doesn't just count the calories to decide when you've had enough, and some foods leave you feeling satisfied for much longer than others.

In a test at Sydney University, Dr Susan Hood fed a variety of foods to volunteers in portions that provided 1000 kilojoules (or about 240 calories) of energy. In the following two hours the volunteers were free to nibble on other foods and their hunger feelings were monitored. She drew up a 'satiety index' of different foods; the better a food was at keeping hunger pangs at bay, the higher it scored. High-fat snacks like croissant, cake and chocolate bars had much lower satiety scores than popcorn, porridge, pasta and potatoes. Wholemeal bread and pasta kept hunger at bay longer than white varieties.

Of course, as a calorie-conscious dieter you will ask only two questions about your food: "Does it taste good?" and "How many calories is it?" Balance doesn't come into it and the daily calorie allowance is often made up of the most unhelpful foods – ones that leave you asking, "Now what can I eat next?"

So you see, science continues to unearth reasons why the high-fat diet of a westernised population is such a disaster – reasons that go far beyond the simple fact that fat is the most energy-dense foodstuff available.

Table 18 Foods to avoid and enjoy

Foods to avoid	Foods to enjoy
Whole milk, cream Imitation cream Coffee whitener	Skimmed milk, fat-free fromage frais
Full-fat yoghurt	Very low-fat yoghurt Buttermilk
Full-fat and reduced-fat cheeses	Cottage cheese, quark
Ice cream	Very low-fat ice cream, frozen yoghurt, sorbet (watch sugar!)
Egg yolks	Egg whites
Butter, margarine, reduced-fat spreads, cooking fats and oils, suet, dripping	
Fried foods	Grilled and 'dry-fried' foods
Nuts including coconut	Chestnuts
Avocado pears	All other fruit and vegetables (fresh, frozen and dried) Unsweetened tinned fruit
Mayonnaise, salad cream, all fatty sauces and dressings	Fat-free sauces and dressings
Peanut butter, chocolate spread, etc.	Reduced-sugar jams
All fatty meats; duck; goose; poultry skin Meat products: sausages, pies, pâté, salami, pasties, samosas, scotch eggs, burgers, luncheon meats	Skinless chicken/turkey breast, game, veal, rabbit, fish, shellfish Soya protein, tofu, Quorn Beans, peas, lentils, chickpeas
Standard cakes and biscuits; croissants, pastries, puddings; chocolate, toffee, fudge Cream crackers, cheese biscuits; crisps and other high-fat savoury snacks	Fatless cakes (watch sugar!) Crispbreads, matzos, bread, pasta (especially wholemeal), Rice (especially brown), Wholegrain cereals, muesli (without nuts), breakfast cereals (low sugar), wholemeal flour, oatmeal
Any processed food with more than 4 g fat per 100 g	

These recommendations are for those who need to lose weight, or have difficulty preventing weight gain. There is no reason why others should avoid nuts or avocado pears, for example. Try to avoid products marketed as 'low-fat' if they are loaded with sugar; their high calorie content won't help you lose weight. Favour products containing less than 10 g/100g sugar.

We have seen in other chapters how important it is for everyone to minimise consumption of saturated and trans fatty acids, which play a key role in the development of heart disease. Those who have no trouble keeping their weight down can be much more relaxed when it comes to good sources of mono-unsaturates (such as hazelnuts, almonds, avocados, olives, olive oil and rapeseed oil) and polyunsaturates (such as walnuts, oily fish, sunflower oil and corn oil). If you need to lose weight, or you have trouble keeping your weight down, you must remember that all fat is equally fattening.

Table 18 shows some of the high-fat foods that will prove most unhelpful if you are trying to keep your weight down.

- Avoid the high-fat foods such as those shown in Table 18.

- Cook and serve food without adding any fat.

- Eat lots of fruit and vegetables (5–9 portions a day).

- Fill up on starchy foods with a low glycaemic index (see Table 10), such as pasta. Choose wholegrain varieties.

- Use lots of beans, peas, lentils and chickpeas to supplement the protein from fish, lean poultry and game.

- Have plenty of skimmed milk dairy products.

Do all this and you will enjoy a very low-fat diet that is bound to help you control your weight. But it won't be a no-fat diet. You would become very ill on a totally fat-free diet, but the cereal grains, poultry and fish in this balanced diet are all providing some fat, including essential fatty acids.

Even so, it is vital to ensure that you don't go short on the fat-soluble vitamins, A, D and E. Vitamin K is the other fat-soluble vitamin but, not only is it obtained from low-fat foods like potatoes, tomatoes, green vegetables and soya beans, it is also manufactured for you by bacteria in your intestine. It would be possible to become deficient in vitamins A, D and E on a very low-fat diet if you were careless. Remember to include generous quantities of skimmed milk powder fortified with vitamins A and D. Have at least two fish meals a week and include some oily fish. This could still leave you low in the crucial antioxidant, vitamin E. On a very low-fat diet, in which you are not using vegetable oils, you might consider taking a supplement of vitamin E, but very high doses may not be safe (see page 96).

If you are an overweight vegetarian, the chances are that high-fat dairy products, cooking oils, fat spreads, cakes, pastries, biscuits, confectionery or nuts are your downfall – unless you are a closet avocadoholic. Making the adjustments indicated in Table 18 will no doubt solve the problem but, without oily fish or poultry, it could leave you uncomfortably low in fat and fat-soluble vitamins. So, even as an overweight vegetarian, it is advisable to include *tiny* quantities of olive oil or rapeseed oil, and a few nuts (e.g. hazelnuts, almonds, walnuts) and seeds (e.g. sunflower and sesame) in your regular diet.

Get wise to GIs

Get to know which carbohydrate foods have low GIs (Table 10) and make them work for your waistline. Foods with a high gly-caemic index are rapidly digested, producing high blood glucose and insulin levels. Persistently raised insulin levels lead to more fat round the tummy. Insulin also makes you hungry. A low-GI diet keeps insulin levels down, so you feel satisfied for longer and you store less fat.

So having more pasta and fewer baked potatoes could work wonders – unless you serve it with a fatty sauce.

Eaten plenty? Give it twenty

If you've finished your meal and still feel hungry, have a glass of water and do something else before you have another helping. It could be that your body needs a little more time to send all the signals to your brain that say you've had enough. Twenty minutes after that last mouthful, you may find the hunger's gone – and you'll be glad you didn't squeeze in another plateful!

Feast, don't fast

If you try going hungry, you won't last long. Foods rich in complex carbohydrate or protein (such as pasta or pulses) will keep hunger pangs away more efficiently than high-fat foods – but don't add fat! A bowl of muesli or cereal with skimmed milk makes a quick and easy pudding – but make sure you stick to low-sugar, low-fat varieties. If you make your own muesli, you can leave out the nuts and keep sugar to a minimum.

Finish meals with fruit and always have fruit or vegetable snacks to hand. A banana in the handbag or briefcase, or prepared carrot and celery sticks in the fridge, could save you from that chocolate éclair. In fact, *healthy* snacking throughout the day will help you control weight and cholesterol much better than going for long periods without food.

Don't skip breakfast and lunch. Have three meals a day.

Size doesn't matter. Or does it?

So portion size doesn't matter as long as you eat the right foods. Well, not quite. Certainly you can eat fruit and vegetables freely and you are unlikely to overdo it as long as they are not cooked or served with fat. And we've seen that choosing foods high in starch and fibre, in place of high-fat foods, means you can eat more and still lose weight, but there is a limit. There is some connection between the size of the portion and the size of the person.

Switch to the right foods, prepared in the right way, and you're more than half way there, but if you persistently eat too much of the right foods you will never reach your ideal weight. As we get older, and less active in most cases, we burn up fewer calories. If you keep on eating at 50 exactly the same as you were eating at 20, 'middle-age spread' is inevitable.

Certainly, one of the great things about getting the balance right, and eating far more vegetables and starchy foods but much less fat, is that you can enjoy a full plate of food and still control your weight. Even so, particularly if you are not very active, there's a lot to be said for getting smaller plates as you get older.

On your marks. Get set . . .

Sprinting is not always advisable, but exercise is essential. You cannot hope to control your weight permanently without including some form of exercise in your routine. If this is a completely novel concept for you, don't start running; it's best not to take the body by surprise.

Walking is ideal, if you have working legs. Start from your present level of activity and build up gradually. This may mean walking to the TV set to turn it on instead of using the remote control. Soon you could be doing half an hour's brisk walking a day and this will make a real difference. It's not so much that the pounds drop off with a little bit of exercise. They don't. But regular exercise increases your metabolic rate – not only while you're exercising but also when you're not.

It also helps to build up muscle tissue as you lose weight. And, as we've seen, muscle burns calories more efficiently than fat does.

Congratulations!

If you've discovered the benefits of healthy eating and you're including aerobic exercise in your daily routine, you might well congratulate yourself. But, as you raise that glass of celebratory champagne, it's worth remembering that alcohol has seven calories in every gram – calories you could well do without if weight is a problem.

Light drinking can have its benefits (see Chapter 10) but a **heavy** drinker may well become just that – and much of the extra weight is often carried in a 'beer gut'. Alcohol, it seems, increases the storage of fat on the abdomen where it is particularly linked to coronary risk.

Keeping it up

Or should that be down? Having lost some weight, it's all too easy to find it again. You are discovering that a really healthy diet is delicious, varied and satisfying. You are finding that exercise can be enjoyable. It can make you feel good about yourself. So this is not a weight-loss programme of so many weeks before returning to normal life. This **is** normal life – a much more satisfying life because you are in control. Here are a few extra tips to help you stay that way:

- Remember that when you weigh less you need less food, unless you increase your activity enough to compensate.

- Recognise the danger times and work out a strategy to deal with them. If you tend to overeat at the end of a stressful day (and then feel guilty or depressed), do a relaxation exercise when you get in or go for a short walk or pedal your exercise bike for 20 minutes. Don't worry about exercise making you hungry; it will often take the edge off your appetite if you exercise before eating.

- If you do overeat, or slip up and eat a high-fat meal, simply go back to your normal, low-fat way of eating straight away (i.e. at the next meal). You are not 'on a diet', so there's no need to overreact and give up as if you had 'broken the diet'.

- Sort out a dozen very low-fat, quick and easy recipes that you (and your family) enjoy. Always keep the ingredients in stock. Fall back on these old favourites whenever you're not sure what to cook.

- When cooking your favourite recipes, make extra portions and keep them in the freezer as a standby.

- Sit at the table to eat meals. Don't watch TV at the same time: tests show this can lead to overeating. Relax and enjoy your food. But stop eating before you feel absolutely full. Round off the meal with fruit. Treat yourself to varieties of fruit that you really enjoy.

Summary of the successful long-term weight control plan

- ◆ Set realistic goals

- ◆ Lose 1–2 lbs/week (0.5–1 kg) at most

- ◆ Reduce fat intake: choose low-fat foods; – with meat, remember: slim, trim and skim (Chapter 4); – grill, bake, boil, steam, poach or microwave, but don't fry

- ◆ Eat more low-GI foods, particularly pasta, pulses and whole grains such as barley, rye and oats

- ◆ Eat more fruit and vegetables

- ◆ Don't go hungry. Have three meals a day

- ◆ Always have healthy, low-fat snacks to hand

- ◆ Include regular exercise in your routine

- ◆ Go easy on the alcohol, but drink plenty of water (six or more glasses a day)

- ◆ Keep going. Once your low-fat lifestyle becomes a habit, you'll find that you prefer it. And that'll be a big weight off your mind

Chapter 18

Controlling cholesterol

'The lard starts forming on the guest even before he gets out of his car, and by the time he rises flushed from the table, he can be used to baste an ox.'

S.J. Perelman (1904–79) *Letter*, 1975

In Chapter 3 we saw how countries with high total cholesterol levels have high rates of heart disease, and how your personal risk of having a heart attack is reduced by getting your cholesterol down. Remember that LDL-cholesterol is the 'bad' one while HDL-cholesterol is 'good'. We learnt that:

LOW-density lipoprotein (LDL) cholesterol should be LOW

HIGH-density lipoprotein (HDL) cholesterol should be HIGH

In this chapter we find out how to achieve it.

Checking your cholesterol

You could check your cholesterol level with a fingerprick test at your doctor's surgery, on the high street or even at home with a d.i.y. test kit. The accuracy of these tests is variable and it would be unwise to base the whole direction of your life on a single reading of this kind. You can be more confident about accuracy if your doctor arranges for a blood sample to be taken from a vein and analysed in a hospital laboratory.

◆ Total cholesterol can be measured without fasting

◆ An overnight fast is needed to tell you triglyceride and HDL levels

◆ Recommended levels:

   – Total cholesterol less than 5.0 mmol/l

   – LDL-cholesterol less than 3.0 mmol/l

   – HDL-cholesterol more than 0.9 mmol/l

Samples taken when you haven't fasted are suitable for measuring total cholesterol (but not for telling you how much of it is HDL-cholesterol or LDL-cholesterol). The total cholesterol is not significantly altered by a 12-hour fast and a non-fasting or 'random' level is useful as a screening test to pick out people at high risk.

Triglycerides are quite different. The level of these fats in the blood shoots up and down according to what you've been eating in the last few hours. So measurement of triglycerides is pointless unless you've been fasting for 12 hours. This is one of the easiest fasts you could do. You can finish a banquet at 9 o'clock in the evening, have blood taken at 9 o'clock the following morning and tuck into breakfast immediately afterwards. You can drink water during the fast, but avoid other drinks.

Measurement of triglycerides and HDL-cholesterol on a fasting blood sample allows the LDL-cholesterol to be calculated (in mmol/l) with this formula:

$$\text{LDL-chol} = (\text{total chol} - \text{HDL-chol}) - \frac{\text{triglycerides}}{2.19}$$

This formula is not accurate if the triglyceride concentration is above 4.5 mmol/l.

So, if your doctor arranges a fasting lipid profile, it will usually tell you your blood levels of the following:

• Total cholesterol;

• HDL-cholesterol;

- LDL-cholesterol;

- Triglycerides.

Some laboratories do not measure the HDL-cholesterol unless the total cholesterol is above 6.5 mmol/l. This policy may be acceptable for general screening but there are circumstances in which the doctor will want to know the HDL-cholesterol level, even if the total is not raised. For example, the doctor may specifically ask the laboratory to measure the HDL-cholesterol if:

- You have a significant family history (e.g. brother died of a heart attack aged 45);

- You are taking certain beta-blockers (such as propranolol) that could reduce the HDL-cholesterol and raise triglycerides;

- You are already on a strict diet or taking a drug to lower cholesterol.

There are times when measuring cholesterol levels can be misleading; for example, it is advisable to wait **three months** after pregnancy, surgery or serious illness, including a heart attack, before having a cholesterol test. (Levels measured just after a heart attack, within 24 hours, are usually considered reliable.) Similarly, you should not have your cholesterol checked within **three weeks** of having flu or a similar illness because the result may be artificially low (unless this is for an insurance medical in which case perhaps it is the ideal time to have the test).

ACTION POINTS

Before having a cholesterol check:

◆ Wait at least 3 weeks after flu

◆ Wait at least 3 months after surgery, major illness, or pregnancy

---

On the level

When your cholesterol result is available, no doubt your doctor or practice nurse will give you individual advice. Here are some guidelines on the level.

Total cholesterol less than 5.0 mmol/l

If you are in this group, you are the proud owner of a 'normal' cholesterol level. But wait. Before you order that Indian takeaway to celebrate, remember you are not immune to heart disease. For a start, your
cholesterol level goes up and down a bit and you might have caught it
at a low point. And heart disease does strike some people in this group;
you need to consider the other risk factors discussed in this book. Some
people imagine that it doesn't matter what they eat because they have
had a normal cholesterol reading. They're wrong. This book explains
how a good diet will protect you – or a bad diet will put you at risk – in
a number of ways that are nothing to do with your cholesterol level.

Total cholesterol 5.1–6.4 mmol/l

This is too high. Mind you, if you're in this group, you're in good
company: the average cholesterol level for the UK population is
about 5.9 mmol/l (5.8 for men and 6.0 for women). And about two-
thirds of the population have undesirable lipid profiles! But you
don't want to be among them. You're reading this book because
you want to escape the epidemic of heart disease. Of course, you
may not have escaped; you may already have heart disease. In that case,
even a mildly raised cholesterol level must be taken very seriously;
there is a strong argument for taking a cholesterol-lowering drug
(see page 306) as well as changing your diet and lifestyle.

If you are overweight, that's the first thing to put right (see
Chapter 17). In many cases, making the changes that bring you
gradually down to your ideal weight will sort the cholesterol out as
well. Avoid all unnecessary fat, have lots of cereal grains and
starchy foods, feast on fruit and vegetables, include fish at least
twice a week and you will do well.

If you are on the skinny side, you should still keep saturated fat
intake as low as possible but there's no need to be afraid of olive
oil, rapeseed oil, hazelnuts, almonds, walnuts, avocados and oily
fish. I wouldn't recommend a high-fat diet, though, as this may
raise the risk of thrombosis.

Total cholesterol 6.5–7.8 mmol/l

This is significantly raised but if you come into this group you are
not a freak: levels in this range are very common in the UK (but,
then, so are heart attacks). It's definitely time to tackle all your risk
factors and adopt a healthy lifestyle.

Total cholesterol above 7.8 mmol/l

Don't panic. Calmly and rationally check that your will is in order. No, I'm not serious – although this is always worth doing if you haven't done it. If your cholesterol level is in this range, it is certainly very high but it doesn't mean you will necessarily die young (as you will realise if you are already 85). Indeed, if you were to check cholesterol levels among the residents of an old folks' home, you would find a good few with levels around 8 mmol/l. Just how serious this is depends what other risk factors are present. If the high cholesterol is your only risk factor, you may well make it to the old people's home; but if you smoke and have high blood pressure as well, you probably won't (unless you make some changes).

Whatever the case, attaining your ideal weight and adopting the diet and lifestyle recommended in this book will significantly reduce your risk of heart disease. If you already have heart disease and a very raised cholesterol, then it's essential to get it down – right down (preferably below 5 mmol/l). Most people will need drug treatment, as well as a good diet, to achieve this.

If your cholesterol level turns out to be something like 10 or 11 mmol/l, then it's just as well you had it measured. You may well have the genetic disorder called familial hypercholesterolaemia (FH), which affects about 1 in 500 of the population. Untreated, most of these people will develop heart disease at a young age. Drug treatment to lower cholesterol is life-saving and other members of the family should have their lipids checked.

Before making any drastic decisions like taking a cholesterol-lowering drug for the rest of your life, you should have at least two measurements including a full fasting lipid profile. Your doctor will also want to use some of the blood to check liver, kidney and thyroid function to make sure your raised cholesterol is not the result of some other disease. You should normally spend at least three months trying to lower your cholesterol by changing your diet although people with familial hypercholesterolaemia will need drug treatment as well.

There are multitudes who do not have a serious metabolic disorder and yet have cholesterols above 7 mmol/l. They will not solve the problem by making a few sensible changes like switching to sunflower spread. Most could achieve a spectacular reduction by following the advice in this book.

> ◆ Some people have inherited disorders that cause very high cholesterol levels and need drug treatment as well as diet
>
> ◆ People who already have heart disease should get their total cholesterol level below 5 mmol/l – with drugs if necessary
>
> ◆ A good diet is essential, whether drugs are used or not
>
> ◆ The importance of a high cholesterol depends on the other risk factors present

Getting the low down

You will remember that the aim of the game is:

To get the LOW-Density Lipoprotein (LDL) down LOW.

Because most of the blood cholesterol is LDL-cholesterol, it is generally the case that if your total cholesterol level is too high, so is your LDL-cholesterol; reducing the total cholesterol will bring down the LDL-cholesterol as well.

How low should you go? Aim for an LDL-cholesterol of 3.0 mmol/l or less; if you have other risk factors such as high blood pressure, this is all the more important. Those who already have heart disease should get it down to well below 3.0 mmol/l – with the help of a statin drug in most cases.

Some people, mostly women, have a raised total cholesterol reading even though their LDL-cholesterol level is satisfactory. This is because they have extra high HDL-cholesterol levels and in these cases it doesn't matter that the total is a little high.

Want to get the low down? Here's the plan:

Keep saturated fat intake as low as possible

Avoid: fatty meats and poultry skin; meat products (e.g. sausages, luncheon meat, beefburgers, pies, pâté, etc.); full-fat dairy products (use skimmed milk products instead); manufactured cakes, biscuits and puddings; dressings and sauces (unless very low-fat); fried foods; lard, suet, dripping, ghee, palm oil, coconut oil and 'vegetable oil'; crisps and similar savoury snacks; chocolate, fudge, toffee and butterscotch; coconut, etc.

Favour friendly fats

Use olive oil or rapeseed oil for dressings and cooking, including home-made cakes and biscuits. Avoid 'vegetable oil', e.g. buy sardines in olive oil. If nuts are called for, favour chestnuts, hazelnuts, almonds and walnuts. If you use a fat spread, consider changing to one fortified with plant sterols or stanols (Flora pro.activ or Benecol). Some olives, avocados, sunflower seeds and sesame seeds are allowable but keep the overall fat intake very low unless you need to gain weight.

Eat fish at least twice a week

Include oily fish (e.g. salmon, sardines, pilchards, mackerel, herring) but have any fish you fancy. Every time fish replaces fatty meat or meat products, it's helping to keep the LDL-cholesterol low (not to mention the effect of fish oil on triglycerides and thrombosis risk). If you don't fancy any fish, try recipes that disguise it.

FISHING FOR ALTERNATIVES

I have recommended that you eat fish – preferably, at least twice a week. If you hate fish, you are not impressed with my advice.

Of course, if you hate fish as a rule, you may find the odd exception to prove it. It could be tuna salad that's uniquely acceptable, or perhaps monkfish kebabs. (Never tried them? Then how do you know you don't like them?) If you're finicky about fins, you can have a well-disguised fillet. A fish cake or pie or casserole could throw you off the scent. Or it may be that nothing less than very strong curry is adequate to disguise its fishy origin for you.

If all these strategies disgust you – if you feel you could never enjoy any form of fish – what then? Of course, you will choose other foods from the high-protein group, such as beans, pulses, nuts, tofu, Quorn and, if you're not a vegetarian, lean meat. But what about those valuable fish oils that supply essential omega-3 fatty acids?

Unless you're a vegetarian, you might choose to take a supplement of fish oil (see page 84). Valuable plant sources of omega-3 (in the form of alpha-linolenic acid) include walnuts, pumpkin seeds, linseeds, flaxseed oil and rapeseed oil.

Eat at least five portions of fruit and vegetables a day

Five is the minimum; nine is fine. You needn't really limit yourself (unless you've added any fat to the vegetables) except in the case of olives and avocados. Large amounts of soluble fibre will help to lower LDL-cholesterol but, more to the point, you'll be eating the fruit and vegetables in place of something containing saturated fat, which would raise it. And beans (including soya products), peas, lentils and chickpeas are high-protein foods that can be used in place of meat.

Eat plenty of complex carbohydrate

The complex carbohydrate (starch and fibre) provided by foods like breakfast cereals, bread, rice, pasta and potato is an important part of the cholesterol-lowering plan. Getting more of your energy from these foods instead of foods high in saturated fat lowers your LDL-cholesterol. Choose plenty of wholegrain and low-GI foods (see Table 10) such as wholewheat pasta and mixed grain breads. Oats, beans, barley and rye are low-GI foods that supply helpful soluble fibre.

Maintaining the high

If you have changed your diet radically, you may be quite elated on re-testing to find your cholesterol has come crashing down. Well done, but spare a thought for your HDL-cholesterol. What's happened to that? Remember, your aim is:

To keep the HIGH-Density Lipoprotein (HDL) up HIGH.

It may be that your doctor is unable to tell you your HDL-cholesterol level because, now that your total cholesterol is below 6.5 mmol/l, the laboratory hasn't measured it. This really is unsatisfactory and, if you have made a drastic change to your diet (just as if you had taken a drug to lower cholesterol), you need to check your HDL. Most laboratories will measure it if the doctor specifically requests it.

It is likely that, if you have switched to a very low-fat diet with a very high carbohydrate intake, your HDL-cholesterol will have dropped a little. (There may also be some rise in the triglyceride level but this usually falls again after several months on this sort of diet.) In addition, you may remember that polyunsaturated fatty acids are helpful in lowering total cholesterol but, unfortunately, tend to push down the HDL-cholesterol too.

Aim to keep your HDL-cholesterol at 1 mmol/l or above. If it has dropped to, say, 0.8 mmol/l because of your low-fat, high carbohydrate diet (and you've got everything else in your diet and lifestyle right) and you've brought your LDL-cholesterol down as well (to, say, 3.0 mmol/l) then you probably don't have much to worry about. People in some parts of the world have low levels of HDL-cholesterol because most of their energy comes from carbohydrate; they have very low saturated fat intakes, low levels of LDL-cholesterol, and low rates of heart disease. Indeed, as a group, vegetarians in westernised societies have lower HDL-cholesterol levels than meat eaters – and lower rates of heart disease.

Here are some tips worth trying if your HDL-cholesterol is struggling to get above 1 mmol/l:

- Add some good sources of mono-unsaturated fatty acids to your diet, such as olive oil, rapeseed oil, olives, avocados, hazelnuts and almonds.

- Cut down any unnecessary sources of polyunsaturates, e.g. sunflower, safflower, soya or corn oils; sunflower spread or sunflower seeds.

- Eat a low-GI diet (see page 60). Cut down on foods with a high glycaemic index such as baguettes, white bread and instant rice. Eat more foods with a low GI, such as pasta and pulses. Spaghetti tossed in a little olive oil (delicious with garlic) would be a better choice than baked potato with sunflower spread.

- If you smoke, you must stop. Apart from all the other harmful effects, smoking depresses HDL-cholesterol.

- Take more exercise. Aerobic exercise raises HDL-cholesterol levels. 20 minutes three times a week is better than nothing, but you may need a lot more than this to make a significant impact on your HDL concentration.

- A little alcohol (e.g. one or two units a day) can help to lift drooping HDL levels.

- If you are a post-menopausal woman and not taking hormone replacement therapy, have a look at Chapter 23. Oestrogen can help to lift HDL- and lower LDL-cholesterol.

- If you are taking a non-selective beta-blocker
  (such as propranolol), it may be reducing your
  HDL-cholesterol and raising your triglycerides.
  This would be something to discuss with your doctor.

We noted that someone who has a very low-fat, high-carbohydrate diet and a healthy lifestyle need not be too concerned about a rather low HDL-cholesterol level. If you are an overweight, inactive smoker with a low HDL-cholesterol, that's quite different. Urgent action is needed.

If your HDL-cholesterol is below 0.6 mmol/l, and especially if you have a family history of heart disease, you should have specific medical advice about this.

Where do triglycerides fit in?

We've seen that triglycerides are fats. They are to be found in our food and in our flab. If we want a meaningful measurement of the level in our blood, the sample must be taken after a 12-hour fast.

Fasting triglyceride levels above 2.3 mmol/l are considered abnormal, but the link between raised levels and coronary heart disease is not as clear-cut as it is with cholesterol. For one thing, high triglyceride levels are commonly found in people who have other problems that raise their risk of heart disease (such as obesity, diabetes, and high blood pressure). There is no doubt that the combination of high triglycerides and low HDL-cholesterol, which is often seen in people with diabetes, is undesirable. Some families have a hereditary metabolic disorder that results in high cholesterol and triglyceride levels (familial combined hyperlipidaemia) and a high incidence of heart disease.

Heavy drinking is a common cause of raised triglycerides and many people could rapidly bring their level down to normal by cutting alcohol consumption.

Triglyceride levels above 5.0 mmol/l are very high. As levels rise above 11 mmol/l the blood plasma looks like milk and there is a risk of pancreatitis – a life-threatening illness.

If your fasting triglyceride level is above 2.3 mmol/l:

- Get down to your ideal weight (see Chapter 17);

- Stay on the healthy diet described under 'Getting the low down' (page 182);

- Eat more oily fish. Fish oils help to reduce triglyceride levels;

- Eat a low-GI diet (see page 60);

- Cut alcohol consumption down to a maximum of one unit a day;

- Keep up a regular aerobic exercise programme;

- Have your blood glucose level measured to exclude diabetes;

- Get your blood pressure checked.

If your triglyceride level is above 5.0 mmol/l, you need specific medical advice.

◆ It's sensible to be settled on an improved diet for 3 months before rechecking your cholesterol

◆ Once you've established a normal lipid profile by changing your lifestyle, there's no need to keep checking your cholesterol level – as long as you keep checking your lifestyle (see Action Plan)

◆ If you are taking a drug to lower your cholesterol, your doctor may wish to do a blood test every 6–12 months

---

What about all the cholesterol in my food?

Frankly, there isn't much. In an average day of munching your way through all those grams of carbohydrate, protein and fat, you will eat less than half a gram of cholesterol. Let's suppose you are eating 400 mg of cholesterol a day and, without making any other changes, you cut that in half to 200 mg a day. We would expect that to reduce your blood cholesterol by about 0.2 mmol/l. Impressed?

Now perhaps you can see why all that talk of a 'low-cholesterol diet' is rather silly. And those eye-catching food labels saying 'Low in cholesterol' are playing on the fact that people don't understand this.

How much of the cholesterol that we eat ends up in the blood? This varies. If you were to eat a whole plate of triglycerides, they would all be digested and absorbed from the intestine into the bloodstream (if you didn't vomit before they had the chance). Only 30–60% of the cholesterol in food is absorbed and this may be influenced by other foods in the diet. For example, the gel-forming fibre in beans and pulses reduces absorption of cholesterol from the intestine.

Despite all this, it is recommended that a cholesterol-lowering diet should contain no more than 300 mg of cholesterol a day. So why have I hardly mentioned ways of cutting down dietary cholesterol in this book? That's simple. Much of the cholesterol is found in foods rich in saturated fatty acids. By cutting down your saturated fat intake, you will automatically reduce your consumption of cholesterol.

Here are some foods with a particularly high content of cholesterol:

- All offal such as liver (including liver pâté);

- Fish roe (including taramasalata);

- Egg yolk;

- Egg mayonnaise;

- Some shellfish such as shrimps, prawns, crayfish, lobster, squid and cuttlefish.

I can't get my cholesterol down

You've made radical changes to your diet. The healthier lifestyle is beginning to be second nature and you're feeling better for it. Three months on, you wait eagerly for the result of your cholesterol test. What a terrible disappointment, then, when it turns out to be much the same as the last one. You pick yourself up and go away for another three months. When the next test is no better, despite every effort to get your cholesterol down, it gets you down instead.

I hope this is not your experience. I hope you are one of the majority of people who can make very satisfying reductions in cholesterol levels as long as they make big enough changes to diet and lifestyle.

If you are having difficulty, it is very helpful to keep a dietary diary for a week. Write down *everything* you eat and drink for seven days. I sometimes ask patients to do this and it often shows up areas that can be improved. Your doctor, practice nurse or dietitian would probably be happy to go through it with you.

There will always be some who have a genuine 'metabolic resistance' to cholesterol reduction. Oh yes, many who are placed in this category are deluding themselves and their physicians and, if they were actually to follow the recommendations in this book, their cholesterol levels would come tumbling down. Others, though, are battling with a genetically programmed overproduction of cholesterol, which cannot be fully controlled by changing the diet.

If you are one of these people, I have something very important to say to you: don't get despondent and decide that the healthy diet is a waste of effort. It isn't.

Firstly, if you achieve even a small reduction in your cholesterol level, this is worthwhile. Remember that every 1% reduction in total cholesterol results in *at least* a 2% (probably 3%) reduction in risk of coronary heart disease.

Secondly, even if you were unable to bring about any reduction at all in your cholesterol level, the healthy diet and lifestyle would still be vital. Cutting down saturated fat and eating more fish will reduce the risk of thrombosis (which can cause a heart attack); the diet and lifestyle recommended in this book may help to control blood pressure (and raised blood pressure makes a high cholesterol more dangerous); antioxidants from fruit and vegetables can stop fatty plaques forming in arteries. These are just a few of the ways in which a healthy diet can protect you even if it doesn't bring down your cholesterol.

Your doctor may recommend drug treatment to lower your cholesterol if it stays high on a good diet – especially if you have other risk factors or have already developed heart disease. Some people imagine that the drug does all the work and a healthy diet is no longer needed. You know better.

- ◆ Cut down saturated fat and you needn't bother about the cholesterol content of most foods
- ◆ Avoid large quantities of offal, fish roe and egg yolk, which have a very high cholesterol content
- ◆ A healthy diet will help to protect your heart even if it has a disappointing effect on your cholesterol level

Chapter 19

Exercise

'I like long walks, especially when they are taken
by people who annoy me.'

Fred Allen

Why bother?

OK, so regular, vigorous exercise might add four years to my life-span. What's the point when I'll have spent those four years doing vigorous exercise? So says the cynic.

Is there any scientific evidence that exercise can help us to avoid heart disease – and perhaps prevent the heart attack that could shorten a life, not just by four years, but by 40 years in some cases?

- ◆ Physically active people are much less likely to have a heart attack than inactive people

- ◆ Being athletic in your youth doesn't protect you in middle age

- ◆ Fitness has a short shelf life. You need to stay active

- ◆ Exercise: raises HDL-cholesterol; reduces thrombosis risk; strengthens bones, muscles and the heart; reduces stress

- ◆ When you are unfit, strenuous exercise can be dangerous

- ◆ It is more dangerous *not* to exercise than to take regular exercise of the right intensity

Are you a sitting duck?

It was half a century ago that Morris and his colleagues presented some early evidence. In 1953 they published a paper in the *Lancet* drawing attention to the fact that bus drivers, who spent all day sitting down, had more heart attacks than bus conductors who ran up and down stairs collecting fares. Similarly, when they investigated postal workers, they discovered that clerks had more heart attacks than postmen who delivered mail.

Twenty years later, Morris and his team were investigating the leisure time activities of male civil servants aged 40–64 (or, at least, the activities they would admit to). Men who reported taking part in vigorous physical activity on the initial survey (1968–70) suffered less than half the coronary heart disease of their less active colleagues over the next eight and a half years.

Dock workers in San Francisco were monitored for 22 years by Paffenbarger and Hale, during which time 11% died of coronary heart disease. The risk of dying from heart disease was 80% higher for those with the less energetic jobs compared with the men doing heavy work (which was defined as using up more than 8500 calories a week at work).

A very different social group, graduates from Harvard, were also studied by Dr Paffenbarger and his colleagues. Those who expended less than 2000 calories a week on leisure time activities had a 64% higher risk of a first heart attack than their more energetic contemporaries.

An interesting discovery was made about the graduates who had been keen athletes at college: they were just as likely to get heart attacks in middle age as their sedentary classmates. To protect against heart disease, regular exercise had to be continued through adulthood. The inactive student who took up regular exercise after leaving college had a lower risk than the college athlete who rested on his laurels (or anything else comfortable he could find to sit on).

This observation – that only continuing exercise protects against heart disease – was confirmed by Morris and his colleagues in a later report on the British civil servants. So, if you think you've done enough exercise to last a lifetime, think again!

Pooling the results of the many studies on this question that have now been published, it looks as though not exercising will more or less double your risk of dying from a heart attack.

The object of the exercise

What can we hope to achieve by exercising? Staying alive by avoiding a heart attack is a pretty good start. It is likely that exercise reduces coronary risk in a number of ways, such as:

- *Reducing blood pressure*
  A number of research groups have shown that regular exercise can lower blood pressure.

- *Raising HDL-cholesterol*
  Many investigations have shown that aerobic exercise raises the level of protective HDL-cholesterol and lowers triglycerides. This probably results from increasing the amount of an enzyme called lipoprotein lipase in trained muscle. The changes are small and a lot of regular, vigorous exercise is needed to make a significant impact.

- *Preventing thrombosis*
  It is likely that regular exercise reduces the risk of blood clots forming in the circulation. This may result partly from changes in platelets and also from reduction in levels of the clotting factor, fibrinogen. The finding that exercise must be continued to protect against heart attacks would be explained by an effect on blood clotting.

- *Exercising the heart muscle*
  Like other muscles, the heart benefits from training. A fit person has a slower heart rate because the heart beats more efficiently. As a result, when extra demands are made during exertion, the heart can cope without straining.

The benefits of exercise don't end with the cardiovascular system. Here are some of the other objectives we can expect to meet with a regular exercise programme:

- *Weight control*
  Exercise is an essential ingredient in any weight-loss programme and helps you to stay at your ideal weight. It increases the metabolic rate, not just while you are exercising, but for some hours afterwards as well.

- *Increased lean body mass*
  If you exercise regularly while losing weight, things are
  even better than your scales would have you believe.
  You will be losing fat and gaining muscle; muscle is
  heavier than fat (but much better at burning calories).

- *Reduced diabetes risk*
  Type 2 diabetes – the sort that usually comes on after
  the age of 40 – is caused by 'insulin resistance' (see
  page 232). Blood glucose levels rise because the body
  doesn't respond properly to insulin. Regular exercise
  helps to prevent insulin resistance and reduces the risk
  of developing diabetes. If you already have diabetes,
  exercise will help to control it.

- *Giving up smoking*
  Several studies have indicated that a regular exercise
  programme helps smokers to quit.

- *Improved mobility*
  Keeping fit is good for all of us but maintaining the
  mobility of muscles and joints is especially helpful for
  older people.

- *Stronger bones*
  Exercise can help to protect bones against osteoporosis –
  the brittle bone disorder that causes fractures in so many
  post-menopausal women.

- *Reduced stress*
  Exercise is a good stress reliever.

- *Improved sleep*
  Vigorous physical activity can help to promote sound
  sleep (but you should avoid exercise just before bedtime
  or it may have the opposite effect).

- *Feeling good*
  Getting physically fit can increase your vitality and sense
  of wellbeing, and help you to work more efficiently.

Running the risk

You may remember Jim Fixx, the American jogging enthusiast who dropped dead while doing his daily run. So, what are the risks of running and other forms of vigorous exercise?

An investigation by Siscovick and colleagues in Seattle, Washington, was reported in the *New England Journal of Medicine* in 1984. The researchers interviewed the wives of 133 men (aged 25–75) who had suffered a cardiac arrest (which means that the heart suddenly stopped beating). They recorded what the men had been doing at the time of the cardiac arrest and their normal pattern of vigorous exercise. Exercise patterns in the community were established by interviewing the wives of a random sample of healthy men.

The conclusions were alarming. Men who were normally inactive were over 50 times more likely to die during vigorous exercise than at other times. The men who took regular exercise were also at increased risk while exercising but for them the risk of dying during exercise was only five times greater than at other times. Perhaps you think that exercise sounds pretty dangerous even for the man who takes it regularly, but the overall risk for the active men in the study was only 40% of that for the inactive ones.

The message is clear. Vigorous exercise is dangerous for middle-aged and older men who aren't used to it. No doubt the same goes for women. Of course, if you never take any vigorous exercise at all, your risk of dying during vigorous exercise is zero. Indeed, it is safer not to take any exercise than to surprise the body occasionally with a burst of vigorous activity. This is especially dangerous when there is added stress; it's just not worth running for that bus unless you are used to running.

The balance of risks is firmly in favour of taking regular exercise. In other words, your risk of heart disease and sudden death is substantially reduced by regular exercise – as long as you take sensible precautions.

What precautions should I take?

Take it gradually

This is particularly important if you are over 40. Walking is a good way to start if you have not been exercising. Gradually increase the distance and pace. If you want to progress to jogging, start with one-minute jogs, followed by a few minutes of walking. If you use an exercise bike, start on an easy setting and be content with a few minutes at first.

Take it easy
Your exercise session should make you puff and pant a *little*, but you should not get so breathless that you are unable to carry on a normal conversation.

Take notice of your body
If it hurts, don't do it. When your body gives warning signals, slow down or stop. Particularly if you have any chest pain, nausea, palpitations or dizziness, ease off. In fact, Jim Fixx was suffering from coronary heart disease and had been ignoring warning symptoms.

Take time to warm-up and cool-down
Starting your exercise slowly and gently allows muscles to become more flexible and less liable to injury. Cool-down by reducing your exercise intensity for some minutes before stopping. It's as simple as walking around after running or pedalling slowly on your exercise bike. This gives your circulation time to readjust after sending extra blood to working muscles.

Take your pulse
Your heart rate can tell you whether you are exercising too hard for safety or not hard enough to get fit. You should aim to keep your heart rate in the target range for your age once you have warmed-up. The cool-down will allow your heart to settle gradually towards its normal rate.

You can feel your radial pulse on the thumb side of your wrist. Alternatively, the carotid pulse is easily felt by pushing the index and middle finger of one hand gently into the neck beside the larynx (voice box). If you count the number of beats in 10 seconds and multiply by six, it will tell you the number of beats per minute (Figure 10).

Your 'maximum heart rate' is calculated by subtracting your age from 220:

Maximum heart rate = 220 – age.

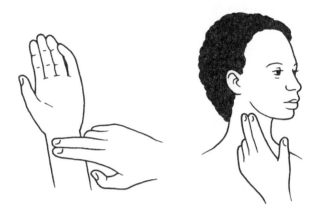

Figure 10 Taking your pulse at the wrist and the neck.

For example, if you are 40 years old, your maximum heart rate is 180 beats per minute. Your target heart rate for exercise is 70% of this (126) and the target range is 65–75% of the maximum heart rate (117–135). I am sure you will have no difficulty following this example to calculate your own target range but Table 19 gives you an indication.

Table 19 Target heart rate for exercise

Age (years)	Target range (beats/min) 65–75% max. rate
20	130–150
30	123–142
40	117–135
50	110–127
60	104–120
70+	97–112

If you are very unfit, you will get your heart rate into the target range just by walking. Having said that, remember that if you are just starting an exercise programme, there is no hurry to get up to the target range. It is more important to ease yourself in gently. Don't go above your range.

For those who like gadgets and have money to spare, an electronic heart rate monitor could be a good investment. This saves inter-

rupting your exercise session to feel your pulse, and can be programmed to tell you whenever you go outside your target range.

Take plenty of fluids

Doctors are always telling people to drink plenty of fluids – to
which you would be entitled to reply, "What else would I drink?"
Of course, to a physicist or chemist, a fluid is a liquid or a gas; but
we are definitely talking about liquid here. In fact, water is hard to
beat. You can lose an awful lot of fluid (including water vapour
from your lungs) during half an hour of exercise. Drink plenty of
water before, after and, if necessary, during exercise. This is even
more important in hot weather.

Take your doctor's advice if you have a medical problem

Any exercise video will tell you to see your doctor before doing the
exercises. That lets the video company off the hook if you do yourself in. Of course, doctors would be overwhelmed if everyone went
for a check-up before doing any exercise. Everyone should take
exercise of some sort and you're more likely to need medical attention
if you don't.

If you have a medical problem – such as asthma, bronchitis,
emphysema, high blood pressure, heart disease, back pain or
arthritis – the right exercise will be positively helpful but it's wise
to check whether your doctor has any specific advice for you.

Take the right equipment

I suppose this is obvious if you exercise by rock climbing, but even
for walking you need a decent pair of shoes. It is particularly
important to have good exercise shoes to cushion the impact for
activities like jogging and step aerobics.

Take a couple of hours to digest your lunch

By all means take exercise shortly before meals; this can take the
edge off your appetite and help you to avoid overeating. Don't take
vigorous exercise straight after meals. Extra blood is diverted to the
gut for digestion and your heart won't welcome the increased
demands of exercise.

Take a break if you're unwell

Don't undertake energetic exercise if you have a fever or flu-like illness. Your heart will already be working harder as a result of the fever and some viruses affect the heart muscle.

If you have to take a break for more than a week, remember to ease yourself in gradually when you start exercising again.

Well, if that's about as much as you can take, why not take five?

Take heart

Although it is wise to take all these sensible precautions, we must return to the fact that the risks of not exercising are much greater than the risks of taking regular vigorous exercise. Occasionally, someone dies of a heart attack while jogging; but he might have died ten years earlier without exercise. And think of all the people who die while lying in bed: nobody seems concerned that that's dangerous (although it is if you do it for days on end).

Death during recreational exercise is very uncommon. It has been estimated to account for 4.46 deaths per 100,000 of the male population per year in Rhode Island. Most of these deaths are due to coronary heart disease and, of course, this book is all about preventing that.

How much exercise do I need?

This apparently simple question has generated much debate among researchers. Does the exercise have to reach a particular intensity before it does any good? Or can you make up for low intensity by doing it for longer? What's the minimum you can get away with?

I mentioned that heavy work, in Dr Paffenbarger's study of San Francisco dock workers, was defined as using more than 8500 calories a week at work. Well, you would need to walk or run over 85 miles (137 km) a week to burn up all those calories. Could you fit that into your leisure time? Don't worry. Other studies have shown much more realistic schedules to be beneficial.

Your aim should be to get fit and stay fit. By doing this, you will significantly reduce your risk of coronary heart disease.

Two scientists (Wenger and Bell) tested a range of different exercise programmes to see how good they were at getting people fit. The programmes differed according to the intensity, frequency and duration (in minutes) of the exercise sessions, and the length (in weeks) of the programme. Monitoring the heart rate (as described above) is a simple means of measuring intensity. Their findings suggest that there is steadily increasing benefit as the schedule is stepped up as follows:

Frequency   2–4 times a week

Duration   15–45 minutes

Length   5–11 weeks

ACTION POINTS

◆ Take 20–30 minutes exercise a day (e.g. brisk walking)

◆ Always increase exercise time and intensity *gradually*

◆ Don't get too breathless to carry on a conversation

◆ Stop exercising if you get pain, nausea, dizziness or palpitations

◆ Stay within your target range

◆ Warm-up and cool-down

◆ Drink plenty of water

◆ Don't take vigorous exercise straight after a meal

◆ Avoid strenuous exercise while you're unwell

Does a half-hearted effort do any good?

Wenger and Bell found that the intensity of the exercise had to be at least 50% of the individual's maximum capacity to provide effective fitness training. As long as this minimum intensity is reached, it looks as though you can make up for a lower intensity of aerobic exercise by doing it for longer.

A sensible aim would be to spend half an hour a day, on six days of the week, on an activity that gets your heart rate into your target range. Apart from all the benefits of being fit, you would cut your risk of heart disease in half – and that's nothing to be half-hearted about!

What sort of exercise should I do?

You should do some form of *aerobic exercise* that you can keep up for at least 20 minutes without stopping. Aerobic exercise is any activity in which the large muscles in the arms and legs are moving rhythmically; the muscles use more oxygen so you have to breathe more frequently and deeply to get extra oxygen into the blood; the heart works harder to increase the delivery of oxygenated blood to the muscles.

'Anaerobic' exercise refers to 'static' or 'isometric' muscular effort: instead of moving rhythmically, the muscles strain against resistance. Examples are weight-lifting and tug of war. This sort of exercise can increase muscle strength but is no help to you in the prevention of coronary heart disease. It should never be done instead of aerobic exercise but is an optional extra for fit people. Those who already have coronary heart disease should avoid anaerobic exercise.

Exercise your choice

There is a wide range of aerobic activities for you to choose from. Here are some examples.

- Walking
- Running/jogging/running on the spot
- Climbing stairs
- 'Aerobics' and 'step aerobics'
- Cycling/using a stationary exercise bike
- Swimming
- Rowing
- Dancing
- Tennis/squash/soccer/rugby football/basketball, etc.
- Skating
- Skiing

To be effective, your aerobic exercise needs to be done several times a week and kept up. It clearly helps if you enjoy it but it also needs to fit into your daily routine. There aren't many people in a position to go skiing that often.

Swimming is excellent if you can do it; drowning is not helpful. It's never too late to learn. A supervised swimming pool is, of course, safer than rivers, lakes or the sea. Because of the support provided by the water, swimming is particularly useful for people with problems such as back pain, arthritis or obesity. It's a great family activity too. Mind you, unless you have your own swimming pool, you need to be well organised to go often enough to make this your main form of exercise.

Dancing could be anything from a slow waltz to an all-night party. Ballroom dancing can provide useful exercise, especially for older people; unless you are very unfit, you will need something more vigorous than a waltz to stretch your cardiovascular system. I used to like disco dancing but would rarely be seen at a club these days. I will confess, strictly in confidence, that I enjoy dancing to disco music in the privacy of my own home – often using a step to increase the intensity.

Music certainly makes any repetitive movement more fun. Avoiding monotony in your exercise routine is more than half the battle. For some people an aerobics class is the answer. Others, like me, prefer to strut their stuff away from the public gaze. There's no shortage of workout videos; my wife seems to have most of them. To be fair, she uses them. I've no objection to watching American fitness guru Kathy Smith in her leotard, but I prefer a less structured workout. Do what suits you.

Sex? Yes, even sexual intercourse is exercise. But remember: you're aiming for at least 20 minutes of rhythmic activity. In fact, the average union of a married couple is considered equivalent to no more than climbing two flights of stairs. That won't satisfy the heart.

Squash is not a game for the unfit. Once the competitive spirit takes over, you don't realise how hard you're pushing yourself. An investigation into 60 sudden deaths connected with squash playing, reported in the *British Heart Journal* in 1986, showed that coronary heart disease was the certified cause of death in 51 cases. You may have been a superb squash player in your youth but fitness has a short shelf life; by the time your racquet has collected dust gradual retraining is due.

Fit in 30 minutes a day?

So, having chosen my aerobic exercise, I could get fit in 30 minutes a day; but how can I fit in 30 minutes a day? Days are too short.

This can be a real problem. Usually, though, once you've decided that exercise is important to you, you can work out ways of fitting it into your schedule.

In the first edition I explained how I would get home from work in the evening, put the kettle on, and pedal the exercise bike for 20 minutes or so while watching TV. Well, since then we've invested in a high-quality treadmill and I've changed my routine. I get up earlier and do over 30 minutes' brisk walking on the treadmill (watching early morning TV) before having my shower. I find it easier to keep going energetically for half an hour on the treadmill than on the exercise bike. This routine works better for me because I can keep to it seven days a week (and still get up later at weekends).

Sometimes I use the exercise bike as well, doing intermittent upper body exercises while pedalling. (Yes, I can ride my exercise bike 'no hands'.) I'm under no illusion: this routine won't turn me into an athlete; but, so far, it's been enough to keep me alive.

Do you remember the study by Wenger and Bell that showed increasing benefit as the frequency and duration of exercise were stepped up? Aim for half an hour a day; if you can do more, so much the better – 20 minutes three times a week is the bare minimum.

Now it may suit you better to do your exercise in the evening. Or perhaps you have exercise facilities at work and you can go in your lunch hour. If you stay in hotels a lot, there may be a gym or swimming pool but you can always dance, skip or run on the spot in the privacy of your room. The important thing is to find a formula that suits you. If you choose something that is extremely inconvenient or unpleasant, there is very little chance that you will keep it up. That's pointless.

If you stick to your routine, your brain will assist by producing morphine-like hormones (endorphins), which can help to get you hooked on exercise. There are a few people for whom exercise has become the sole purpose of their existence, resulting in social dysfunction. I'm not advocating that!

In addition to my exercise bike routine, I try to snatch a few minutes of activity here and there throughout the day. After all, our bodies are designed to move but modern technology – which provides us with cars, escalators, washing machines and remote controls – spares us (or denies us) activity at every turn. There are lots of ways that you can put some movement back into your life. Here are some of them.

- Use stairs instead of lifts and escalators. If you must use an escalator, walk as well.

- If it's not far, forget the car.

- When you do use the car, park and stride: park well away from your destination (which is often easier) and walk the rest.

- When you use public transport, ride and stride: get off a stop earlier, or forget the taxi from the station.

- Go to work on your legs, not on an egg. (Sorry if I've baffled younger readers.) Walk to work if you can.

- Buy a large dog and train it to throw sticks for you.

- If you have children, prise them away from the TV or computer and play energetic games with them. Children, too, are suffering the consequences of inactivity these days.

I won't suggest that you do all your washing by hand or generate your electricity with a treadmill; but you can use your ingenuity to put technology in its place. It is an irony that technology contrives to spare us our every move with no end of labour-saving schemes, yet bids to save us from decaying through disuse with high-tech exercise machines.

Exercise is easy: you can walk it

Unlike me, you may be able to get all the vigorous activity you need without any exercise machines. (As well as the bike and treadmill, we have a huge 'multi-gym' at home; you wouldn't believe the exercise I get dismantling it and humping it around every time we move house.)

Brisk walking is hard to beat. Although many of us have forgotten this, it can actually be used as a means of transport. Make sure you have

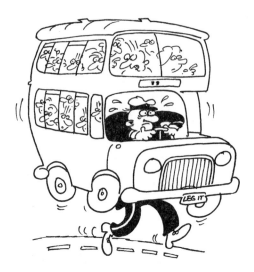

You can use your ingenuity to put technology in its place.

good, comfortable shoes. Aim for a speed of four miles per hour (6.4 km/h) if you are able-bodied. Start at a very gentle pace if you are unfit and gradually increase the Frequency, Intensity and Time of your walks until you are **FIT**.

How can you tell how fit you are? Well, for a start, if you haven't been physically active in your job or your leisure time, you can confidently say you are unfit without doing any sort of exercise test. On the other hand, if you are a keen athlete doing regular training, you will be fit and no doubt have a slow resting heart rate to confirm it. A 'normal' resting heart rate is around 72 beats per minute; very fit people may have a rate below 50 beats per minute. (If you have a resting pulse of 40 beats per minute but get tired walking from the kitchen to the lounge, your slow pulse is unlikely to mean you are fit; it's more likely you have 'heart block' and might benefit from a pacemaker. See your doctor!)

There are various standardised exercise tests designed to measure your fitness level. For example, the Canadian Home Fitness Test involves stepping up and down two 10 cm (4 in) steps at a speed that depends on your age. Either a metronome or a pre-recorded audiotape giving one beat per step is used to set the pace. The pulse is taken after three minutes and very unfit people have to stop then; others continue for a further three minutes and the fitness rating depends on the pulse at that stage.

Most readers attempting this would probably have to make do with steps of the wrong height and, without an age-appropriate pre-recorded tape, it would be impossible to get the speed right. These factors would completely invalidate it as a standardised fitness test and I think it would be positively unhelpful to provide you with a score table.

What you can do, though, is to document your improvement as you train. Using any steps that you have at home (such as the bottom two stairs or a proper aerobics step) and stepping up and down at a fixed rate (such as the beat of a particular piece of music) you can take your pulse after three and six minutes. As always, stop if you have any warning symptoms, become too breathless to converse, or find your pulse above your target range after three minutes. As long as you keep the conditions exactly the same on each occasion, you can make a valid comparison of your fitness level at different times. As you train, your resting pulse – and your pulse after a standard amount of exercise – will slow down.

Yes, getting fit and staying fit can be a walkover. Learn complicated exercises and sports physiology if you wish, but all you need to *learn by heart* is your *target range*. No matter what your walk of life, if you can include 30 minutes of brisk walking in your daily routine, you'll soon be there.

ACTION POINTS

◆ Choose an enjoyable aerobic exercise that fits into your daily routine

◆ Use stairs, not lifts and escalators

◆ Use legs more and wheels less

Chapter 20

Smoking

'A custom loathsome to the eye, hateful to the nose, harmful to the brain, dangerous to the lungs, and in the black, stinking fume thereof, nearest resembling the horrible Stygian smoke of the pit that is bottomless.'

James I (James VI of Scotland) (1566–1625)
A Counterblast to Tobacco, 1604

Like the 'wisest fool in Christendom', as James I was dubbed, most people realise that smoking is bad for you. Few understand how bad.

◆ Everybody knows smoking is bad for you; few understand how bad

◆ Smokers have more heart disease, artery damage, strokes, cancer, bronchitis, emphysema, osteoporosis and wrinkles

◆ Smoking in pregnancy harms the baby

◆ Smoking doesn't just increase risk; it is always harmful

◆ Pipe smoking is a bit less dangerous than cigarette smoking – but only if you've never been a cigarette smoker

---

Smoke alarmism?

If you are a smoker, you may feel persecuted. Non-smokers, like me, constantly bemoaning the social evils of the weed make it ever harder to have a relaxing cigarette in public without sensing the icy glare of someone's disapproval. We fill people's heads with the notion that even passive smoking is more dangerous than bungee jumping. In pursuit of our moral crusade, you tell yourself, we dramatise the dangers of this time-honoured pleasure.

After all, it was back in the sixteenth century that Sir Walter Raleigh came across those fine flowering plants from the genus Nicotiana. What was anyone supposed to do with a find like that? Isn't it only sensible to take a bunch of the dried leaves, roll it in a piece of paper, stick it in your mouth, and set fire to it – then inhale the smoke?

The truth is that, with approximately 4000 different chemicals now identified in that smoke, it would be a hard job to exaggerate the ill effects of smoking. They are so far-reaching. Here are a few facts:

- About 100,000 deaths in Britain each year are related to smoking.

- Approximately half of these 100,000 deaths are caused by damaged arteries.

- Smokers are much more likely to die of a heart attack than non-smokers. The more you smoke, the bigger the risk. The British Doctors Study included an interesting comparison of men in different age groups who smoked 25 or more cigarettes a day:
  (a) the under-45s were **15** times more likely to die of a heart attack than non-smokers in that age group;
  (b) those aged 45–54 had treble the risk, and those aged 55–64 had double the risk of non-smokers in their age band.

- At first glance, it might look as though smoking gets safer as you get older but this is not the case! Heart attacks are far more frequent in the older age groups anyway. Remember that risk factors multiply: raised blood pressure or high cholesterol are much bigger hazards in a smoker.

- Smokers are more likely to have a stroke.

- The death rate from aortic aneurysm (weakness in the wall of the body's main artery, which can result in fatal haemorrhage) is ten times higher in men smoking more than 25 cigarettes a day than in non-smokers.

- Blockage to arteries in the legs leading to pain, and even gangrene and amputation, is not an uncommon problem – but it rarely arises in those who have never been smokers.

- Women over 35 taking the oral contraceptive pill have a very low risk of suffering a heart attack or stroke – unless they smoke!

- Like heart disease, cancer (of which there are many types) is a major killer. Lung cancer is one of the commonest forms and is caused by smoking; it's very rare in non-smokers.

- Apart from lung cancer, smoking is to blame for many other cancers as well. Cancers of the lips, mouth, throat, larynx (voice box), oesophagus (gullet), bladder, kidney, and pancreas are all more common in smokers.

- Chronic bronchitis and emphysema – serious lung diseases that can lead to sufferers fighting for breath – are caused by smoking in the great majority of cases.

- Smoking in pregnancy is extremely harmful; it results in a smaller baby with a reduced chance of survival.

- Osteoporosis, in which the bones become brittle, is made worse by smoking. A study published in the *British Medical Journal* in 1997 concluded that women who continued to smoke after the menopause were more likely to break their hips; by the age of 80, the risk was 71% higher in smokers.

- Digestive problems in smokers range from reduced ability to smell and taste food through to difficulty healing duodenal ulcers.

- Wrinkles are an outward sign of the accelerated ageing processes throughout a smoker's body. In fact, 'smokers face' has been described in the *British Medical Journal*; it features increased wrinkling and wasting of the skin together with grey discoloration.

Are you putting up a smoke screen?

Sometimes smokers say they enjoy smoking and don't want to stop. After all, this sounds better than admitting that you can't stop. Unfortunately, when you hide behind a smoke screen, you end up fooling yourself.

There are lots of other arguments that smokers put forward in the hope of convincing others, and themselves, that it's reasonable to continue smoking.

Any smoker will draw comfort from the sprightly 85-year-old who smokes 20 a day and still outwalks his old dog on the way to the pub. No wonder this exceptional example is imprinted on the memory and invoked whenever the hazards of smoking are raised. It's far more comfortable, of course, to forget all those who died in their fifties or spend the last miserable year of life attached to an oxygen cylinder. I would like to make two additional observations: (a) this fortunate pensioner would have been fitter still without cigarettes – perhaps running the marathon, and (b) the dog has very little incentive to get to the pub.

Understandably, many smokers are concerned that they will put on weight if they stop smoking. A small weight gain may occur initially (both because of a change in metabolism and because some people eat more). Weight gain is certainly not inevitable, even though you may find food tastier and more enjoyable as a non-smoker; following the advice in this book will allow you to control your weight – permanently. But to suggest that you might as well keep smoking rather than put on weight is complete nonsense. You'd have to gain about ten stone before it started to match the risk of smoking 20 a day!

Then there's the argument that says: "I might be knocked over by a car tomorrow, so why worry about the dangers of smoking?" Of course, it's true that any of us could be killed on the roads but, as a smoker, it's overwhelmingly more likely that your death will be caused by smoking; you may even combine the two spectacularly and have a heart attack while driving.

This idea that smoking is a risk but it's a gamble you're prepared to take is another piece of self-deception. Smoking is often depicted as a game of Russian roulette: if you're unlucky you get lung cancer, but, if fate smiles on you, you get off scot-free. Rubbish. The smoker always incurs a penalty; damaged health is a certainty.

We cannot predict which smokers will die before the age of 60 from a heart attack or a stroke or cancer. But you don't need a crystal ball to see that any smoker's body would function better if it weren't being poisoned.

It's an unfortunate fact that many people do give up smoking – after they've had a heart attack. Many others don't get the chance to think again at that stage. Bismarck wisely said, "Only a fool learns from his experience: I learn from the experience of others."

The age of innocence

I have every sympathy with older folk who took up smoking at a time when the dangers weren't appreciated. Although James I had made an accurate assessment almost 350 years earlier, it wasn't until about 1950 that science made the connection between smoking and lung cancer. Since then, so much more has been learnt about the deadly path that smokers are on. What a tragedy that young people still flock like lemmings to join them!

"I never smoked a cigarette until I was nine," protested W.C. Fields, apparently.

Children, of course, will always experiment. I cannot have been more than nine myself when I acquired a plastic pipe from a Jamboree Bag and thought what fun it would be to smoke tea leaves in it. I only tried it the once. Young people often find their first cigarette unpleasant, but peer group pressure ensures they persist until they've mastered the weed – or rather, it's mastered them.

Meanwhile, the cigarette makers hide behind platitudes about the individual's right to choose. They shield themselves with spin-doctors (medically qualified in some cases) employed to conceal or confuse the conclusions of research. This smouldering fuse is running out: surely manufacturers are soon to be smoked out to face an army of the aggrieved, all making claims for compensation.

To the young, though, middle age and ill health seem remote. If you tell a teenaged girl that smoking will kill her, she'll probably laugh a lungful of smoke in your face; but if her boyfriend tells her he'd rather kiss an ashtray, that'll get her worried.

Don't the young and impressionable deserve protection from the greedy – from those who glamorise this ghastly deathtrap? Why would legislators hesitate?

'This vice brings in one hundred million francs in taxes
every year. I will certainly forbid it at once – as soon as you
can name a virtue that brings in as much revenue.'

Napoleon III (1808–73). French emperor

Just a pipe dream?

If you've been smoking cigarettes for years, becoming a non-smoker may seem an unrealistic aim. Perhaps you've thought about changing to a pipe to reduce your risks. It is true that pipe and cigar smokers who have never smoked cigarettes have a lower risk of heart disease than cigarette smokers. That's because those who've always smoked cigars or a pipe usually don't inhale the smoke; not surprisingly, they still have high rates of mouth cancer.

Perhaps you've already made the change from cigarettes to a pipe and now congratulate yourself on doing what you could to help your heart. Unfortunately, pipe smokers who've switched from cigarettes continue to inhale. And a scientific paper on the risks of 'secondary pipe smoking' would give you no comfort at all. Put that in your pipe and smoke it.

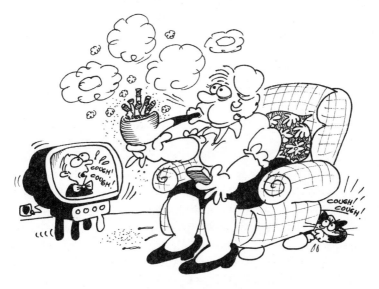

Changing to a pipe is not the answer.

The big smoke

Whatever you choose to put in your pipe – and even urban atmospheric pollution – will be hard-pressed to beat the range of toxins released by burning tobacco. Of course, I don't really recommend changing to a different fuel; at least the tobacco smoker has the benefit of intensive research into the diseases he is inducing.

The 4000 or so different chemicals in tobacco smoke include minute quantities of well-known poisons such as arsenic and DDT. **Free radicals** speed up ageing processes (such as thinning and wrinkling of the skin) as well as damaging the lining of arteries and triggering production of cancer cells. Quite a number of **carcinogens** (cancer-producing substances) have been identified in tobacco smoke, not to mention the many chemicals with unknown effects.

Some ingredients of the smoke act as **irritants** in the lung, provoking increased mucus production and paralysing the lungs' self-cleaning mechanism. Other chemicals are absorbed into the bloodstream and carried all round the body. Two of these – **nicotine** and **carbon monoxide** – are known to be particularly important.

Nicotine is a poison that can be used as an insecticide. Equally, it could be used for homicide but you'd need to administer a smoker's total daily dose as a single shot. (People are bigger than insects.) Nicotine reaches the brain within a few seconds of inhaling tobacco smoke and is largely to blame for a smoker's dependence on cigarettes. Nicotine also has damaging effects on the heart and circulation. It constricts blood vessels, including the coronary arteries that supply the heart, and at the same time stimulates adrenaline, which makes the heart work harder. Blood pressure rises, and irregularities of the heart rhythm may be provoked.

Carbon monoxide, of course, is the silent killer that strikes when the flue on a domestic gas appliance malfunctions; people just wake up dead. It is now removed from car exhaust fumes, which are no longer used for suicide (except in soap operas). No doubt it plays a key role in the deaths of millions of smokers. Oxygen is carried round our bodies by the red pigment in blood called haemoglobin. Carbon monoxide can combine with haemoglobin more easily than oxygen can (to form carboxyhaemoglobin). As a result, the blood is able to carry less oxygen to organs such as the heart and brain.

The combined effects of nicotine and carbon monoxide increase the heart's requirement for oxygen while reducing the supply. In addition, the clogging of arteries with fatty deposits is accelerated and (because of effects on platelets and fibrinogen) the blood clots more easily. It would be difficult to design a drug that paved the way for a heart attack more efficiently.

Do unto others . . .

Roy Castle, the much-loved entertainer, died of lung cancer. He was not a smoker. During his years in show business, he'd been subjected to an awful lot of smoke from other people (especially in smoky clubs).

'Passive smoking', or involuntary smoking, is dangerous. A Japanese study published in the *British Medical Journal* in 1981 showed that the non-smoking wives of heavy smokers had an increased risk of lung cancer. Since then, many research teams have confirmed the higher rate of lung cancer in non-smokers living with smokers. An analysis of 37 published studies was reported in the *British Medical Journal* in October 1997. The conclusion was that living with a smoker increases a non-smoker's risk of lung cancer by 26%. In addition, cancer-producing substances from tobacco can be found in the blood and urine of these involuntary smokers.

Coronary heart disease, too, is commoner in passive smokers. It is true that there is more nicotine and carbon monoxide in the 'sidestream' smoke (which comes off the end of the cigarette) than in the 'mainstream' smoke (which is drawn through the cigarette by the smoker). Even so, the extent of the risk to non-smokers has been an unwelcome surprise.

The evidence from 19 published studies of heart disease risk in lifelong non-smokers who live with a smoker was analysed in the *British Medical Journal* in 1997. The risk of coronary heart disease in these involuntary smokers was 30% higher than the risk in non-smokers who did not live with a smoker. Some of this extra risk (about 6%) results from the fact that non-smokers in smoking households eat poorer diets, with less fruit and vegetable. The increased risk of heart disease *caused* by passive smoking is about 23%. The percentage rise in risk is very similar to that found for lung cancer; but the number of extra deaths from heart disease will be far greater because heart disease is so much more common. One estimate blames passive smoking for 62,000 heart disease deaths a year in the USA.

Despite the inevitable bleating of the tobacco industry, the dangers of environmental tobacco smoke are established beyond doubt. Employers have a clear duty to provide a safe working environment for their employees. They can either ban smoking in the workplace or provide properly separated (and ventilated) smoking facilities. Not only is it cheaper to go for a total ban, it is kinder to smokers in the long run. Smoking in designated areas, densely filled with smoke, can only add to the dangers. And some people have found it easier to stop smoking altogether after a ban at work. Dangers aside, most non-smokers find it very unpleasant, or even disgusting, to breathe in second-hand tobacco smoke. When asked if he minded if someone smoked in the non-smoking compartment, Sir Thomas Beecham, the English conductor, replied, "Certainly not – if you don't object if I'm sick."

Smoking parents put their children at risk. Smokers' children are more likely to suffer sudden infant death syndrome ('cot death'), respiratory infections, asthma attacks and middle ear problems. Children with a smoking parent are also more likely to become smokers themselves.

◆ The 4000 chemicals in cigarette smoke include nicotine, carbon monoxide, free radicals and substances that cause cancer

◆ Living with a smoker increases a non-smoker's risk of lung cancer by 26%, and of heart disease by 30%

◆ It has been estimated that passive smoking causes 62,000 deaths from heart disease every year in the USA

◆ Smokers' children suffer more asthma attacks, respiratory infections, ear problems and cot deaths; they are more likely to become smokers

---

Is it too late to stop?

No. It's never too late to give up smoking. Perhaps you think the damage has already been done and, yes, if you've been smoking for years, a lot of damage has been done. But a lot can be undone. In the British Doctors Study, the increased heart disease risk from smoking was cut in half in the first two or three years after stopping; after 10 years the risk had returned to that of a non-smoker! Some benefit is immediate. For a start, you'll be supplying the blood with oxygen instead of carbon monoxide. And the increased risk of blood clots is soon reversed.

If you have already developed chronic bronchitis or emphysema, you can't undo the lung damage; but it is essential to stop smoking immediately or you will go downhill fast.

Smokers who already have coronary heart disease have everything to gain by giving up (cigarettes, I mean, not the will to live). If you have already had a heart attack, you are much less likely to have another one if you stop smoking.

Kicking the habit

If you are a smoker, and in your right mind, you want to kick the habit before you kick the bucket. Most smokers would like to stop. But it's not that easy, is it? Millions have done it, though, and there's no reason why you shouldn't join them.

Here is a plan that can help you do just that. This approach has already helped thousands to become successful ex-smokers.

Ready . . .
So, you're ready to stop smoking. Congratulations. Realising that smoking is bad for you and deciding that you'd like to stop just won't do. You must decide that you are *going to stop* and that you are ready to do it now.

Steady . . .
Hold it right there. Don't throw away your cigarettes just yet. I know. Once you've made the decision to stop, you want to get on with it right away, before you change your mind. If you prepare yourself properly before you stop, you are much more likely to succeed.

Fix the date when you will become a non-smoker – one or two weeks ahead. It could be an ordinary working day or at a weekend. Don't choose a day when you will be under extra pressure.

Tell people about your decision, especially friends who don't smoke; they can be a great support. The more people you tell, the more committed you will feel. If a friend or colleague wants to give up with you, so much the better. A smoking partner will make life much more difficult for you and it really is ideal to give up together. Joining – or even setting up – a self-help group and working through this programme with others is often more successful than going it alone.

Make a list of all the benefits you will enjoy as a non-smoker. Put it on your dressing table or by your dentures or wherever else you can read through it every day. This should be your own personal list but it might include any of these:

- I will age less quickly – inside and out;
- I will be putting oxygen into my blood, instead of carbon monoxide;
- I will feel generally more healthy;
- I will be better at sport;
- I will reduce my risk of heart disease, cancer, stroke, bronchitis and emphysema;
- I won't have bad breath, yellow fingers, smelly hair and smelly clothes;
- I will have less trouble with catarrh, coughs, and chest infections;
- I will be able to smell and taste my food better;
- I will have more money to spend on other things;
- I will no longer be a nuisance and a health hazard to others;
- I will not damage my unborn child;
- I will not provoke asthma attacks, catarrh and ear infections in my children;
- I will no longer be encouraging my children to smoke;
- I will be more attractive;
- I will feel more in control.

Keep a 'smoking diary' – a record of every cigarette you smoke – for one week before you stop. This can be either a little notebook or simply a piece of paper but it must be kept with your cigarettes.

It is helpful to make out a chart for each day (Figure 11). Whenever you reach for a cigarette, simply note the time, what you are doing, who you are with, and how much you feel you need that cigarette. Complete this before you smoke the cigarette.

No.	Time	Activity	Who with?	Need? (+,++ or +++)

Figure 11 A smoking diary. Keep a record of every cigarette for a week before you stop.

It will soon become clear if you smoke every time you have a coffee, or go to the pub, or meet your lover. Work out how you will avoid each of these situations when you stop smoking. Rating the importance of every cigarette shows you where you will need to be extra careful.

Try to analyse why you have smoked each cigarette. Is lighting up a pure habit – something you do automatically? Or is there a real craving, which starts soon after the last cigarette? Perhaps tension is a trigger and you use cigarettes as a way of trying to calm yourself down.

During this week or two of preparation, you can start cutting out the cigarettes that are easy to avoid. I'm not recommending cutting down as a way of giving up; it usually fails. After all, you are going to become a non-smoker on the chosen date. In the meantime, when you are offered cigarettes, you can practise refusing and explaining what you are doing. Anyone who teases you or tries to force cigarettes on you is someone to avoid. You may find it helpful to put an elastic band round your cigarette packet, possibly retaining your smoking diary, so you have to think twice before taking a cigarette.

You can collect your cigarette ends in a glass jar (but make sure the marmalade is finished). Each evening hold the jar, have a good smell, meditate on the disgusting contents, and rejoice that you will soon be rid of all this.

Stop!

When your chosen day arrives, your waking thought will no doubt be "What's that strange bleeping noise?" Once you've realised that it's the alarm clock, and it really is time to get up, your next thought should be "I'm a non-smoker now!" Yes, this is your first day as a non-smoker. Of course, that's not strictly true: you were actually born a non-smoker. (If God had intended anything else, why would he surround us with water in the womb?) Today you will return to your natural state.

Bleary eyes permitting, read through the list of benefits you will now enjoy as a non-smoker. Have a good stretch and tell yourself that you don't need to smoke, and you don't want to.

Perhaps the postman will bring you some cards from supportive friends, congratulating you on becoming a non-smoker or, at least, from yourself, if you were thoughtful enough to post some the day before.

You must now live as a non-smoker. Rid your house or flat of cigarettes, lighters and ashtrays. Ask other people not to smoke in your home.

If you get a strong craving for a cigarette, don't worry. That intense feeling won't last very long. Go and get a glass of water or a raw carrot, or mow the lawn, or take the tortoise for a walk. Take a long, deep breath and think of all the lovely oxygen you're getting into your lungs; breathe out slowly and dwell on the deadly carbon monoxide you're getting rid of. Repeat the deep breathing until the craving has passed.

You are expecting some withdrawal symptoms; you know that your body has got used to a regular supply of nicotine. Cravings, irritability, headaches and sleep disturbance are all common but settle as the body readjusts itself over a couple of weeks. Some people don't notice any withdrawal symptoms.

What about nicotine patches? Nicotine replacement therapy, with skin patches, chewing gum, nasal spray, or inhalator, can be very helpful – especially for heavy smokers with strong cravings. For many years, smokers who wanted to use these preparations had to buy them, but it is now possible to obtain them on an NHS prescription. All that nicotine patches can do is to smooth out the physical withdrawal from nicotine. Plenty of people who are determined to stop smoking sail through the nicotine withdrawal without patches. On the other hand, those who think the patches will be a simple solution often fail. Don't expect them to patch up worn-out will-power. They won't.

Zyban (bupropion) won't give up smoking for you either, but it is proving extremely helpful for some smokers who are determined to stop. It works on chemical pathways in the brain that are involved in nicotine dependence. Zyban isn't suitable for people with epilepsy, eating disorders or certain psychiatric conditions. The tablets are normally taken for two months and smoking is continued until the 'quit date' – usually the eighth day. It's essential that drug treatment is combined with some form of emotional support.

Apart from nicotine dependence, you are dealing with a habit – a behaviour that has been automatic for some years. The habit can still haunt you long after you've got through the physical withdrawal from nicotine. This is where your smoking diary comes in. Avoid activities and situations that were strongly linked with smoking.

Here are some guidelines that are particularly important in the first two weeks after you stop smoking:

- *Avoid alcohol.* You probably think this is a really rum suggestion. Your spirits need lifting more than ever, now that you're coping with nicotine withdrawal, and I suggest going without alcohol as well! The long and the short of it is that most smokers light up when they drink alcohol. Going to a smoke-filled pub is asking for trouble. Also, alcohol anaesthetises the will-power.

- *Avoid coffee and tea.* This might seem to add insult to injury, but check your smoking diary. How often do you drink tea or coffee without smoking? If you have reached for your cigarettes every time you've had a coffee, day after day, year after year, you'll be making it very hard for yourself if you keep drinking coffee while adjusting to life as a non-smoker.

- *Drink plenty!* There are lots of suitable drinks – such as water, fruit juice, diluted fruit juice, squash, and herbal tea. You must keep well hydrated.

- *Change your ways.* Use your smoking diary to avoid being trapped by routines that were strongly linked with smoking. If you would normally light up at the end of your evening meal, get up; wash up, if necessary, but don't sit there missing your cigarette. If you normally eat lunch in a canteen with smoking colleagues, go somewhere else for a while.

- *Weigh your change.* Or, at least, collect the money you would have spent on cigarettes – perhaps in a glass jar. You'll soon have enough to treat yourself to a celebratory meal out – but make sure you sit in the non-smoking section!

- *Change your weight.* Yes, if you need to lose weight, there is no reason why you shouldn't do so after giving up smoking by making sensible changes in your diet (see Chapter 17). Above all, there is no need to succumb to the weight gain that everybody fears. Have plenty of healthy snacks to hand (such as raw carrots, celery sticks, sugarsnap peas, apples) and avoid comforting yourself with sweets and biscuits. Whenever you're not sure what to do with your hands, get a glass of water.

- *Wait, you'll change!* At this stage, you may think "I can't go on like this, craving after cigarettes for months on end". But it's not like that. If you can get through one day as a non-smoker, you can get through every day. Just take one day at a time. Like Old Nick himself, nicotine holds many in bondage; but you are breaking free, and you'll soon change from being an addict to being in control.

You've given up now. Don't give up now

It was Mark Twain who pointed out that it was easy to give up smoking – and that he had done it hundreds of times.

Now you've come this far, the last thing you want is to throw it all away. There's far too much at stake. You are a non-smoker now. Here are a few filtered tips to help you stay that way:

◆ The sooner you stop smoking, the better. But it's never too late to stop

◆ In the British Doctors Study, the increased risk of heart disease in smokers had disappeared 10 years after stopping

◆ If you already have bronchitis, emphysema or heart disease, stopping is even more urgent

◆ Benefits of giving up include: ageing less quickly; feeling better; reducing the risk of cancer, heart disease, stroke and chest problems; being more attractive; tasting food better; having less catarrh; saving money

◆ If you follow this programme, you could join millions of successful ex-smokers

Avoid smoky social situations. Alcohol makes things worse by lowering your resistance. A party is a recipe for disaster. And beware the temptress, sending smoke signals across the room.

Brush up daily on your list of the benefits that are building up now you've become a non-smoker. Brush your teeth thoroughly each morning – if you have any (teeth, I mean, not mornings) – and bethink how beautifully fresh your breath is becoming.

Contracts can help to strengthen resolve when cravings or irritating symptoms such as coughing come along. Consider a contract with yourself or a colleague, confirming your commitment to remain a non-smoker, come what may. Coughing can be a nuisance when you stop smoking but don't be tempted to treat it with a cigarette! Cilia are the microscopic hairlike growths that normally keep the lungs clean but have been crippled for years by smoke. Clearance of conglomerated muck commences as the cleaning system gets to work again; coughing is a sign of recovery.

Distance yourself from smokers, now you are a non-smoker and always dine in designated non-smoking areas. Don't despise smokers, but do consider developing a discussion group for those who decide to drop the habit. Don't duck the issue, but decline cigarettes decidedly by declaring "I don't smoke" and don't dither with "Er, well, I'm trying to give them up".

Exercise regularly (but not excessively). Exacting experiments have exposed the fact that those who exercise are extra likely to remain ex-smokers.

Failure frequently follows from falling for 'just one fag' – perhaps as a reward for giving up so successfully. Five cigarettes later, all your good intentions have gone up in smoke!

Chapter 21

Blood pressure

'I do apologise for writing by hand – and so badly. I shall soon be like Helen Thomas, notoriously illegible. In her last letter only two words stood out plain: "Blood pressure". Subsequent research demonstrated that what she had actually written was "Beloved friends".'

Sylvia Townsend Warner (1893–1978), *Letter*, 21 June 1963

Friend or foe?

Could blood pressure turn out to be a beloved friend, much misunderstood, or is it, in fact, a deadly foe, which should be feared?

It is essential for the blood in our arteries to be under pressure: blood has to travel from the largest artery (the aorta), through branches of ever decreasing diameter, until it reaches blood vessels of microscopic width (capillaries). It would never make it without pressure. Just as you could never sprinkle your lawn without water pressure, so your circulation would come to a standstill without blood pressure. Water pressure must overcome the resistance of the hose, and a kink in the hose may leave much of the lawn dry; blood pressure must rise above the resistance of arteries, and narrowing of arteries by fatty deposits of atheroma calls for higher pressure to refresh the parts lower pressures cannot reach.

Now, if you have a steeply sloping garden and you run the hose from the tap at the bottom to the vegetable patch at the top, the water pressure must also overcome gravity; if it does not, your cabbages will become compost. In the same way, when we stand up, our blood pressure must overcome gravity to get blood up to the brain; if it did not, our brains would end up like those cabbages. Your blood pressure is constantly regulated by the body's intricate system of sensors and adjustment mechanisms. Without these split-second changes, the gravity of a simple manoeuvre like getting out of bed would soon become apparent; the consequences would indeed be grave.

If you are reeling at the prospect of maintaining an adequate blood flow to your brain, spare a thought for the giraffe. You won't be surprised to learn that his blood pressure is sky-high (and, if it weren't, his brain would be high and dry).

How can I tell if I've got blood pressure?

Well, of course, if you're alive then you must have blood pressure. The question is whether or not your blood pressure is too high. Some people assume their blood pressure is OK because they feel fine. Others think their blood pressure must be high because they have headaches or feel hot or get flushed. The inconvenient truth about blood pressure is that it's very discreet, or shy, or downright deceitful: it simply doesn't declare itself like that. Going red in the face might indicate all sorts of things but is often, quite wrongly, taken to be a sign of high blood pressure.

> 'I always take blushing either for a sign of guilt,
> or of ill breeding.'
> _____
>
> William Congreve (1670–1729)
> *The Way of the World*, 1700, act 1, sc. 9

You can have a very high blood pressure with no symptoms. You can have a normal blood pressure and feel terrible. The only way to find out your blood pressure is to measure it; everyone should have this done.

Perhaps it would be more convenient if we could monitor our blood pressure by the way we were feeling, but measurement of blood pressure these days is not nearly as inconvenient as it used to be. The first recorded measurement of blood pressure was carried out by an English clergyman called Stephen Hales in 1733. He connected a main artery from a horse to a vertical glass tube, using the windpipe of a goose. Blood rose to a height of eight feet three inches. I've seen some pretty antiquated surgeries in my time, but I'd be very surprised if your doctor has ever suggested doing this to you. Measuring blood pressure still involved cutting an artery right up until 1896 when Scipione Riva-Rocci introduced the arm cuff.

Nowadays, of course, checking your blood pressure couldn't be more straightforward. It's simpler than checking your cholesterol level – or even your bank balance in many cases. It's quick and cheap – and could save you, and the Health Service, a lot of trouble and expense in the future. It's painless: all you feel is a brief squeeze on the upper arm. And, at a time when the Health Service is feeling the squeeze, that seems a small price to pay.

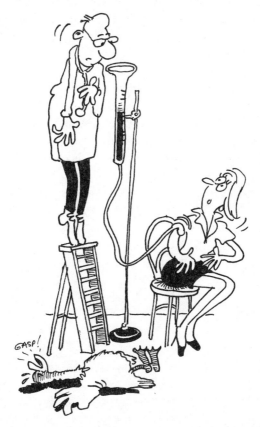

I'd be very surprised if your doctor has suggested doing this to you.

> ◆ Blood has to be under pressure in order to circulate
>
> ◆ High blood pressure increases the risk of strokes and heart attacks – the higher the pressure, the higher the risk
>
> ◆ You might feel fine with a high blood pressure or terrible with a normal blood pressure
>
> ◆ All adults should have their blood pressure checked

Measurement of blood pressure

Your blood pressure results from the pump at the heart of your circulation forcing blood through a network of narrowing arteries. Your heart is a muscular pump that squeezes blood through one-way valves with every beat. It's a thankless task. Anyone who had a heart would feel at least a wave of sympathy on reflecting that it beats about 100,000 times a day, but if it so much as rests for just a few seconds, all hell breaks loose. Imagine trying to work the muscles in your legs this way. It takes a dedicated muscle to keep going like that – for life – and the heart muscle is specially adapted to the task.

This kind of pump could not maintain a completely steady pressure. Blood pressure rises to a peak level as the heart contracts, and falls to a minimum as the heart relaxes to refill with blood. Of course, the heart's one-way valves prevent any backward flow. You can feel for yourself the surge of pressure with every heartbeat; it is felt as the pulse in one of your arteries. So your blood pressure rises

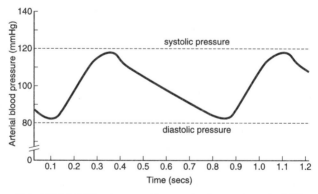

Figure 12 Arterial blood pressure. Pressure rises to a maximum (systolic) and falls to a minimum (diastolic).

and falls as a wave – constantly varying between peak and trough (Figure 12). The **squeezing** phase of the heart's cycle is called **systole**; the **downbeat** phase in which the heart relaxes and **draws** in more blood is called **diastole**.

What does all this have to do with measuring blood pressure? Everything. You can now understand why two numbers have to be noted, and why the peak pressure is called the *systolic* and the minimum pressure the *diastolic*. The instrument you see at your doctor's that is used to measure these pressures is called a *sphygmomanometer* – at least, by those who can say it (Figure 13).

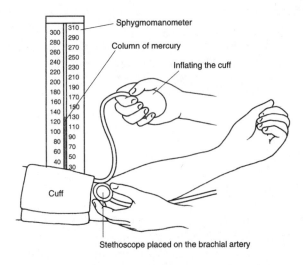

Figure 13 Getting your blood pressure checked in the surgery.

A cuff of cloth, which is wrapped around your upper arm, contains a tubular balloon that can be blown up, applying pressure to the brachial artery in your arm; this pressure is measured by the mercury column (in 'millimetres of mercury' or mmHg).

The doctor or nurse taking your blood pressure will blow up the cuff enough to squeeze the walls of the brachial artery together so that no blood flows past that point. Don't worry. The cuff is then slowly deflated – long before your arm turns black – while any noises in the artery are detected with a stethoscope. The moment the cuff pressure falls below the systolic pressure in the artery, blood will push audibly past the cuff, and the operator will note the level of the mercury column at that moment – the systolic pressure in mmHg.

As the cuff pressure is gradually reduced further, the tapping sound of blood forcing its way through the squashed artery will continue to be heard through the stethoscope. After all, as long as the cuff pressure is greater than the minimum artery pressure (the diastolic), the artery walls will be squeezed together between heartbeats – only to be forced apart again as the pressure rises in systole. The moment the cuff pressure falls below even the diastolic pressure, the artery will remain open all the time; the tapping sound of blood forcing the artery open disappears. At this point, the height of the mercury column is noted – and that gives the diastolic pressure in mmHg.

The systolic pressure reading (the high number) is written on top and the diastolic pressure reading (the low number) underneath. So, if your systolic pressure were 120 mmHg and your diastolic 80 mmHg, your blood pressure would be written down like this:

$$\text{Blood Pressure (BP)} = \frac{120}{80} \text{ mmHg}$$

Your doctor or nurse would say that your blood pressure was '120 over 80'.

Safety in numbers?

Can a couple of numbers really be so important to our health and safety? Yes, they do matter, and matter a lot.

Back in 1948, about 5000 men and women in the American town of Framingham, near Boston, Massachusetts, agreed to be examined every two years. The now famous Framingham Study has provided a lot of information over the years and has shown that higher blood pressures go with higher rates of heart disease and stroke.

An analysis of nine studies involving a total of 418,000 people was published by MacMahon and colleagues in the *Lancet* in 1990. Again, heart disease and strokes occurred more frequently among those with higher blood pressures. When people with an average diastolic pressure up at 105 mmHg were compared with those who had a diastolic of 75 mmHg, they were found to have between 10 and 12 times the risk of stroke and 5 to 6 times the risk of coronary heart disease. These two studies show beyond doubt, the importance of lowering your blood pressure if it is raised.

Which number is the important one?

Clearly, lower numbers are safer. But, bearing in mind the analysis by MacMahon and colleagues, should we just concentrate on the diastolic pressure? No. Early research on treating raised blood pressure focused on the diastolic but later studies have consistently shown that both numbers are important. In fact, systolic blood pressure is slightly better at predicting the risk of coronary heart disease and stroke.

Some people have 'isolated systolic hypertension' (ISH), in which the systolic pressure is raised but the diastolic is not. When a doctor's records say 'BP = 190/75 ISH', it probably doesn't mean that the doctor couldn't be bothered to specify exactly what the blood pressure was; ISH is a common abbreviation. Even ISH is associated with an increase of major health problems.

Choose any number

If a doctor tells you that you have 'hypertension', he means that you have high blood pressure, and not that you are a bag of nerves (although, of course, you might be after he has told you this).

But how can you say whether someone has hypertension? I mean, we all have blood pressure; it's just a question of degree. It's like height. If you were to take the shortest person in the world and the tallest, you could find people of every conceivable height in between. In just the same way, blood pressure in any group of people varies along a scale. What's more, the lower your blood pressure on that scale, the better. The risk of stroke and heart disease gradually rises as blood pressure rises. It's not as if the risk begins at a certain level of blood pressure.

Hypertension can't be a disease like, say, cancer. You either have cancer or you haven't. You can't have 'a touch of cancer'. Blood pressure's different. So, is there really such a thing as hypertension or is it just a load of hype – attention-grabbing propaganda?

There is a condition in which blood pressure is so high that swelling may occur round the optic nerve at the back of the eye, so-called 'malignant hypertension'. Before treatment for high blood pressure became available, 80% of people with this condition died within a year of diagnosis. Now that effective drugs are available, it's definitely better to be diagnosed and treated. Clearly, these people have a severe problem but, as we move down the blood pressure scale, where should we draw the line with our diagnosis of hypertension?

The late Professor Geoffrey Rose came up with a practical approach, defining hypertension as 'the level of blood pressure above which treatment does more good than harm'.

An alien concept

So, risk rises continuously up the blood pressure scale, but we choose a certain level of blood pressure and call it 'hypertension'. You may find this a difficult concept.

You could think of it this way. Returning to our height analogy, imagine that we are living on a planet plagued by low-flying alien spacecraft. I'm talking about very small aliens, piloting very small craft – no bigger than a football. When touring our planet, the aliens fly their vehicles six or seven feet above the ground. Their detection devices help them to steer clear of buildings and other obstacles but, unfortunately, they seem to have a complete blind spot where people are concerned. They are forever crashing into people's heads. The usual flight paths are over six feet above the ground and you will hardly ever see one below four feet. They travel at variable speeds but, in general, the lower they go, the slower they go.

If you are struck on the head by one of these visiting space vehicles, you might make a full recovery (as people do after a mini-stroke); this largely depends on the speed of the craft at impact. After a series of such knocks, most people will become 'punch-drunk', showing signs of permanent brain damage. On the other hand, a high-speed collision will kill you outright (like a massive stroke).

It turns out that the taller you are, the greater your risk of being struck – and struck at high speed too. Someone over six feet six inches tall will almost inevitably be dead within a year of attaining that height. But someone under five foot is unlikely to run into any trouble at all.

Imagine the only treatment we can offer (perhaps because no one has come up with the idea of a crash helmet) is an operation to shorten the legs. This surgery is unpleasant and not entirely without risk but anyone over six foot is definitely better off having the treatment. If you are just five foot four, even though you have a slightly higher risk of head injury than your five-foot neighbour, the hazards of surgery would not be justified.

Everyone has height (just as everyone has blood pressure) and, naturally, extends a certain distance above the ground on standing.

We could choose to define the medical condition of 'hyperexten-sion' in the same terms as Rose defined hypertension: the height above which treatment does more good than harm.

Mercifully, the medical treatments for hypertension are far less dramatic and hazardous than leg shortening. As with any drug therapy, side effects may arise. A drug that's marvellous for one person will not be right for another. But we have a good range of drugs for controlling blood pressure and can normally find a treat-ment that does the job without unwanted effects. Even so, you wouldn't want to take a drug unless your blood pressure was putting you at significant risk.

Solving this problem by shortening legs would be a tall order – long on cost and short on common-sense. It would, of course, be short-sighted to concentrate on shortening people's legs while doing nothing to make the environment safer – as bad as giving people drugs to lower blood pressure while doing nothing to reduce the sodium content of processed foods.

Mystery numbers?

Can doctors say why one person has high blood pressure readings while another is blessed with low numbers? Is it a complete mys-tery – just a game of lucky numbers – or do we know what causes high blood pressure?

In some ways, asking what causes high blood pressure is like asking why some people are tall. You understand now that it's not a case of most people having 'normal blood pressure' while a few are afflicted with 'high blood pressure'; it's a continuous spectrum from low to high. Genetic factors, of course, are very important in determining somebody's height – and some people come from tall families – but so too are environmental influences such as nutri-tion. It's the same with blood pressure.

Very rarely, an underlying disease is responsible for extra growth or lack of it. In most cases, it wouldn't cross your mind that a person was tall as a result of some disease. Similarly, doctors can search high and low for a disease to explain someone's high blood pressure and in 95–98% of cases they will draw a blank; the patient is said to have 'essential hypertension'. (Just occasionally it turns out that a disease of the kidneys or adrenal glands is pushing up the blood pressure.)

Control is essential

The body has intricate control systems that are remarkably good at balancing many variables to keep the blood pressure within an appropriate range. Without any disease being present, a small shift in the balance could result in high blood pressure (essential hypertension). Here are some of the more important factors that influence blood pressure.

Hormones, enzymes and nerves

Renin-angiotensin system
In the kidney an enzyme called renin sets off a chain reaction that produces a protein named angiotensin II. Production of more angiotensin II raises the blood pressure because the arteries constrict (narrow) and the kidneys keep more sodium in the body.

Insulin
Insulin is the hormone produced by the pancreas to help glucose in the blood get into the liver and muscles. Diabetes mellitus occurs when the pancreas produces too little insulin (Type 1 diabetes) or when the body is resistant to the action of insulin (Type 2 diabetes). What has this to do with high blood pressure? Possibly not a lot. But doctors have noticed that some people, who do not actually have diabetes, have high blood glucose readings with high insulin, high triglyceride, and low HDL levels together with raised blood pressure and a tendency to a tubby tummy (central obesity). This combination has been called 'syndrome X' or 'metabolic syndrome'. It is linked with an increased risk of coronary heart disease. The underlying problem is 'insulin resistance': if organs are reluctant to respond to insulin, the pancreas has to produce extra insulin to get the blood glucose level down. Some scientists think insulin resistance is an important cause of hypertension. Research continues.

Other chemical messengers
Scientists continue to discover more chemical messengers (such as bradykinin, endothelin and atrial natriuretic peptide), which influence blood pressure by regulating the width of blood vessels or the transport of sodium.

Nervous system

The part of the nervous system that automatically regulates body functions (the autonomic nervous system) is constantly adjusting blood vessels and heart rate, for example in response to stress.

Part of this system called the sympathetic nervous system (well, it's nice to know that someone cares) is responsible for adrenaline release.

Output and resistance

'Ponderous and uncertain is that relation between pressure and resistance which constitutes the balance of power.'

Sir Harold Nicholson (1886–1968), English diplomat,
Public Faces, 1932, ch. 6

Blood pressure depends upon the rate at which the heart pumps blood (cardiac output) and the resistance to flow within blood vessels (peripheral resistance). Most people with essential hypertension have a normal cardiac output but an increased peripheral resistance – mainly due to contraction of muscles in the small arteries (arterioles).

Sodium

The link between eating a lot of salt and having high blood pressure has now been proved by medical research. The world-wide Intersalt project was particularly revealing. It found that, in parts of the world where people eat high-salt diets, blood pressure increases with age; but the study revealed that this doesn't happen where the normal diet is very low in sodium. Other studies have found that when rural Africans move to cities and adopt the higher salt diets of urban life, their blood pressures rise within months of migration. Clinical trials have shown that reducing salt intake lowers blood pressure. A recent study on chimpanzees with ideal blood pressures showed that their blood pressure kept on rising as more and more salt was added to their diet. (No wonder they drink so much tea.) Blood pressure returned to normal when they went back to their original diet with no added salt.

Potassium, calcium and magnesium

The Intersalt project showed a link between high-potassium diets and lower blood pressure. Clinical trials have shown that some reduction in blood pressure can be achieved by raising potassium intake. In real life, a high-potassium diet will often be a low-sodium diet.

There is also some evidence that maintaining a good intake of calcium and magnesium helps to lower blood pressure.

Alcohol

Heavy drinking is a cause of high blood pressure. A graph relating blood pressure to alcohol consumption is almost J-shaped – more like a tick really. Some researchers have found slightly higher average blood pressures in teetotallers than in those who drink one or two units a day. But as alcohol consumption increases beyond moderate levels, so does blood pressure. Of course, these are trends within a population; some light drinkers will have higher blood pressures than some heavy drinkers. If you are unsure whether drinking is pushing up your blood pressure, a period of alcohol restriction should settle it.

Weight

Measurement of blood pressure in a big arm requires an extra large cuff to wrap around it. A standard sized cuff cannot apply even pressure to the brachial artery. How much difference does this make? Off the cuff it's hard to be precise, but there's no doubt that an undersized cuff can result in a significantly higher reading. Doctors are well aware of this. Even when correct cuff sizes are used, bigger bodies (bigger BMIs) tend to have bigger blood pressures. In fact, many people with high blood pressure can bring it down to normal just by losing weight.

Exercise

Exercise raises blood pressure, but only while you're doing it. Regular exercisers have lower blood pressures than those who conserve their energy. Of course, the exercisers probably smoke less, drink less and eat better too, and working out how much is down to physical activity itself has certainly exercised the scientists. We now have evidence that regular exercise does indeed help to control blood pressure. It isn't just that active people have fewer bad habits; exercise adds to the benefit of other lifestyle changes.

Stress

If you are the best man at a wedding ceremony, and you can't find the ring when it's called for, your blood pressure will go up. But it should be well settled by the time the groom kisses the bride. Stressful events will raise your blood pressure, but whether the ongoing stresses of life are a significant cause of permanently raised blood pressure is far less clear. Certainly our blood pressure goes down when we get really relaxed, but not necessarily down to normal levels. Patel showed that a six-week programme of relaxation aided by biofeedback (in which a signal told the person when his or her blood pressure went up or down) could achieve substantial reductions in blood pressure. Unfortunately, the effect did not last for the follow-up period of one year but some studies have reported more sustained benefit from relaxation techniques. So, relax! It may bring down your blood pressure.

Genes
You may think my fable of flying aliens is a tall story but, just like height, blood pressure is determined by genetic as well as environmental factors. There are tall families but that doesn't mean that every individual in such a family will necessarily be tall; there are hypertensive families but some members may have normal blood pressures.

And how does race affect blood pressure? Again the genes and the environment are found vying for the last word. In Western societies, hypertension is commoner among black people than white people. But in the environment of rural Africa, black people have low blood pressures. Asians, on the other hand, who migrate to Western countries from the Indian subcontinent, are plagued by coronary heart disease, although their blood pressures are not high compared with those of their white neighbours.

◆ The maximum pressure is called *systolic* and the minimum is called *diastolic*

◆ Both systolic and diastolic pressures are important

◆ Most cases of *hypertension* are 'essential' – no cause is found

◆ Sometimes high blood pressure runs in families

◆ Hormones and the nervous system are constantly regulating blood pressure

◆ Blood pressure is raised by eating too much salt, drinking excess alcohol, being overweight and not exercising

What if my number's up?

At last you get round to seeing your doctor to have your blood pressure checked, only to be told "It's a bit up, I'm afraid". If your reading's up, don't let it get you down. And don't give up. It's not over yet!

For a start, Table 20 will help you figure out your numbers.

Table 20 Blood pressure measurement

	Systolic pressure (mmHg)	Diastolic pressure (mmHg)
Ideal	under 120	under 80
Normal	120–129	80–84
Borderline	130–140	85–90
Raised	over 140	over 90
High	over 160	over 100
Very high!	200+	110+

Could it be a wrong number?

Phoney numbers are all too possible if careful attention is not paid to maintenance and correct use of the sphygmomanometer. The mercury column has been used to measure blood pressure for over a hundred years and I've seen a few instruments that looked as if they were there at the beginning. It's impossible to obtain accurate readings if the manometer is not properly calibrated or if the top of the mercury column is hidden behind oxidised mercury on the inside of the glass.

Electronic instruments that bleep and flash may seem more state-of-the-art but that doesn't automatically make them more accurate. If you are thinking of buying one of these devices to check your own blood pressure, choose one that has been validated according to standards set by the British Hypertension Society (BHS) or the Association for the Advancement of Medical Instrumentation (AAMI). You can find information about validated instruments on the BHS website (www.hyp.ac.uk/bhsinfo).

Automatic electronic blood pressure recorders are extremely easy to use and they eliminate the 'observer error' that occurs with mercury manometers. No doubt electronic devices will soon replace mercury instruments altogether, not least because mercury is considered an environmental hazard.

Even the most accurate of blood pressure readings is merely a snapshot – a record of one moment in a constantly changing scene. Your blood pressure varies throughout the day and probably falls to its lowest level while you're asleep. Anything from being in a hurry to having a very full bladder will push it up temporarily. It's the 'resting blood pressure' that counts; try to arrive in plenty of time for an appointment at the surgery so you can sit calmly for a few minutes before your blood pressure is taken. Of course, if you sit there fuming because the doctor's running late, this won't help at all.

You can see how misleading a single measurement of blood pressure could be. A series of readings, taken on different occasions, allows decisions to be based on the average or mean blood pressure.

The mean machine

Think how useful it would be if there were a machine that would tell us the mean blood pressure over a 24-hour period of normal activity. There is.

The computerised ambulatory blood pressure monitoring machine is worn, usually for a period of 24 hours, while getting on with normal life. It automatically records the blood pressure at programmed intervals – usually every 30 minutes. Not only does this provide the mean systolic and diastolic pressures, it also allows analysis of the pattern of blood pressure variation during the 24 hours. For example, it seems that people who do not show the normal drop in blood pressure overnight ('non-dippers') are at increased risk.

24-hour blood pressure monitors are particularly useful for identifying those with so-called 'white coat hypertension'. These people have normal blood pressures most of the time. But as soon as someone comes along to measure the pressure, it shoots up. For most of these people, the blood pressure will go up whether the doctor is actually wearing a white coat or not, although it is said to occur a little less often when nurses take the reading (but I'm sure it all depends on what gets you going). It's completely normal to be a little apprehensive about seeing a doctor or having your blood pressure checked and this certainly doesn't mean that your blood pressure will necessarily be high. Even so, it may be that up to 20% of those with high readings actually have 'white coat hypertension'.

Those clever 24-hour machines cost around £2000 each so don't be surprised if your doctor isn't using one on everybody.

Cost is not the only good reason for restricting the use of these machines at the moment. Another problem is that most of the research that has enabled us to decide what levels of blood pressure are risky enough to require treatment has relied upon the conventional method of measuring blood pressure. We cannot assume, for example, that someone who always has high blood pressure readings at a clinic is necessarily at very low risk simply because a 24-hour record looks fine. When 24-hour recording has been used in more long-term studies, we will be clearer about its value in assessing risk. In all probability, as more data are gathered, this high-tech investigation will become routine.

Are you due for an age rise?

When you get to a certain age, lots of things start dropping. Blood pressure isn't one of them. I recall being told at medical school that the normal systolic blood pressure was given by 100+the person's age (120 mmHg at age 20; 160 mmHg at age 60). This rise in blood pressure with advancing age is so common in our society that we have come to regard it as normal.

Rural communities that have not adopted a westernised lifestyle escape this age-related rise in blood pressure. Their low-salt diets can take much of the credit.

◆ A blood pressure of 120/80 mmHg or less is ideal; 160/95 mmHg is high

◆ Blood pressure tends to rise with age but not in communities with extremely low salt intakes

◆ Readings on at least 3 separate occasions are needed to indicate the average blood pressure

◆ A 24-hour blood pressure monitor can help to identify 'white coat hypertension' (in which readings are only high in the surgery/clinic)

What does high pressure do to you?

We have seen that people with high blood pressure are more likely to suffer a stroke or heart attack. Why?

The wall of an artery is made up of three layers: a tough, fibrous, outer sleeve; a muscular, elastic middle layer; and a smooth inner lining. This smooth, low-friction lining is delicate; it can easily be damaged by the wear and tear of blood flow under pressure. Minor scuffs are soon put right by the body's maintenance service. But constantly raised blood pressure is more punishing and cholesterol builds up on damaged areas of the artery lining. When this process affects the coronary arteries, angina and heart attacks may follow. Narrowing of arteries in the brain can lead to a stroke; a haemorrhagic stroke, in which a damaged artery bleeds, is more likely when the pressure is high.

There are other ways, too, in which constantly high blood pressure can damage organs. After years of working extra hard, the heart's main pumping chamber (the left ventricle) can become enlarged and, eventually, heart failure may occur. Eye damage can result in impaired vision or blindness. Long-term effects on the kidneys may lead to kidney failure.

Can treatment really help?

We know that strokes and heart attacks are more common among those with high blood pressure. But do we have evidence that lowering blood pressure reverses the risk? The prevalence of train spotting may be higher among men wearing anoraks; but we cannot be sure that keeping them dressed in suits will reduce their train spotting. Treatment of blood pressure could be very disappointing. Raised blood pressure could be an anorak – an outward sign of a deeper problem within. Suppose it reflected a hidden metabolic disturbance, such as insulin resistance, which was the real cause of strokes and heart attacks.

In 1990, the *Lancet* published an analysis by Collins and colleagues of *observational studies* on hypertension. These studies provide evidence of risk because they observed what happened to people with various levels of blood pressure over a number of years: they don't prove that treatment would have helped. Having analysed the data, it was possible to calculate the theoretical benefit of treatment – the number of strokes and heart attacks that would have been prevented by treatment if, indeed, you can undo the risks of hypertension by reducing the pressure.

The conclusion was that a sustained reduction of 6 mmHg in diastolic pressure should result in a 35–40% drop in the number of strokes, and a 20–25% decrease in heart attacks. When they analysed data from *intervention studies*, which do provide direct evidence on the effect of treatment, it turned out that treatment had actually reduced the risk of stroke by 42% and of heart disease by 14% (but this rises to 16% if the results of more recent trials on older people are included in the analysis).

It seems that drug treatment of blood pressure prevents *all* the strokes that theory predicted it should, and *some* of the heart attacks.

We have clear evidence, then, that lowering blood pressure does reduce risk. Why weren't more heart attacks prevented? This may have something to do with the fundamental influence of cholesterol on heart disease and the fact that the drugs used (beta-blockers and diuretics) can have unwanted effects on lipid and glucose metabolism.

It's likely that, while reducing blood pressure cuts strokes rapidly, only about half the benefit on heart disease will be seen within a five-year trial.

To treat, or not to treat?

That is the question being asked by doctors in every surgery up and down the land. The patient has returned for a fourth blood pressure check and, yet again, the reading is high. Should drug treatment be started?

If you have a mean blood pressure of around 200/110 mmHg, your doctor will, quite rightly, want to get it down quickly. You are likely to need drug treatment and it should not be unduly delayed.

On the other hand, if your blood pressure is more moderately raised, you may be able to avoid the need for drug therapy by making the right lifestyle changes (see below).

When there is no urgency about the situation, your doctor is likely to let you try to reduce your blood pressure without drugs for at least three months. If some progress has been made in that time, it's well worth trying for longer.

If your systolic pressure remains above 160 mmHg, or your diastolic above 100 mmHg, your doctor will probably recommend drug treatment. When raised blood pressure has already caused heart, kidney or eye problems, treatment would be started at lower levels of blood pressure (systolic 140 mmHg; diastolic 90 mmHg). If your blood pressure is staying between 140/90 mmHg and 160/100 mmHg, but you have no problems with your kidneys, eyes, heart or circulation, and no diabetes, your risk of getting heart disease is now used to decide whether or not to prescribe blood pressure treatment. Current guidelines recommend drug treatment if your coronary heart disease risk is at least 15% in ten years (see Chapter 24).

What difference does diabetes make?

If you have diabetes, it is even more important to avoid high blood pressure; your doctor will be trying to keep your reading below 140/80 mmHg. Diabetes is bad for the arteries, and one of the main aims of managing diabetes is to reduce the risk of heart disease. There is now strong evidence that people with diabetes do better if blood pressure is well controlled.

Managing high blood pressure

Management of blood pressure is not, in fact, just a numbers game – even though it was sometimes seen that way in the past. High blood pressure is a very important risk factor but it's not the only one. The aim is to treat the whole person – not the numbers on a mercury manometer. Doctors realised a long time ago that high blood pressure is not a disease of the left arm. All risk factors need to be addressed.

Whether you need drug treatment or not, you must also change your lifestyle. Not only does this make your drug treatment more effective, and perhaps limit the dose you need, it also works in other ways to protect your heart and circulation.

Once you have started drug treatment of high blood pressure, you will normally need to continue for good. It's not a cure. You don't take a drug for a couple of months and settle your blood pressure forever. Occasionally, though, if significant lifestyle changes are made after treatment has been started, the drug can be stopped without your blood pressure returning to its previous high level. Of course, you must not stop your medication on your own because that is highly dangerous. Discuss it with your doctor who will want to keep an eye on your blood pressure, especially if any change in treatment is advised.

◆ Constantly high blood pressure is bad for arteries, and can damage your heart, brain, kidney and eye

◆ Lowering raised blood pressure reduces strokes dramatically and heart attacks significantly

◆ If you have diabetes, it is even more important to control high blood pressure

◆ Very high blood pressure should be controlled quickly and drugs will be needed

◆ Mildly raised blood pressure may respond to lifestyle changes without drugs

---

Drugs used to treat high blood pressure

Doctors today have a wide variety of drugs (see Table 21) that bring down blood pressure.

In fact, the first four letters of the alphabet could provide a useful mnemonic if you wanted to remember all the important classes of drugs used to treat high blood pressure:

ACE inhibitors
Angiotensin receptor antagonists
Alpha-blockers

Beta-blockers

Calcium channel blockers

Diuretics

◆ Lifestyle changes reduce the risks, whether drugs are used or not

◆ Drugs have side effects, but it is usually possible to find a treatment that controls blood pressure without side effects

---

Table 21 Classes of drugs

Class of drugs	Examples
ACE inhibitors (angiotensin converting enzyme inhibitors)	captopril, cilazapril, enalapril, fosinopril, lisinopril, moexipril, perindopril, quinapril, ramipril, trandolapril
Angiotensin receptor antagonists	candesartan, irbesartan, losartan, valsartan
Alpha-blockers	doxazosin, indoramin, prazosin, terazosin
Beta-blockers	acebutolol, atenolol, betaxolol, bisoprolol, celiprolol, metoprolol, nadolol, oxprenolol, pindolol, propranolol, sotalol
Calcium channel blockers	amlodipine, diltiazem, felodipine, isradipine, lacidipine, nicardipine, nifedipine, verapamil
Diuretics	bendrofluazide, hydrochlorothiazide

Diuretics

Thiazide diuretics lower blood pressure by encouraging the kidneys to excrete more sodium and water, and by relaxing the muscle layer in artery walls

Beta-blockers (beta-adrenoreceptor blockers)

The eminent Nobel Prize winner, Sir James Black, has made several landmark contributions to medicine. After all, he was my professor of pharmacology when I was an undergraduate at University College London. Not only that, but he developed the brilliant idea of beta-blockers while he was working at Imperial Chemical Industries. Propranolol was the first one that could be taken by mouth and it is still in widespread use today. Since its birth in the sixties, there has been a beta-blocker baby boom. (I am referring to the many new beta-blockers, and not suggesting that these drugs boost fertility!)

These drugs block some of the body's responses to adrenaline and similar chemical messengers; they slow the heart rate but also lower blood pressure by reducing the output of renin.

Calcium channel blockers

This is not a reference to chalk cliffs collapsing into the Channel Tunnel. It's the name given to a group of drugs that block the passage of calcium through channels in cell membranes. The effect of this is to relax the muscle in artery walls, making the arteries wider and reducing resistance to blood flow.

ACE inhibitors

Don't get this term confused with the ACE *vitamins*: any drug that inhibited the action of those vital antioxidants would be little help to us in our battle against coronary heart disease. No, the full name of this family of drugs is *angiotensin converting enzyme inhibitors*. They hinder the activity of the renin-angiotensin system. As a result, artery walls become more relaxed and the kidneys allow more sodium into the urine.

Angiotensin receptor antagonists

This novel class of drugs was launched in 1995. Like ACE inhibitors, the new drugs work on the renin-angiotensin system but they block the angiotensin receptor instead of interfering with the production of angiotensin II.

Alpha-blockers (alpha-adrenoreceptor blockers)

These drugs make blood vessels dilate (get wider) by relaxing muscle tissue in their walls.

Side effects

All these drugs cause side effects in some people. Beta-blockers can trigger wheezing and must be avoided by people with asthma. Diuretics sometimes provoke gout and, like certain beta-blockers, can have unwanted effects on the lipid profile. Calcium channel blockers may cause ankle swelling. Some people get a dry cough when using ACE inhibitors. Sometimes drugs used to treat blood pressure make it more difficult for a man to get an erection. Why suffer in silence? In fact, if you think your treatment is causing any side effects, please tell your doctor; it may well be possible to change to something that suits you better.

How does a doctor choose a drug?

Confronted with a patient with high blood pressure, and such a wide choice of drugs, how can a doctor make a rational choice? Let me immediately assure you that this is not merely a question of which pharmaceutical representative has just taken your doctor out to lunch. These days, most GPs are very well informed about the therapeutic options.

Diuretics and beta-blockers are the traditional first choices and, it must be said, most of the evidence that treating raised blood pressure is beneficial comes from research using these drugs. The traditional approach to rational treatment was 'stepped care' – starting with a diuretic or beta-blocker, combining the two if necessary, and adding in a third drug if that wasn't adequate.

Frequently, though, it is a matter of tailoring the therapy to fit the patient. In many cases, a diuretic or a beta-blocker will still be a good first choice. If you have high blood pressure and angina, a beta-blocker may deal with both. A beta-blocker would be less suitable for some people with diabetes and positively dangerous for someone with asthma. For a man with high blood pressure and prostate symptoms, an alpha-blocker would be a rational first choice. Where high blood pressure is combined with heart failure an ACE inhibitor would be the best bet. Black people often have low renin levels and respond less well to an ACE inhibitor (unless it's combined with another drug).

If your blood pressure is poorly controlled on the most appropriate dose, or if side effects occur, it will be necessary to change to another drug and, perhaps, to a different class of drugs.

The intention is to control your blood pressure with a single drug if possible. But often a second drug has to be added and some people need three or four. An ACE inhibitor and a calcium channel blocker often work well together.

Good control of blood pressure without side effects can normally be achieved.

Should I take aspirin?

Aspirin reduces the risk of forming a blood clot in the circulation (thrombosis) and that's why a low dose (75 mg a day) is recommended for those who already have heart disease or have had a stroke caused by a blood clot in the brain. Also, some research suggests that aspirin can reduce the chances of developing certain cancers.

A lot of people have heard these claims and take an aspirin with their cornflakes just to be on the safe side. The trouble is that taking an aspirin every day increases the risk of bleeding – particularly from the stomach. If you have already suffered a thrombosis in an artery, the small risk from taking aspirin is overshadowed by the benefit. But if you've never had a problem with your circulation, the risk from taking the aspirin might be bigger than the risk you're trying to reduce. Wearing a steel bucket over your head could reduce your risk of being killed by a freak missile, but that's no use if you get run over because you can't see where you're going.

What if your only problem is high blood pressure – which does raise that risk of having a stroke or heart attack? You may have been confused by media coverage of one study showing that people with high blood pressure were protected by aspirin, followed by reports highlighting the risk of brain haemorrhage when people take aspirin if they have high blood pressure.

Well, aspirin is hazardous if the blood pressure is poorly controlled. The thing to do is to weigh up the risks and tip the balance in your favour. Above all, get high blood pressure (and other risk factors) under control. If you have high blood pressure, it's a good idea to take aspirin (75 mg daily) if *all* of these are true:

- you are at least 50 years old;

- your blood pressure is now well controlled (below 150/90 mmHg);

- you have diabetes OR there are already signs of blood pressure affecting your heart, kidneys or eyes OR your heart disease risk is at least 15% in ten years (see Chapter 24);

- aspirin doesn't upset you.

It's possible that the beneficial effects of aspirin on the circulation are cancelled by taking the anti-inflammatory drug ibuprofen at the same time. The Medicines Monitoring Unit at the University of Dundee reported an increased risk of death among those taking ibuprofen as well as aspirin; they found no evidence of the same problem when other anti-inflammatory drugs were combined with aspirin.

A lifestyle to lower the pressure

Making the right changes to your lifestyle may avoid the need to take blood pressure-lowering drugs altogether. If your blood pressure is normal now, the healthy lifestyle will help to keep it that way. When drug treatment is necessary, lifestyle remains crucial: getting it right helps the drugs to work better and protects your heart in other ways. If your doctor has prescribed a drug for your blood pressure, you must never stop it without medical advice.

Here is the **SAFE** way to lower your blood pressure. There are now many good studies to show that each of these changes can reduce blood pressure:

Salt

Cut down gradually and your palate will adjust to not adding salt in the kitchen or at the table. Season well with herbs, spices, pepper, garlic, mustard powder, vinegar, lemon, etc. Watch out for high-sodium seasonings like soy sauce. Remember that most of the salt consumed by the nation comes in processed foods. Read those labels and use fresh ingredients when possible (see Chapter 6).

Every day, eat at least four portions of fruit and four portions of vegetables (including plenty of pulses) to boost potassium and magnesium intake. Have two or three servings a day of very low-fat dairy products (see Chapter 4) to keep up your calcium.

Alcohol

Excess alcohol raises blood pressure; cutting down reduces it. The maximum allowance on any one day is 4 units for a man and 3 for a woman. But 1 or 2 units (e.g. 1 or 2 glasses of wine) on most days would be better (see Chapter 10).

Fat

Losing that fat can lower your pressure. In fact one analysis predicts that a weight loss of 12 kg (less than 2 stone) will produce a fall in blood pressure of 21/13 mmHg – a very significant reduction. Of course, in any individual, the actual change in blood pressure will be influenced by other factors (such as salt and alcohol intake) which are changing at the same time (see Chapters 6 and 10).

To reduce body fat, the first move is to eat less fat (see Chapter 17). For the sake of your arteries, avoid saturated fat wherever you can.

Exercise

Move your body and master your pressure. Studies have now confirmed that when physical activity is increased, the resting blood pressure is reduced. Remember to increase very gradually from your present level of activity (see Chapter 19).

The DASH diet

This may sound like fast food for the gulp-and-go gourmet, but the DASH (Dietary Approaches to Stop Hypertension) trial was an American research project that investigated the effects of different diets on blood pressure. Published in 1997, the study showed that a diet including 8–10 servings a day of fruit and vegetables (much richer in potassium, magnesium and fibre than the typical American diet) could lower blood pressure significantly. And when the calcium content of this diet was boosted by the addition of 2 or 3 servings a day of low-fat dairy products, the reduction in blood pressure was almost doubled. A follow-up study published in 2001, the DASH Sodium Trial, confirmed that the DASH diet lowered blood pressure most efficiently when combined with a low salt intake.

To improve your blood pressure now and in the future, follow this **SAFE** plan for salt, alcohol, fat and exercise. Don't forget to include at least eight servings of fruit and vegetables, and three servings of very low-fat dairy products, every day for maximum benefit.

Of course, it's important to support the **SAFE** plan to lower your pressure with the other recommendations in this book to protect your heart. In particular:

- Eat oily fish at least twice a week (but watch out for the added salt content of tinned fish). There is evidence that high doses of fish oil can reduce blood pressure and, in one study, giving fish oil was more effective when combined with salt restriction.

- Don't smoke! Your blood pressure goes up when you smoke a cigarette and, of course, the long-term effects of habitual smoking are disastrous.

And, if the pace of life is a problem, the next chapter, which deals with stress, should help to ease the pressure too.

ACTION POINTS

◆ Have your blood pressure checked (unless you have had a normal reading in the last year)

◆ Follow this SAFE plan for salt, alcohol, fat and exercise

◆ Eat at least eight servings of fruit and vegetables (including plenty of pulses) every day

◆ Have three servings of very low-fat dairy products a day

◆ If you have been prescribed a drug for high blood pressure, take it regularly and never stop it without medical supervision

Chapter 22

Stress

'Stress . . . The overpowering pressure *of* some adverse
force or influence.'

The Shorter Oxford English Dictionary

Is stress a cause of heart disease?

What is stress and how do we know whether one man's stress is
bigger than another's? How do we measure it?

Is the busy business executive more stressed than the dustman –
or is the executive thriving on challenges while the dustman is
frustrated by lack of control over his life? Clearly, if you can't measure stress, or identify those with a lot of it, you can't tell whether
the more stressed get more heart disease.

An early attempt to resolve this was made by Friedman and
Rosenman in the 1950s when they developed their famous theory
of personality types. The classification was simpler than ABC – just
A and B, in fact. The type A person is hard-working, competitive,
aggressive, impatient, never satisfied and always in a rush. He's
the guy who finishes all your sentences for you because you take
too long to find the right word. And he always turns the toilet roll
to face the 'right' way. On the other hand, the Type B personality is
non-competitive, easy-going and relaxed.

Of course, this classification is a little too simple to accommo-
date the full range of humanity: most of us will display both type A
and type B behaviour at different times. Even so, you can probably think
of people who fit firmly into one category or the other.

250

A study of 3524 men aged 39–59 classified them according to personality type and studied the history of their heart disease over eight years. This was reported by Rosenman and colleagues in 1975 as the Western Collaborative Group Study. The researchers made an adjustment for the main risk factors (such as smoking) and concluded that those with a type A personality had double the risk of heart disease.

Later research found a much weaker link between type A personality and heart disease. Out of twelve studies reviewed by Kornitzer in 1992, seven showed no connection between type A personality and coronary heart disease.

A follow-up on the men in the Western Collaborative Group Study, after 22 years, in 1988, is astonishing. As a risk factor, type A personality appeared to have done a U-turn. The men who had developed heart disease in the first eight and a half years of the investigation had a lower death rate – one third lower – if they had been labelled type A rather than type B at the outset!

What could have changed since the 1970s? In some studies, different methods of identifying type A behaviour may be relevant but this would not apply to the Western Collaborative Group Study. It could well be that the no-nonsense, high-achieving type A people have taken messages about healthy living to heart and been more successful at making lifestyle changes.

◆ Aggressive type A behaviour is bad for your heart but you can change this behaviour and reduce your risk

◆ Achieving goals, including lifestyle changes, can help your heart

◆ Psychosocial stress – such as lack of job control – increases heart risk

---

It probably is bad for your heart (not to mention your social life) to be aggressive, hostile and impatient, but some positive type A characteristics, such as devotion to work, do not appear to raise the risk of heart disease. A certain level of stress is quite normal and healthy, if balanced with relaxation; it can help you to achieve satisfying goals. So don't worry yourself sick about a little bit of stress.

Lifestyle changes can more than compensate for the risk attached to the 'wrong' personality. And, while you cannot transform yourself to become a different personality, you can certainly change the more destructive elements of type A behaviour.

Psychosocial stress

This is nothing to do with a gathering of Alfred Hitchcock fans. It's the term used to refer to stress that results from a person's *psychological* response to difficult *social* circumstances.

Among the women followed for 20 years in the Framingham Study, heart disease was linked with low educational level, low pay, and lack of holidays (even after physical risk factors had been allowed for).

The Scottish Heart Health Study found higher coronary rates in areas of high unemployment.

Having a job can be stressful too. The Whitehall II study reported in the *British Medical Journal* in 1997 involved 10,308 male and female civil servants aged 35 to 55.

The researchers concluded that those with little control over their jobs were significantly more likely to develop heart disease. The findings applied equally to men and women. This helps to confirm the conclusions of other investigators. In fact, in a 1994 review, 17 out of 25 studies found a significant link between job control and cardiovascular risk.

It seems that giving employees more variety in their duties, and a bigger say in decisions about work, could be to the benefit of public health.

- ◆ Stress releases adrenaline, speeds up the heart and primes the body for 'fight or flight'
- ◆ Some stress is normal; too much is damaging to health
- ◆ Stress reduction can help to lower blood pressure

How does the body respond to stress?

Faced with a hungry wolf at the entrance of his family cave, primitive man immediately produced a surge of adrenaline. His heart rate increased and he started breathing faster. This, together with diversion of blood from the skin and gut to the muscles, ensured all muscles were well supplied with oxygen – ready to fight a ravenous predator. No doubt, sudden confrontation by a fierce caveman produced the same stress response in the wolf, boosting its performance for a speedy getaway. Both wolf and caveman released extra fats and sugar into the blood to fuel fast-working muscles.

If he happened upon stampeding elephants, on the other hand, our courageous caveman did not confront them; he used his stress response to effect an escape. Even so, if it came to the crunch, his body had prepared by increasing the clotting power of the blood to minimise bleeding.

You can see why this stress response is called the 'fight-or-flight' reaction and how useful it is for avoiding disasters. Even in modern life we are occasionally faced with a challenge requiring an immediate physical response; it could be anything from a mugger to a volcanic eruption. But your body may have the same fight-or-flight reaction when you serve a cantankerous customer in a department store. In this case, fighting or running away, or even moderate bleeding, won't be very helpful.

And when you are sitting in a traffic jam – adrenaline and cortisol coursing your arteries, fat and glucose mobilised, muscles primed for action – what is your body to make of it when, half an hour later, the only sign of physical activity is your turning of a few pages of the road atlas in the vain search for a short cut?

Frequent arousal of the stress response, especially without appropriate exercise, will take its toll on health and, in the long term, raise the risk of heart disease. Of course, the risk will escalate if stress provokes heavy smoking, overeating or excess alcohol consumption. Chronic stress – that is, stress which continues over a long period – can lead to anxiety, depression and a very wide range of physical symptoms (such as palpitations, chest pain, headaches, muscle pains and bowel upsets).

Can stress reduction lower the risk of heart disease?

Raised blood pressure is, of course, one of the main risk factors for coronary heart disease. We know that acute stress pushes up the blood pressure temporarily; it is not so clear whether chronic stress is an important cause of permanently raised blood pressure (hypertension). Several studies have used relaxation techniques, breathing exercises or biofeedback while monitoring blood pressure. Typically, up to ten people would attend sessions for ten weeks, each session lasting an hour or so. A review in the *Drug and Therapeutics Bulletin* in 1989 concluded that these methods could lower blood pressure and that, in some cases, the benefit could be sustained for years.

A study by Friedman and colleagues on people who had survived a heart attack was published in the *American Heart Journal* in 1986. The people who were given special counselling sessions to modify their type A behaviour (in addition to routine care) were less likely to have a further heart attack.

Stress busting

There's no need to be a victim of stress. You're the boss. Don't be fooled into smoking, eating all the wrong things, drinking too much alcohol, or overdosing on caffeine in response to stress. That's letting it get the better of you.

The positive 'arousal' that gives you the energy to achieve your best is good. Negative, energy-sapping anxiety is not. Here is a plan to turn the turmoil of stress into **REST**.

To conquer stress you need:

RELAXATION	Respiration. Breathing is essential
	Relaxation of muscle and mind
	Replay. Got it taped?
	Recreation
	Retiring – to bed, I mean
EXERCISE	
STRATEGIES for STRESS REDUCTION	Stress diary
	Solving problems
	Social skills training
	Sex
	Stroking a pet
	Saving time
TALK	Talking it through
	Taking advice
	Talking therapy

Relaxation

Rest and relaxation are essential. If you don't recharge your batteries, they go flat. This may happen insidiously until you suddenly discover that there's no juice left – just like the car that won't start one winter's morning.

Winston Churchill regularly made time for a rest – even when he had the Second World War to run. The **rest** is history.

"Just relax," says the doctor, as he approaches you with a long shiny metal thing. It's rather difficult to relax to order, isn't it? Sometimes, the harder you try to relax, the more wound up you become – especially when relaxation is a matter of urgency, so you can fit in a few hours' sleep before making an early start the next day.

Relaxation is a technique that can be learnt. With practice, you get better at switching to relax mode whenever it's called for.

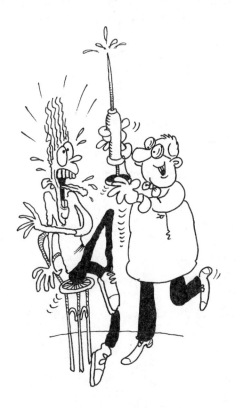

"Just relax!"

Respiration. Breathing is essential

Of course, those of us without respiratory diseases take breathing for granted. You just do it (about 17,000 times a day). You don't need to be told. But the way you breathe directly affects the way you feel – and vice versa. At times of stress, you take rapid, shallow breaths; you sigh and gasp. Regular, leisurely, 'abdominal' breathing helps you to unwind and feel relaxed.

Try placing your right hand on your abdomen – below the rib cage – and your left hand on your chest. Breathe out with a leisurely sigh, allowing all tension to flow away from you, and see the hand on your tummy move inwards. Breathe in through your nose and see how your tummy moves out while the hand on your chest stays still. Your diaphragm is doing its job. Keep breathing through your nose now, gently and calmly. Don't force extra-deep breaths. Let your tummy rise and fall with your body's natural rhythm. Feel the calm come over you as tension drains away.

Now you've got the idea of abdominal breathing, you can do it with your hands in any relaxed position – by your sides or on your lap. A few minutes of breathing like this is a good start to any relaxation exercise but you can also do it on the train, or at the dentist, or waiting for a job interview.

Relaxation of muscle and mind

'Damn braces: Bless relaxes.'
_____

William Blake (1757–1827)
The Marriage of Heaven and Hell, 1790–3, Proverbs of Hell

Stress tenses muscles and primes them for action; releasing muscle tension tells the brain that all is well and allows your mind to become relaxed.

For a successful relaxation session you need a comfortable, warm room where you will be undisturbed for at least 20 minutes. You can do it sitting down but it is usually helpful to lie on the bed or floor, with your head supported by a pillow or cushion. If it's at all chilly, you should cover yourself with a blanket.

A relaxation session

Lying on your back, feet apart, arms relaxed at your sides, close your eyes and begin your abdominal breathing. Feel the tension leave you as you breathe out. Imagine the warmth of the sun caressing you as your body becomes heavy and limp. Your breathing becomes naturally slow and peaceful.

Now clench your right fist and tense the muscles of your right arm. This is what tension feels like; concentrate on it for a few moments. Release the tension, let your fingers go loose and feel how warm, limp and heavy the arm is becoming. Repeat this for your left arm.

Tighten the muscles in your right leg, lifting the knee a little. (Don't overdo it if you get cramp easily!) Concentrate only on your right leg. Feel the discomfort of tight muscles. As you breathe out, let the tension go. Feel the leg become heavy and warm as every part of it relaxes. Repeat this with your left leg.

Say 'relax' as you breathe out, and think of the tension ebbing away with each breath.

Lift your shoulders up – right up to your ears. Hold them there. Feel the tension in your chest, your neck and your head. Then, as you breathe out, let more and more of the tension go. Let the full weight of your head and neck sink into the pillow. Relax.

Tense your neck and throat muscles by pushing your head down into the pillow. Hold it for a few moments, then gently let the tension go, bit by bit, until it's all gone.

Pull your shoulders back a little, towards the floor. Notice the tension in the muscles of your back. Let the tension go again, sinking into the floor as you breathe out. Feel warm and heavy.

Pull your tummy in – right in – tensing the muscles of your abdomen. Note how your breathing is pushed up into your chest. Feel the tightness. Then, as you breathe out, let the tightness go. Relax. Let your breathing become calm and natural once again.

Tighten all the muscles in your face. Screw up your eyes, frown and clench your teeth. Feel the tension all over your face, in your jaw and in your head. How uncomfortable this is.

*How unnatural. Gradually, let all the tension go. Feel the
warmth of sunshine on your face as your brow becomes quite
smooth again. Let your mouth fall slightly open as every muscle
is released.*

*Let your whole body feel heavy, warm and limp – sinking into
the floor. Feel completely relaxed as you breathe gently and
calmly, your tummy rising and falling. Now that you are relaxed,
let your thoughts take you to a beautiful walled garden. As you
enter the garden, smell the sweet aroma of the flowers. Feel the
gentle, warm breeze on your face. Hear the birds singing and the
brook babbling. Bask in the sunshine. There's nothing to trouble
you here. You can come here whenever you want, once you've
become relaxed.*

*When you are ready to leave, let your thoughts take you out of
the walled garden. Slowly open your eyes and become aware of
your surroundings. Have a really good stretch. Roll onto your
side for a little while before getting up.*

Replay. Got it taped?

Once you've learnt a relaxation exercise of this sort, you don't need
any special equipment to practise it. To begin with, though, it's best
to use a relaxation tape and these are widely available. You could
even record the above text onto an audio cassette if you like listening to your own voice (sad). A calm, soothing voice is much more
helpful than a squeaky, tense one. A good professional tape would
be a sound investment.

Doing relaxation exercises once or twice a day gives you the
best results. You soon become more aware of the tension that
creeps into muscles at times of stress – and you know how to
release it, with or without a tape.

Talking of audiotapes, it's worth mentioning that anxiety is
often provoked by playing back a sequence of negative thoughts –
over and over again. Do you sometimes catch yourself thinking
"I'll never cope; it's going to be awful . . ."? You need to stop the
'tape', take the cassette out of your head, and replace it with one
full of positive thoughts: "Of course I'll cope; I'll enjoy it; I've met
bigger challenges than babysitting a hamster." I realise that your
worries may not be trivial at all. You may be worried sick about

coping with disability or bereavement or about how you will support your family after redundancy. Just the same, the constant
playing of negative thoughts feeds anxiety that can well up and hit you
in surprising ways. Change the tape.

Recreation

'He who laughs, lasts.'

_____

Mary Pettibone Poole, *A Glass Eye at the Keyhole*

Whether your hobby is gardening, playing Monopoly or rearing
stick insects, the diversion is very refreshing and helps to trickle
charge your batteries. Listening to music can be very relaxing and
if you play an instrument, so much the better. (But, if you're a
beginner, a soundproof room could save some stress in other members of the family.) Where there's life there should be laughter, and
a really good giggle is a great boost.

Retiring – to bed, I mean

'I love sleep because it is both pleasant and safe to use.'

_____

Fran Lebowitz, *Metropolitan Life,* **1978**

Sleep is the ultimate rest (excluding death). If you can sleep like a
log it's a great blessing. Sometimes, when stressed, the most we can
manage is a few splinters. If you haven't yet twigged the root cause
of your insomnia, these tips may help:

- Sleep requires a noise-free environment. If your
  neighbour uses a chain saw all night, trying to sleep
  like a log is bound to go against the grain. Talk to your
  neighbour (when he hasn't got his chain saw). If this
  fails, talk to your local Environmental Health Officer.

- It's difficult to sleep if you're uncomfortable. If you
  are around six foot six, and trying to sleep in a six-foot
  bed, is it any wonder you feel a bit hung over in the
  morning? Is your room too hot or cold? If it's pain
  that keeps you awake, a painkiller would be more

appropriate than a sleeping tablet. (Just a small
appendix to that point: I'm assuming here that you
know the cause of the pain. But if it's appendicitis,
appendicectomy would be more appropriate still.)

- Too much caffeine won't help, so watch the cola, coffee
  and tea – especially coffee in the evening if you're not
  used to it.

- You may drop off easily after a few alcoholic drinks –
  only to wake early, unable to get back to sleep.

- Regular physical exercise can help you sleep better,
  but taking it late in the evening can keep you awake.

- An afternoon cat nap of a few minutes can be refreshing.
  But, just as eating between meals can cause trouble,
  so daytime sleeps can spoil your 'nappetite' at night.
  Try to limit them to 20 minutes maximum.

- Going to bed at wildly different times every night
  doesn't give your body clock a chance to settle down.
  Try to establish a routine.

- Don't necessarily expect eight hours' sleep a night.
  Didn't Mrs Thatcher thrive on four? Some people need
  more than others but we all need less as we get older.

- If an active mind is keeping you awake, do your
  relaxation exercise (unless the active mind is not your
  own, in which case ask your partner to stop talking).
  End up in your beautiful walled garden, or on the beach
  listening to the breaking waves. It beats counting sheep.

Exercise

Regular physical exercise is a vital part of your stress-busting programme. You can never really rest unless you've been active, any
more than you can wake up unless you've been asleep.

An exercise session gives you an important break and perhaps a
change of scenery but, as an antidote to stress, it goes much further than
that. Aerobic activity, such as brisk walking for half an hour a day,
deals with those stress hormones and burns off the extra fuel

released for fight or flight. It also stimulates release of the body's natural tranquillising proteins – endorphins – which help to bring about a feeling of wellbeing. Whatever you do, build up gradually from your present level of activity (see Chapter 19).

Strategies for stress reduction

There are various steps you can take to reduce the stress in your life.

Stress diary

You may find it helpful to keep a diary for a few days to identify your main sources of stress. Is your relationship with a particular person causing trouble? Or are there certain events or tasks that you find especially stressful? Of course, on really stressful days, which could provide a lot of information for your diary, you'll be far too stressed to bother with a diary on top of everything else.

Solving problems

Once you've identified the problems, you can set about finding some solutions. A wise friend might see an answer that hasn't occurred to you.

If your wife is always in the bathroom just when you need to shave, getting up 15 minutes earlier could save a lot of frustration.

Or it may be that your husband snores – loudly. In some cases, simple measures such as taking less alcohol, or using a nasal appliance from the pharmacy (for the snorer), or ear-plugs (for the partner), or separate rooms (for the snorer, at least, even if everyone else has to share) will be satisfactory. If not, it's well worth seeking medical help before you end up in separate houses (or get serious complaints from the neighbours).

> 'Laugh and the world laughs with you, snore and you sleep alone.'
> _____
>
> Anthony Burgess, *Inside Mr Enderby*, 1968

Perhaps your journey to work winds you up, setting you off on the wrong foot. Leaving the house half an hour earlier could make all the difference. You might even be able to change your hours to avoid peak travel times. Consider using a different route, or changing to public transport, or car sharing or, if at all possible, walking to work.

If you get very edgy at work, your stress diary may help you put your finger on the main causes of tension. It could be one person who irks you. Sometimes a frank discussion will sort things out. On the other hand, working practices could be at fault; you may need the help of your union to deal with that.

The feeling that you have no control over the way you work can be very stressful. Remember that studies have consistently shown a link between lack of job control and coronary heart disease. It's not in anyone's interests to have a demoralised work force with a poor sickness record. The scientific evidence suggests that workers should be given some say in decisions about their work. You are not powerless. A healthy and contented team is a productive team, and everyone wants that.

With any problem, apply the **ABC** of problem solving:

Avoid	*Can I avoid the problem?*	(Avoid rush-hour travel)
Bend	*Can I bend my ways?*	(Wear ear-plugs/get in the bathroom earlier)
Change	*Can I change the problem?*	(Change work practices with the help of the union)

You won't find a perfect solution to every problem but a strategy to handle it better will reduce stress. Don't try to solve everything yourself: the support of friends, self-help groups or professionals can make all the difference.

Social skills training

Have you ever bought a set of encyclopaedias you couldn't afford because the salesman was so persuasive? Allowing yourself to be pushed into unwise decisions can cause a lot of stress. Assertiveness training helps people reduce stress by taking more control of their lives.

Being assertive does not mean being aggressive. Indeed, you will be far more effective if you are calm and polite but unshakeable.

This is one aspect of social skills training. Some people have serious problems when it comes to communicating and dealing with others; they need the special help of a clinical psychologist to learn these skills, but we all have room for improvement.

Do you accept another piece of Auntie Mabel's suet pudding against your better judgement? Many of us become overburdened with commitments because we don't like to say "No". Assertiveness training is founded on learning to value yourself. Role-play is used to practise self-assertion – for example, when complaining about a bad meal at a restaurant.

Sex

Satisfying sex soothes stress. Could sex actually save your life? Of course, if it weren't for sex, you wouldn't have a life to start with but does sexual activity prolong life? The Christmas 1997 edition of the *British Medical Journal* carried a paper by Davey Smith and colleagues suggesting that it does. In their study on middle-aged men, the researchers found the death rate to be 50% lower in men declaring frequent sex (twice a week or more) than in those reporting infrequent sex (less than monthly). Both total mortality and mortality from coronary heart disease were lower among those reporting more frequent sex.

Before I'm held responsible for a national earth tremor, or the inevitable baby boom to follow, I must point out that there are many unanswered questions about this study. It would be quite wrong to assume that frequent sex was the *cause* of the lower death rate. For a start, we would expect older men to have sex less frequently than younger men; they are also more likely to die. Again, being depressed, or extremely stressed, will increase your risk of dying: it will also put you right off sex. Further research is needed here.

In the meantime, let me recommend quality sex, in the safe setting of a committed relationship, as a good stress reliever. On the other hand, an extramarital affair increases stress: research has shown that it places a much greater strain on the cardiovascular system; it could provoke coronary death in those at risk.

Stroking a pet

Well, perhaps not the stick insects, but the companionship and physical contact of an animal friend is an effective stress reliever. Research has shown that single people who have had a heart attack tend to live longer if they have a pet. (A hamster is cheaper than a wife and doesn't answer back.)

Saving time

If only you could – save time, I mean. You know, the way you do with money. "I don't feel like spending this time at the moment," you could say. "I'll put it in the time bank for now and spend it when I feel more motivated."

You could have a time box on the mantelpiece for the odd spare minute; it would soon mount up. And when something had to be done urgently, you'd have all the time you needed put by. As long as you saved time sensibly, and didn't waste time, you could always take time out for leisure activities – just when it suited you.

Sadly, you can't. If you are in full-time employment and have a family to look after, there are never enough hours in the day. If you are unemployed, there may be too many. Both extremes are stressful. The answer is good time management. Here are some simple guidelines.

- Write down a plan for the day, ideally on the previous evening. (I know: you'd write it on a piece of paper.)

- Even if you are unemployed, a structured day is helpful; setting and achieving goals is satisfying.

- If you have too much to do, sort out the priorities. Not achieving goals is stressful.

  1. Some tasks may be important but not at all urgent. Work out the deadlines and plan to do the urgent jobs first.

  2. On reflection, some tasks are unimportant and can be scrapped altogether.

  3. Non-urgent tasks can be extremely important, even though you can't fix a date for the deadline. Making a will is an example; the deadline is very real. Include these tasks in your overall plan or they will always be squeezed out by the urgent things.

  4. Are there jobs on your list that would be better done by someone else? Delegate where appropriate. Hand back the jobs you should never have taken on.

- Make sure you allow enough time to complete each task on your plan for the day. Include time for travel, for the unexpected phone call and for appointments running late.

- Remember that all the routine jobs, such as dealing with your mail, take time and must be allowed for in your plan.

- Set aside time for relaxation and for physical exercise.

- Sometimes you can make better use of time by doing two things at once. While using your exercise bike, you can read a book. I can even play piggy-in-the-middle with my children as I pedal – but I have to put the book down for that. (I prefer to use a soft toy, rather than a ball, as it doesn't bounce all over the room – and it's easier for me to catch.)

- Include time for social activities: playing with your children or grandchildren; sharing with your partner; or, if you live alone, having a drink with a friend or making a social phone call.

- Live a day at a time but have one eye on the longer term so those vital things that aren't urgent don't get left out.

Talk

'The telephone is a good way to talk to people without having to offer them a drink.'

Fran Lebowitz, *Interview* magazine, 1978

Talking it through

Have you ever thought that there's no point in talking about a problem because talking doesn't change anything? It isn't true, is it? It can be surprisingly helpful to talk things through with a friend. Even if your friend can't offer a solution, just talking about it helps to sort things out in your own mind.

And so many relationships break down because people allow feelings to fester instead of talking openly, honestly and kindly to each other. The most important words in the language are not, in fact, 'fatty acid' or 'antioxidant' but "I'm sorry" and "I forgive you". Like all words, their power lies in the sincerity of the speaker.

Taking advice

Whatever the problem you are trying to cope with, there is bound to be a voluntary organisation or self-help group that can give you advice. There are always people who have worked through the same problem; they can be a great support.

Don't forget your local Citizens Advice Bureau. And if you are one of the many thousands of people sinking in debt, debt counselling can help you to surface again. Couples who can't resolve their differences should make a date with Relate, the relationship counselling service.

Talking therapy

Talking things over with friends and colleagues, and taking advice from those in the know, is likely to help. Some problems, however, need more formal talking therapy and perhaps the expertise of a psychiatrist, a psychologist or a psychotherapist. Your doctor will point you in the right direction.

If you follow this plan, you can **REST** assured that stress will be kept in its proper place.

ACTION POINTS

◆ Learn and practise relaxation. This section shows you how

◆ Replace negative thoughts with positive ones

◆ Develop an interesting hobby

◆ Get regular sleep; avoid excess caffeine and alcohol

◆ Exercise daily

◆ Identify your main sources of stress and apply the ABC of problem solving

◆ Plan your day (see 'Saving time')

◆ Talk and listen to the important people in your life

Chapter 23

The truth about women

'A woman who strives to be like a man lacks ambition.'

Graffito, New York, 1982

◆ Heart disease kills 5 times more women than breast cancer in the UK

◆ Over 50,000 women die of heart disease each year

◆ Before the menopause, the low rates of heart disease in women are linked with the 'pear' pattern of fat storage, higher HDL and lower triglyceride levels

◆ Low iron stores in women before the menopause may reduce free radical attack on artery walls

---

Inspired by the suffragettes in the early 20th century, women have protested their right to equality with men ever since. Their demands do not extend to an equal share of heart disease, any more than men have sought a fairer spread of breast cancer. After all, heart disease is a male affliction, is it not? Many women reading this book are concerned about a husband, partner, brother, son or father rather than themselves. And as P.J. O'Rourke observed, "... there is one thing women can never take away from men. We die sooner."

For all that, the truth is that every year in the UK many more women die of coronary heart disease than of breast cancer – about five times as many. Heart disease kills over 50,000 women a year in the UK. No other single disease takes so many female lives. And yet, many people, including some health professionals, see it as a male disease.

True it is that when you hear of a tragic early death – a friend or neighbour struck down by a heart attack before the age of 50 – it is far more likely to be a man. Occasionally, you do hear the shocking news that a very young woman has died of a heart attack; it usually turns out that she was a heavy smoker. On average, heart disease strikes women a decade later than men.

Mind you, the seed of heart disease is sown in childhood, or even before (see Chapter 15), so it's never too early to adopt a healthy lifestyle.

Perhaps you're thinking: "Well, I've got to die of something; it might as well be a heart attack. I'd prefer that to a slow death from cancer." I agree that, given the available options, a quick heart attack seems quite desirable – especially if you could arrange to slip away in your sleep. But we can't make these arrangements and, rather than a quick death, heart disease could bring 20 years of disability. Don't invite it.

Why do women lag behind?

Men often complain that women drive too slowly. They certainly die more slowly – in the sense that, on average, they get round to it later in life than men, and not in the sense that they take longer to do it when the time comes. You could postulate a direct connection between their patterns of driving and dying. I mean, apart from the obvious point about driving more safely, you could focus on the fact that the main reason why women live longer is that they get heart disease later. Could it be that women lag behind both in driving and dying simply because type A behaviour is more prevalent in men behind the wheel, increasing their coronary risk?

It's an attractive theory but it doesn't fully explain all the facts. What about the main risk factors for heart disease? Perhaps lifestyle differences can explain why heart disease hits women a few years later than men. Prepare for a shock. As a sweeping generalisation, compared with men, women:

- Eat more saturated fat (as a percentage of calories);
- Eat less fibre;
- Are less active.

With the passing years, compared with men, women are more likely to:

- Become obese;
- Develop diabetes;
- Have raised cholesterol levels;
- Have high blood pressure.

Once we could at least have pointed to the lower rates of smoking among women. Not now. As the proportion of UK adults smoking cigarettes has dropped, women have clung to their percentage and have just about achieved equality with men – as if bidding for an equal share of smoking-related diseases. And more teenaged girls than boys now smoke.

With all these features pushing up the risk in women, is it not surprising that, on average, they get their heart disease a decade after men? What factors can we find to help explain why women lag behind? Here are some more generalisations about women that will count in their favour:

- HDL-cholesterol levels are higher;
- Triglyceride levels are lower;
- They are more pear-shaped.

We all have some body fat and women have more than men. As well as being an energy store it provides us with thermal insulation like the lagging on a hot-water cylinder. Although most women are very sensitive about the amount of 'lagging' round their bottom and thighs, it's much safer to carry it there; fat round the tummy (central obesity) brings a much higher coronary risk. Now perhaps you understand why women lag behind.

The lipid link

What lies at the bottom of the link between lower body fat and a lower risk of heart disease? Why do those who carry fat higher up have a higher risk? Studies attempting to get to the bottom of this mystery have found that carrying your fat lower down goes together with lower triglyceride levels and higher levels of HDL-cholesterol. This is the typical female pattern. Having a fat tummy – the classic male shape – is linked with the reverse lipid profile (high triglycerides and low HDL-cholesterol), which is much more hazardous for the heart.

The waist–hip ratio (see pages 163–4), which is low if you're pear-shaped and high if you're apple shaped, is related to the lipid profile and risk of heart disease.

Research has also uncovered a link between insulin resistance (in which the body has to produce higher levels of insulin to get a response) and central obesity with high triglycerides and low HDL-cholesterol. When the pancreas is unable to produce enough insulin, or the response to insulin is so poor that blood glucose levels rise, the result is diabetes. Women who develop diabetes as they grow older are often found to have:

- The 'male' body shape with a high waist–hip ratio;
- Raised triglyceride levels;
- Low HDL-cholesterol levels.

These women have also adopted the male risk of heart disease.

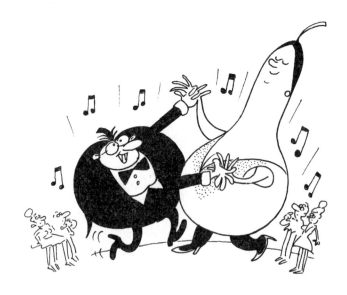

"They say opposites attract."

Don't forget your change

It may be all too easy to walk away from a shop without your change but, for many women, hot flushes and sweats are the frequent reminders that make the change of life unforgettable. This time in a woman's life, during which the ovaries are winding down and a variety of symptoms can result from falling oestrogen levels, is known as the climacteric or perimenopause. The menopause is the point in time when the periods actually stop – or the last menstrual period – but climacteric symptoms can go on for a long time before and after that. Even those fortunate women who sail through the climacteric without any symptoms should not forget that the change is profound.

As oestrogen levels fall, various metabolic changes follow:

- LDL-cholesterol rises at the menopause;

- HDL-cholesterol falls, starting a few years before the last period;

- Changes in fibrinogen and Factor VII make the blood clot more easily.

These changes will all increase the risk of heart disease. However, the idea that the number of deaths due to heart disease *suddenly* increases at the menopause is not correct. There continues to be a steady rise in risk with increasing age.

The Iron Lady?

To leave the role of Prime Minister meant a huge change for Mrs Thatcher, but she had this comfort: her period in office was history – safe in the archives for ever. At the change of life, you have some consolation: your period is now history; you no longer experience the monthly bleed that sapped your strength; your risk of anaemia recedes and your store of iron builds up. But this inner store of strength could make a surprising contribution to your fortunes. It could result in more free radicals (see Chapter 8). Perhaps the slump in oestrogen secretion is the crucial change that pushes up your risk of heart disease. Even so, the danger from free radicals should not be overlooked. Attacking from within, like political rebels reacting to that iron hand, they damage arteries – those vital channels of support – starting a process that could prove fatal.

We all need iron. When you are young, you may lose so much with your periods that you need a supplement to help you to avoid anaemia. After the menopause you can normally obtain all the iron you need from your food, and you'd do well to give iron supplements a miss unless specifically advised by your doctor to take one. Iron shortage can crop up in old age as a result of a poor diet.

◆ Countries with high rates of heart disease in men have high rates in women too; the same risk factors affect both sexes

◆ Angina is as common in women as in men

◆ Women with heart disease are less likely than men to be correctly diagnosed

---

Heart disease in women

Heart disease is killing an alarming number of women in the UK. In fact, we're right near the top of an international league table – nothing to be proud of in this case.

When we compare the death rates for heart disease in men and women in different countries, several points stand out:

- The death rates are much lower in some countries than in others. For example, the problem in Japan is a tiny fraction of that in Scotland.

- In all countries, the death rates for women are lower than for men.

- Countries with high rates of heart disease in men have high rates in women too; the international rank order for men and women is similar.

- **Women** in the UK have **higher** death rates than the **men** in Japan, France and Spain.

Women are different from men. In particular, they get off to a good start with the protection that oestrogen gives them against heart disease. Comparing rates of heart disease in different countries tells us something very important: high rates in men go together with high rates in women; the rate in women always reflects the rate in men (Figure 14). Clearly, the same risk factors affect both men and women. The very low cholesterol levels in Japan make heart disease uncommon in both sexes. In Scotland, high levels of the risk factors result in high death rates in women as well as men.

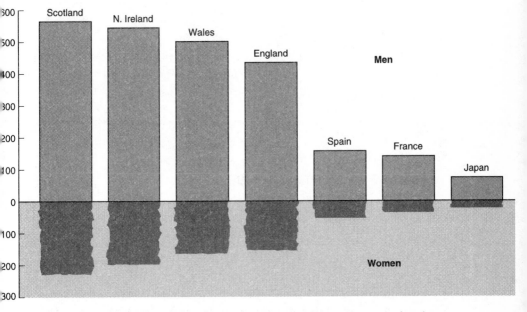

Figure 14 Death rates for heart disease. This chart is like a row of buildings on the water's edge – from the skyscraper full of heart disease victims in Scotland down to the single-storey building in Japan. In every country, the rate of deaths from heart disease in women is a reflection of the rate in men.

This is a vital observation. Even though so much of the research into heart disease has been done on men, we can be certain that women have everything to gain from the advice in this book.

Women who develop coronary heart disease are most likely to get angina. In fact, angina is as common in women as it is in men. Heart attacks occur more frequently in men. Mind you, women often have 'silent' heart attacks: the heart muscle becomes scarred without the normal symptoms of a heart attack.

Women with coronary heart disease actually have a rather worse prognosis than men with the disease. This is partly because the women will, on average, be older and more of them will have complications such as diabetes. It may also have something to do with the widespread myth that heart disease is a male problem. Research has shown that women with heart disease are less likely than men to be diagnosed and treated – even when the symptoms are the same.

◆ Oestrogen replacement therapy relieves symptoms of the change and, when used for long enough, protects against osteoporosis and possibly heart disease

◆ Oestrogen therapy is not suitable for men

◆ Unless a woman has had a hysterectomy, HRT includes progestogen to protect the womb against cancer

◆ Progestogen may undermine some beneficial effects of oestrogen on the circulation

---

Hormone Replacement Therapy

Oestrogen and progesterone – nature's double act

In nature, the opposing actions of these two female hormones produced by the ovaries are finely balanced to regulate the reproductive cycle. After the menopause when the ovaries stop working, reproduction is not an issue (but it might be if a woman ignores the advice to use some form of contraception for a year after the menopause as freak ovulation can occur). At this stage in life, it is the oestrogen that may be sorely missed.

Hormone replacement therapy (HRT) aims to replace the missing oestrogen. If oestrogen is given on its own to a woman who still has her womb, the lining of the womb (endometrium) grows thicker and the risk of cancer (endometrial carcinoma) is increased. This was a problem with early versions of HRT but modern preparations reduce the risk by including a progestogen. (A progestogen is a synthetic version of the natural hormone, progesterone.) If you have had a hysterectomy, you can safely use oestrogen by itself.

Why replace what nature has taken away?

The most effective treatment for women with symptoms of oestrogen deficiency – such as hot flushes, sweats and vaginal dryness – is oestrogen. The natural oestrogens (e.g. oestradiol) used for HRT appear to be safer than the more powerful synthetic oestrogen, ethinyloestradiol, used in the oral contraceptive pill.

Apart from the relief of unpleasant perimenopausal symptoms, another big benefit of taking HRT is the prevention of osteoporosis. This condition, which particularly affects women after the menopause, gradually weakens the bones and often results in fractures. Information from the Framingham study suggests that oestrogen needs to be taken for at least seven years to have a lasting effect on bone strength.

Is HRT good for the heart?

Over the years, a number of large-scale observational studies have concluded that women who take oestrogen after the menopause are less likely to suffer from heart disease than those who don't. Overall, it looked as though women taking HRT enjoyed a 50% reduction in the risk of heart disease.

The Nurses' Health Study monitored many thousands of female nurses in the 1970s. The risk of heart disease in those who were taking oestrogen at the time of the survey was only 30% of the risk in those who had never taken it. Women who had used oestrogen therapy in the past had a 70% risk compared with those who had never done so.

The natural conclusion was that HRT protected the heart. But the problem with these observational studies is that the women who were prescribed HRT might have been healthier in the first place. For a start, health conscious women were more likely to request oestrogen replacement. And a doctor who suspected that HRT could increase risks (like the Pill) would be less likely to prescribe it for a woman with obvious risk factors (such as high blood pressure or obesity).

The only way to eliminate bias of this sort is to conduct huge randomised controlled trials. (These are known as 'prospective' as opposed to 'observational' studies.) The first results from such investigations have caused a few shock waves.

The Women's Health Initiative (WHI) study in America published some findings in 2002. This was a properly controlled trial to investigate the effects of HRT in 16,608 women (aged 50–79) with no history of heart disease. Instead of confirming that the women on HRT were protected from heart attacks, it reported a few extra heart attacks and strokes among those taking oestrogen together with progestogen. (There were about seven extra heart attacks in every 10,000 women taking HRT for one year.)

Another prospective study, dubbed HERS and published in 1998, examined the effects of HRT on women who already had heart disease. HERS stands for Heart and Estrogen progestin Replacement Study ('Estrogen' being the American spelling). In this investigation, the women who were taking HRT had just as many heart attacks as the women who weren't. A closer look reveals that the risk actually went up in the first year of taking HRT and reduced after that. Perhaps starting HRT was linked with an increase in blood clots before a slow protection against the build-up of fatty deposits could show up.

Why should HRT protect against heart disease?

The original idea that oestrogen could protect women from heart disease came from the observation that heart disease is rare before the menopause. But, as we have seen, the risk of heart disease doesn't abruptly shoot up at the menopause; it rises steadily with age.

Observational studies showing that women on oestrogen replacement therapy had lower rates of heart disease seemed to confirm the protective effect of oestrogen. Now, however, the disappointing results from randomised prospective studies have cast considerable doubt on the idea that oestrogen protects the heart.

While these latest investigations have raised doubts, there is certainly no place for dogma just yet.

The HERS and WHI studies both used oestrogen with progestogen. We know that progestogen, which is so important for protection of the womb, could undermine the beneficial effects of oestrogen on the circulation. In the early observational studies, women were taking oestrogen by itself. The WHI study also included women on oestrogen only (those who have had a hysterectomy do not need the progestogen) and results from this part of the trial are expected in 2005. It must also be remembered that several different types and doses of progestogen are used in HRT; we do not know yet whether the findings of the HERS and WHI studies (which both used 0.625 mg conjugated equine oestrogen plus 2.5 mg medroxyprogesterone) will apply to other HRT formulations.

More research is needed. In the meantime, a number of observations suggest that replacing natural oestrogen after the
menopause ought to protect against heart disease:

- Atherosclerosis, the process that clogs up our arteries,
  can be prevented in animals by giving them oestrogen.

- Oestrogen therapy in women has been shown to raise
  HDL-cholesterol and lower LDL-cholesterol.

- A great deal of research has shown that oestrogen can
  relax artery walls and improve blood flow.

It may be that the weak natural oestrogens in soya protein,
which seem to be good for the prostate glands of Japanese men,
are also helping Japanese women to avoid hot flushes and osteoporosis. What part, I wonder, do these food oestrogens play in the
heart protection that is linked with the Japanese diet?

Pause, O men

If oestrogen does have these positive effects on women after the
menopause, perhaps men should take it too! After all, they don't
have a womb so they wouldn't need the progestogen; maybe they
have even more to gain. They also have quite a lot to lose – if they
grow breasts, for example. In 1973, the Coronary Drug Project
Research Group set up an extraordinary clinical trial to compare
four different cholesterol-lowering treatments in men, including
two very high-dose oestrogen treatments. The trial was hampered
by the number of men who dropped out when they developed
breasts. The impotence wasn't very popular either.

Any more bad news?

I haven't given you all the good news yet. In addition to treating
symptoms of the change and protecting bones against osteoporosis and fractures, HRT has been shown consistently to reduce
the risk of developing cancer of the large bowel. There is also some
suggestion that it can protect against Alzheimer's disease but the
evidence for this is not very strong.

Before I leave the subject, though, I must say a little more about
the risks of HRT; you need this information to decide whether you
want to take it and, if you do, for how long.

Does HRT cause breast cancer?

Doctors have been trying to answer this question for many years. Some researchers have reported an increased incidence of breast cancer after long-term use of HRT; others haven't confirmed it. One of the problems is that breast cancer is all too common: up to 10% of women suffer breast cancer at some stage in their lives. Clearly, most women who get breast cancer while taking HRT would have got it anyway.

Following recent research, doctors are now agreed that more cases of breast cancer arise among women who take HRT for more than five years (Table 22).

Think of a group of 1000 women aged 50 who are not using HRT. Over the next 20 years, 45 of those women will have breast cancer diagnosed.

Now think of another group of 1000 women aged 50 who start taking HRT, and continue to take it for many years. After 20 years there will be the 45 cases of breast cancer that would have occurred without HRT. Once the group has been taking HRT for just 5 years, some extra breast cancers will arise. You could expect 2 extra cases of cancer after 5 years, 6 after 10 years and 12 after 15 years.

Table 22 *Extra* breast cancers in women on HRT (in addition to the 45 cases in 20 years per 1000 women not taking HRT)

Length of time HRT taken (years)	Number of cases (per 1000 women)
5	2
10	6
15	12

Five years after stopping HRT, the extra risk of getting breast cancer disappears: your risk becomes the same as it would have been if you had never used HRT.

The Million Women Study published in the *Lancet* in 2003 confirmed that the risk of breast cancer with long-term use of HRT is significantly higher when oestrogen is combined with progestogen than when oestrogen is taken on its own.

Breast cancers linked with use of HRT appear to be easier to treat. In general, the prognosis is better than it is when the disease strikes a woman who doesn't take HRT.

Does HRT cause deep vein thrombosis?

It's important for you to get it clear that we are not talking about arteries here, or all my explanation will be in vain and you'll get very confused.

You will remember that a heart attack results from a blood clot in an *artery* supplying the heart (coronary thrombosis). Whether HRT makes this more or less likely to happen is a complicated question which is still under investigation. It is clear, however, that the oral contraceptive pill does slightly raise the risk of thrombosis in an artery (especially if you are a woman aged over 35 and you smoke).

It has also been known for many years that, in some women, the contraceptive pill can trigger thrombosis in veins. Deep vein thrombosis in a leg causes painful swelling of the calf. There is a risk of pulmonary embolism in which a clot travels up to the lungs causing chest pain and breathlessness: a large pulmonary embolus may be fatal.

We know that the natural oestrogens in HRT are safer than the pill and for some time it was not clear whether HRT increased the chances of having a deep vein thrombosis. Several scientific papers published in 1996 and 1997 have clarified this: taking HRT does raise your risk of getting a deep vein thrombosis but the risk remains low.

The studies suggested that while a woman is taking HRT, she is about three times more likely to have a deep vein thrombosis. As soon as she stops HRT, the increased risk disappears. One study concluded that the extra risk was present only in the first year of taking HRT. It may be that HRT unmasks a tendency to suffer from deep vein thrombosis; if you are susceptible, it is most likely to come to light within the first year of taking HRT.

Some women are much more likely to get a deep vein thrombosis and this should be taken into account when deciding whether to use HRT. These features would raise the risk of thrombosis in a vein:

- Being obese;
- Having severe varicose veins;
- Having a significant past history of deep vein thrombosis;
- Having a significant family history of deep vein thrombosis.

In some cases (for example, if you have had a deep vein thrombosis in the past) it is helpful for the doctor to arrange a special blood test (thrombophilia screen) to see whether your blood clots too easily.

Major surgery, or trauma such as a road traffic accident, and prolonged bed-rest will temporarily increase the risk of deep vein thrombosis.

Should I take HRT?

If you are suffering perimenopausal symptoms such as hot flushes, HRT could make life a lot easier. You are likely to need it for at least a year. If you use it for less than five years, you will not significantly increase your risk of breast cancer.

Vaginal dryness is a common symptom of oestrogen deficiency but, if this is your only symptom, there is no need to treat the whole body with HRT: oestrogen cream or pessaries can be placed directly into the vagina.

To protect your bones you would need to take HRT for longer. This is all the more important if you have an early menopause; if your periods stop at the age of 40, you can take HRT for 10 years before you start thinking about the usual risks of postmenopausal hormone replacement. Your risk of osteoporosis will also be increased by:

- A family history of osteoporosis;

- Taking steroids for over 6 months;

- Six months without periods (before the menopause);

- Thyroid, liver or kidney disease;

- A low calcium intake;

- Too much alcohol;

- Smoking.

Taking regular aerobic exercise and eating plenty of calcium-rich foods (such as low-fat dairy products) will help to protect your bones.

You may find it difficult to decide whether it's worth taking on an increased risk of breast cancer to reduce the risk of osteoporosis.

If very close relatives of yours have had breast cancer, you need to be particularly cautious about using HRT for more than five years; discuss this with your doctor. Sometimes the decision becomes easier after a scan to assess bone mineral density; you may find out that your risk of osteoporosis is very low or very high.

What if you've already been treated for breast cancer? You may then be advised that HRT is too risky for you. But breast cancers are not all the same and there are cases where the specialist is quite happy for a woman to take HRT when the cancer has been treated. This is a matter for individual advice from a specialist. Sometimes 'phytoestrogens' (plant oestrogens) are recommended for women who can't take HRT. Eating plenty of soya, which is rich in plant oestrogens, certainly seems to help Japanese women and they enjoy low rates of breast cancer.

So, if you are suffering from symptoms such as hot flushes and night sweats, or if you have an increased risk of osteoporosis, HRT could be very beneficial. The important thing is to see your doctor so that the risks and benefits can be carefully weighed up in your particular case. If you opt for HRT, this decision should be reviewed at least once a year.

Sadly, on current evidence, HRT cannot be recommended as a way of preventing heart disease. Research continues. In the meantime, don't forget that this book is full of other things you can do to protect your heart – and most of them will reduce your risk of breast cancer too.

◆ **HRT is used to treat symptoms and to prevent osteoporosis**

◆ **Currently, HRT is not recommended for prevention of heart disease**

◆ **HRT helps to protect against bowel cancer and possibly Alzheimer's disease**

◆ **Taking HRT can increase the risk of deep vein thrombosis and breast cancer**

◆ **The balance of benefits and risks should be discussed with a doctor and reviewed annually**

Chapter 24

Assessing your risk

'In America any boy may become President and I suppose
it's just one of the risks he takes!'

Adlai Stevenson (1900–65)
Speech in Detroit, 7 October 1952

Risk is a difficult concept. In this book, I talk about reducing your risk of having a heart attack – and about percentage reductions in risk. How do you assess the importance of a risk and decide whether it's worth changing your life for?

We all know that life is full of risks – such as the risk of being run over by a bus. Most of us will push this right out of our mind so we can get on with everyday life. Some will wear clean underwear, just in case. A few will avoid bus routes altogether.

It's easy to lose our sense of proportion, if we ever had one. A powerful TV programme can leave you anxious about being struck by a meteorite – so anxious, in fact, that you smoke your way to a heart attack. If people generally had a good grasp of risk analysis, the National Lottery would be a flop.

Relative risk

It may sound as though this section is on family history – or heart disease in your relations. Not so. *Relative* risk needs to be distinguished from *absolute* risk.

Let's suppose you normally buy one entry for the National Lottery. One week you decide to splash out and buy two. By paying

◆ A huge increase in *relative risk* (e.g. of being hit by a meteorite) may still leave you with a tiny *absolute risk*

◆ The risk of having a heart attack is high to start with when risk factors (such as high blood pressure and cholesterol) are present; doubling the risk by smoking is extremely dangerous

◆ Risk factors don't just add to the risk: they multiply it

◆ Having a high cholesterol level is far more serious if you have high blood pressure and smoke as well

twice as much, you have doubled your chances of winning the jackpot. You have doubled the relative risk of winning – increased it by 100% – but the absolute risk remains so low it's not worth considering. The following week you go wild: you sell your classic collection of Barbie dolls and buy 100 entries. You've purchased a huge increase in your relative risk of winning top prize; it's now 100 times greater than it would have been with your normal outlay. But, contrary to popular delusion, your absolute risk of hitting the jackpot is still so low it isn't worth a second thought.

And if you were to double your girth – become twice as wide – I imagine that your risk of being hit by a small meteorite would more or less double (excluding complications like the fact that you would move more slowly, cover less ground, and be less likely to be in the 'right' place at the 'right' time). Despite this hefty rise in relative risk, however, you'd have a fat chance of hitting the headlines on that count. The absolute risk would be negligible.

By contrast, if your huge weight gain had also doubled your risk of coronary heart disease, a meteoric passage to the obituary column would be all too likely. Our background risk of heart disease is high in the UK. Anything that doubles the risk is significant.

Indeed, if you were now to take up smoking, further doubling this expanded risk, who knows? The next edition of your local paper could carry your obituary. This is how risk factors multiply. The bigger the risk to start with, the more dangerous it is to magnify it.

This is why some people get away with having one high risk factor – such as raised cholesterol. It is also why many others have heart attacks with 'normal' cholesterol levels – well below the national average of 5.9 mmol/l. An overweight, diabetic man of 40, whose mother developed angina at the age of 54, is off to a bad start. Perhaps his cholesterol level and blood pressure are only slightly raised. Now, if he smokes, he's not so much *adding* to his high risk as *multiplying* it. No wonder he is struck down with a heart attack before his 50th birthday when others, with higher cholesterol levels or blood pressures, go on to enjoy their retirement.

If you are at high risk, like this unfortunate man with diabetes, bringing in any unnecessary risk factors can be disastrous. By the same token, you have even more to gain than the low-risk person by making a few changes. Even a modest reduction in your relative risk can make a significant impact on absolute risk.

Like all family doctors, I have patients who are extremely anxious about their blood pressure. And yet they continue to smoke. A modest reduction in blood pressure, combined with giving up smoking, would cut risk more effectively than controlling blood pressure perfectly while ignoring everything else. As risk factors multiply, tackling them all is far more efficient than concentrating on one alone.

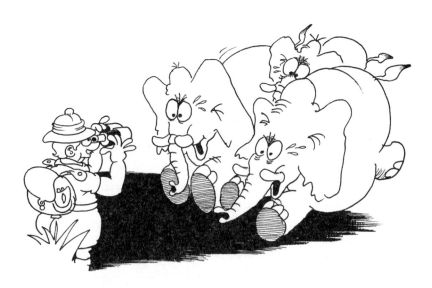

The bigger the risk to start with, the more dangerous it is to magnify it.

◆ If you have a family history of heart disease, it's all the more important to tackle the risk factors you can alter

◆ People with diabetes are more likely to get heart disease; controlling all the risk factors is extra important

◆ Some 'ageing processes' (such as the clogging of arteries and rise in blood pressure) can be prevented by the right lifestyle

Gene genie?

We cannot invoke some supernatural power to change our gene code or our gender. Does that mean that our fate is fixed – our destiny determined in our DNA?

Certainly, we can inherit a high risk of coronary heart disease. If one of your first degree relatives (a parent, brother, sister, son or daughter) developed the disease at a young age (below 50 for a male relative or 55 for a female relative) that gives you a risk factor that you cannot alter. Race, too, could raise your risk. Of the various ethnic groups within the UK population, Asians from the Indian subcontinent are at particularly high risk of heart disease. This seems to be linked with a genetic tendency to insulin resistance and diabetes.

If you're starting off with risk factors like this, which are beyond your control, you may be tempted to give up. What can you do about it anyway? In reality, if nature's dealt you a bad hand, there's everything to play for.

Perhaps you have relatives who developed diabetes in middle age – making them more prone to heart disease. You fear that you are set to suffer the same fate. A good diet and regular exercise could tip the balance in your favour; it might stop you getting diabetes. Even if you do get diabetes, the right lifestyle will limit its effects.

You know how risk factors multiply. You've seen that when the risk is high, changes in relative risk become more important. We have no gene genie (yet). And it doesn't take a genius to see that, when your genes are against you, you have all the more to gain by getting everything else on your side.

The risk factors

We've agreed that you can't do much about your age, sex or family history. You will remember these important risk factors, which are all affected by lifestyle:

- High blood cholesterol;

- High blood pressure;

- Smoking;

- Diabetes;

- Being overweight/obese;

- Lack of exercise.

Looking at the top three will tell you a lot. Supposing there are two men of the same age with no relevant family history. Finding out their cholesterol levels, blood pressures and smoking habits should tell you whether one of them is much more likely to have a heart attack in the next ten years than the other. It would also reveal the major changes needed to reduce that risk.

Simple methods of scoring coronary risk focus on these three top risk factors.

Of course, if one of the two men has diabetes, that will count against him. The metabolic effects of diabetes make heart disease more likely. Subtle changes in clotting factors and blood platelets make it easier for the blood to clot. Blood levels of triglycerides are often raised, while those of HDL-cholesterol are low. Central obesity and high blood pressure are common. Accelerated atherosclerosis may narrow arteries enough to cause angina or a heart attack.

Getting the diet right in diabetes is essential – not just to help control blood sugar but also to protect the arteries. The good news is that, if you have diabetes, you don't have to eat a *special* diet at all. The right diet is the same healthy, balanced diet that we should all be eating. Reducing saturated fat intake helps to prevent blood clots as well as controlling cholesterol. Obtaining more energy from foods high in starch, soluble fibre and mono-unsaturates improves the balance of lipids. Including enough fruit and vegetable provides antioxidants to prevent the oxidation of LDL that leads to atherosclerosis. An adequate intake of oily fish makes platelets less keen to clump together and lowers blood triglyceride levels. Reducing salt consumption helps to keep blood pressure down. I could go on. (No doubt you think I have already.)

In the same way, aerobic exercise, which is so important for all of us, is essential in the management of diabetes. It reduces body fat, keeps up HDL-cholesterol, improves control of blood pressure, and reduces the risk of heart disease.

With a healthy lifestyle, and sometimes a little help from drugs, all the risk factors in this list can be improved.

What about the ones you can't alter? Well, your sex and family history may stay much the same (the latter is more liable to change than the former) but your age is guaranteed to change – for the worse, most readers will think. And, yes, the older you get, the more likely you are to have a heart attack.

Young at heart

The increased risk of coronary heart disease is not the only unwelcome effect of ageing, of course. We'd all like to stop the clock. We can't.

We can stop some of the changes that are just accepted as part of the ageing process. For a start, there's that rise in blood pressure which, you may remember, does not occur in communities that eat very little salt. Then there's the progressive narrowing and hardening of arteries – atherosclerosis – at the heart of Western vascular diseases. We see this insidious process as part and parcel of ageing, but it's quite possible to reach old age with arteries unscathed by atherosclerosis. Some people in the Third World do so. And antioxidants, which have a range of 'anti-ageing' actions, play a vital role in fighting off the ravages of time on arteries as well.

"You're as old as you feel," they say. Many people feel just fine until the silent ageing of their heart becomes apparent. Exercising, not smoking, and eating as this book advises will do a lot to keep you young at heart.

ACTION POINT

◆ Have a well person check to find out your risk factors. You will probably be able to arrange this at your doctor's surgery

The Dundee Coronary Risk-Disk

This is nothing to do with the coronary risk attached to eating fruit cake (which is very low if you follow the recipe in Chapter 27). It's a sort of circular slide rule designed to estimate someone's risk of having a heart attack (Figure 15). The Risk-Disk was developed in Dundee by Professor Hugh Tunstall-Pedoe (try saying that with your mouth full of Dundee cake). Little used now, this ingenious device illustrates how a simple risk score can help people to improve their lifestyle.

A doctor or practice nurse using the Risk-Disk would enter the patient's level of smoking, blood pressure and cholesterol to obtain a relative risk score. If you were the patient, you would be given a rank number between 1 and 100. This allows you to picture yourself standing in a queue of people of the same age and sex, all waiting for a coronary heart attack – as if waiting for a bus. If you're right at the back of the queue, with a number near 100, you're at very low risk: just as you might never get on the bus, you may well escape a heart attack. If you're near the front of the queue with a number between 1 and 10, you're at very high risk compared with others of the same age and sex.

I think this is a very useful picture. It allows you to change your smoking habits, blood pressure and cholesterol level and see yourself move

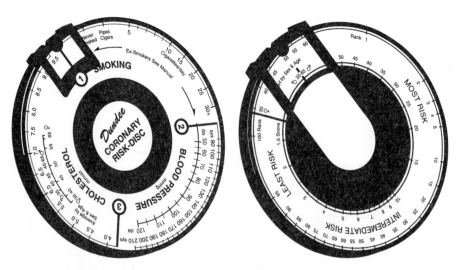

Figure 15 The Dundee Coronary Risk-Disk (Courtesy of Professor H Tunstall-Pedoe).

towards the back of the queue. From the doctor's viewpoint, it's true of heart attacks, as it is of buses, that you wait for ages and then three come at once.

Note that the Dundee Risk-Disk does not tell you your *absolute* risk. An old man near the back of his queue will be at greater risk than a young woman near the back of hers. It does not attempt to state the percentage probability that you will have a heart attack in the next five years.

A doctor will routinely check your smoking habits and your blood pressure; checking cholesterol levels is a little more expensive and involved. The Dundee Risk-Disk could be used to provide a 'provisional rank' when the cholesterol level was unknown. This could even help when deciding whether the cholesterol should be measured or not.

Should I have my cholesterol checked?

By now you understand, I hope, how unhelpful it is when cholesterol gets all the attention. Sometimes people quote their 'cholesterol number' as if it were a complete statement of coronary risk. Knowing how risk factors interact with each other, you will want to avoid focussing all your attention on any one risk factor.

Even so, blood cholesterol level is a key risk factor. We've seen how the very low levels of cholesterol in Japan are responsible for low rates of heart disease. So, shouldn't everyone have a blood test?

Taking and processing blood samples from the whole population would use up an awful lot of time and money. Most experts agree that this would not be the best use of our limited resources. After all, we know that the average cholesterol level for the population is too high and that the great majority of people have a lot of room for improvement.

We have an epidemic of heart disease on our hands and you don't need to measure all those cholesterol levels to see that we desperately need the population to change its ways. If the nation were really to take the message of this book to heart, it would transform the health of our nation and relieve our National Health Service of crippling expenditure on diseases of the heart and circulation (not to mention cancer).

Healthy living is vital for all of us, whatever our cholesterol may be.

If we don't measure any cholesterol levels, though, we won't identify those people who have special lipid problems requiring medical
help. About two in every thousand people have familial hypercholesterolaemia and it takes drugs as well as lifestyle changes to save
them from disaster.

You should certainly get your lipids measured if you have any
of these problems:

- Angina or a previous heart attack;

- Blocked arteries in the legs causing pain on walking
  (claudication);

- Diabetes;

- High blood pressure;

- Fatty lumps under the skin/round tendons (xanthomas),
  fatty deposits in the eyelids (xanthelasmas), or an opaque
  ring round the cornea of the eye under the age of 50
  (juvenile arcus) any of which *may* be a sign of an
  inherited cholesterol problem;

- Family history of high cholesterol levels;

- Family history of coronary heart disease (in a close male
  relative under 55 or close female relative under 65).

Having said all this, I believe one of the main benefits of measuring cholesterol is that it can provide motivation. There's nothing
quite like a cholesterol reading of, say, 7.2 mmol/l for kick-starting
that dietary overhaul that you've been meaning to get round to for
the last few years. By the same token, it is not at all helpful if a
'normal' cholesterol result reassures you that you needn't bother
about a good diet or healthy lifestyle. Remember that, like blood
pressure measurement, because of biological and technical
variations, two readings are better than one.

If you are already taking enough interest in the health of your
heart to be reading this book, your doctor will doubtless be willing to
arrange to check your cholesterol.

◆ The benefit of lowering cholesterol has been underestimated and a 10% cholesterol reduction could mean a 30% drop in risk

◆ An APT diet has major benefits for the circulation, reducing atherosclerosis, pressure and thrombosis – the three big players in the run-up to a heart attack

◆ Cholesterol is only part of the story and two diets might be equally effective at lowering cholesterol but have different effects on risk

APT to underestimate?

There is agreement among experts that the benefit of lowering cholesterol has probably been underestimated. It is generally considered that a 1% reduction in cholesterol results in a 2% reduction in coronary risk – so that, if you reduced your cholesterol level by 10%, you would reduce your risk by 20%. In reality, a risk reduction of 3% for every 1% drop in cholesterol level is probably nearer the mark (that is, 30% reduction in risk for a 10% fall in cholesterol level).

And don't forget that if a change in diet produces a drop in cholesterol, that's only part of the story. The artery-clogging process of atherosclerosis will be affected, not only by the balance of lipids (LDL-cholesterol, HDL-cholesterol and triglycerides), but also by the supply of antioxidants and of folic acid (which lowers homocysteine levels).

The build-up of cholesterol on artery walls is not a passive process like fat clogging up a drain pipe. Artery linings are constantly being damaged and repaired. The importance of inflammation in the growth of fatty plaques is becoming clearer. A blood test for something called C-reactive protein (CRP) is a measure of inflammation. Raised CRP levels (perhaps reflecting inflammation in artery walls) are linked with higher rates of heart disease. No doubt, lots of factors in our diet (such as omega-3 fatty acids from fish oils) influence this inflammation.

Again, the significance of thrombosis is apt to be neglected: heart-attack risk is greatly reduced by cutting the risk of clots forming in the circulation. Your level of the blood-clotting protein, fibrinogen, seems to be an important coronary risk factor but it is difficult to measure so this is usually done only in research or in very specialised clinics. We know that diet has an important influence on blood clotting through effects on platelets, fibrinogen, factor VII and other clotting factors. The crucial importance of thrombosis is not just that a blood clot in a coronary artery is normally the final cause of a heart attack: thrombosis also plays a part in the gradual growth of cholesterol-laden plaques on artery walls. Of course, arteries that have been narrowed in this way are much more likely to be blocked by a clot.

This is how atherosclerosis and thrombosis work hand in hand to pave the way to a heart attack.

A good diet will protect your heart in many subtle ways that will not show up as a change in total cholesterol. It's possible to imagine two diets that offer quite different levels of protection against heart disease even though they are equally effective at lowering your cholesterol. There are three major ways in which a truly **APT** diet slashes your coronary risk.

Atherosclerosis   – furring up of arteries is slowed down, stopped or reversed!

Pressure   – blood pressure is reduced.

Thrombosis   – blood clots are less likely to form in the circulation.

The balanced, varied, delicious and exciting diet you've been reading about in this book does all these things. Table 23 shows some **apt** dietary changes, which help by holding back the three big players in the long run-up to a heart attack.

Table 23 APT changes in diet

Atherosclerosis	Pressure	Thrombosis
↓ Fat	↓ Fat (weight control)	↓ Fat
↓ Saturates	↓ Sodium	↓ Saturates
→ Mono-unsaturates	↑ Potassium	↑ Fish oils
→ Polyunsaturates	↑ Magnesium	↑ Garlic
↑ Starch	↑ Calcium	Moderate alcohol
↑ Soluble fibre	↓ Alcohol	
↑ Antioxidants	↑ Garlic	
↑ Garlic	↑ Fish oils	
Moderate alcohol		

A ready reckoner of risk

Figure 16 shows a chart that can be used to estimate the risk of having a heart attack within the next 10 years. It is based on information gathered in the Framingham study.

Health professionals use a chart like this (or the computer equivalent) to assess your risk of developing heart disease in the future. This can help to decide whether drugs should be used to reduce the risk by lowering your cholesterol or blood pressure. The chart is not designed for people already suffering from heart disease or those with an inherited high cholesterol level or very high blood pressure; where the risk is known to be that high, drug treatment will be offered anyway.

To use the chart, you need to find out your blood pressure and cholesterol level. You probably already know your age and sex (and whether you smoke or have diabetes)! Only the systolic blood pressure (the top figure) is used for the chart; an average of several readings is always better than one. The chart uses the ratio of total cholesterol to HDL-cholesterol (i.e. your total cholesterol divided by your HDL-cholesterol); but, if you don't know your HDL-cholesterol level, you can assume it's 1.0 and simply use the total cholesterol number.

If you stopped smoking today, congratulations, but you should still read the chart as a smoker. And sometimes people have diabetes without realising it, so it's well worth having a urine test at your doctor's surgery if you haven't done so recently.

Once you're clear whether you should be looking under 'DIABETES' or 'NO DIABETES' in Figure 16, you can find the correct square for your sex, age and smoking habits. Now simply find where a horizontal line from your blood pressure on the left meets a vertical line from your cholesterol ratio at the bottom. The point where the two lines meet will fall within one of the three risk zones. Check the shading of your zone against the key to find out whether your 10-year risk is less than 15%, between 15% and 30% or over 30%.

Your risk doesn't actually leap up once a decade, of course, any more than you suddenly become a year older on your birthday.

Where there is a significant family history of heart disease, the chart may underestimate risk. If a close female relative (mother, sister or daughter) developed coronary heart disease before the

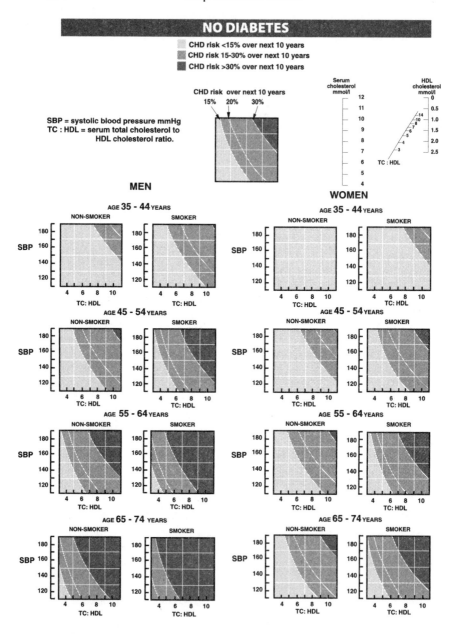

Figure 16 Reading your risks. Find the right section of the chart (according to your sex and whether or not you have diabetes) and select the square that corresponds to your age and smoking habits. Mark the point where a horizontal line from your blood pressure on the left meets a vertical line from your cholesterol ratio at the bottom. Use the key to read your approximate risk of having a heart attack in the next 10 years. © The University of Manchester.

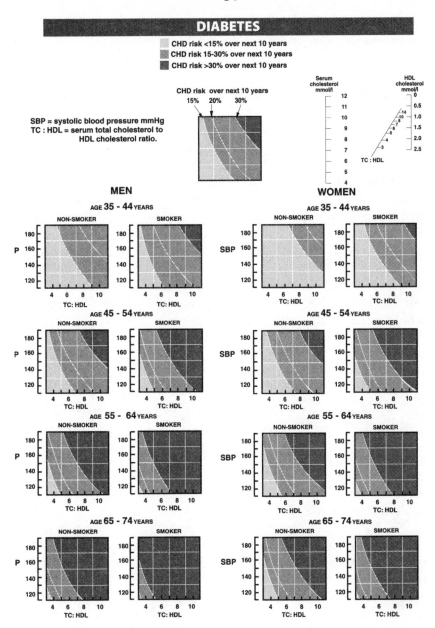

Figure 16 (continued). © The University of Manchester.

age of 65, or a male relative (father, brother or son) before 55, you should multiply your risk score by 1.5.

However high your risk, you can improve it!

A change of heart

A heart transplant is a drastic measure, for people with no other hope. Unless you have a rare kind of heart disease (such as a serious cardiomyopathy) there is a lot you can do to transform the outlook for your heart.

Michael was a 49-year-old bank employee. His wife had been trying to persuade him to have a check-up for some time but it was after a colleague died of a heart attack that Michael came to see me.

He was not a pie-and-chips man. You wouldn't catch him at the greasy spoon. He was well aware that his diet wasn't perfect but he felt he'd made some healthy changes: cooked breakfasts were restricted to weekends; sunflower spread had replaced butter; he would often choose pasta dishes, especially in the staff canteen; chicken was frequently selected in preference to red meat; when convenient, reduced-fat products were included.

In fact, Michael was disappointed that, despite making these changes, his trousers were getting harder to do up. His wife had pointed out that love handles were one thing, but an overhanging balustrade was another.

His 20–30 cigarettes a day had been on the New Year hit list for as many years as he could remember. His busy schedule left no time for regular exercise. There was no history of heart disease in his close family but the sudden death of a colleague, just two years his senior, had really shaken him up.

After a few visits, we established that Michael's average blood pressure was 140/90 mmHg and his average total cholesterol level was 6.9 mmol/l, with an HDL-cholesterol of 0.9 mmol/l. So the ratio of total cholesterol to HDL-cholesterol was 7.7. He did not have diabetes. If you look at Figure 16 you can see that this would have given Michael a 15–20% risk of a heart attack in the following 10 years.

I asked Michael to complete a dietary diary for 7 days. Spurred on particularly, it seemed, by his raised cholesterol level, he and his wife made some really big changes over the following four months. In Table 24 I have shown his entries for just one day on the original diet and, beside it, just one day on his changed diet.

Table 24 Extracts from Michael's dietary diary

	Tuesday (original diet)	**Thursday** (changed diet)
Breakfast	2 cups cafetière coffee (black) 1 slice toast, sunflower spread and marmalade Muesli (probably with coconut)	Shredded Wheat Bitesize with chopped dried apricots, raisins, sliced banana; skimmed milk Instant coffee, skimmed milk
Mid-morning	Coffee, 2 digestive biscuits	Cup of tea, skimmed milk Glass of water
Lunch	Fruit juice Lasagne, small portion chips Treacle tart, ice cream Coffee	2 glasses water Baked beans, 2 slices wholemeal toast (no spread) 1 bowl fruit salad 1 apple Cup of tea, skimmed milk
Afternoon	Cup of tea, whole milk Slice of swiss roll	Glass of water Cup of tea, skimmed milk Banana
Early evening	Bag of crisps (reduced fat)	2 slices wholemeal toast, low-sugar jam (no spread) 2 cups tea, skimmed milk
Dinner	Roast chicken quarter, roast potatoes, cauliflower cheese with 3 glasses red wine Cheese (including reduced-fat cheddar), savoury biscuits, sunflower spread 2 cups cafetière coffee 3 chocolate mints	Salmon steak, broccoli, sweetcorn, peas, jacket potato fat-free garlic and herb dressing (Kraft) 1 glass water 2 glasses red wine Summer pudding (fruit and bread) 1 cup filtered coffee Dates
Late evening	Hot chocolate (whole milk)	Home-made muesli (no coconut), skimmed milk

With the help of the practice nurse, he gave up smoking. By leaving the car at home, and walking to and from the station, he included 40 minutes of brisk walking in his daily routine and bought an exercise bike to use at weekends.

Six months later, Michael told me he didn't feel at all deprived; he was enjoying his food more and feeling generally better. He had lost over one and a half stone in weight. His average blood pressure was now 120/80 and his total cholesterol was down to 5 with an HDL-cholesterol of 1. You will see that his risk of a heart attack in the following 10 years was now well below 15%.

In fact, I am convinced that Michael's real risk reduction is even better than it appears on this chart because he has made so many sound dietary and lifestyle changes that would not necessarily be reflected in this simple score based on the Framingham study.

It just doesn't add up

Imagine a man who, like Michael, makes a series of lifestyle changes to reduce his coronary risk. Taking into account his age and the number of cigarettes he was smoking a day, we estimate that giving up smoking has reduced his risk by 50%. He then takes up an exercise programme that brings him another 50% reduction in coronary risk. Changes in his diet result in a 15% drop in cholesterol level, conferring a risk reduction of at least 30% (probably 45%). If we add these up, we're well over 100% already and there are other factors we haven't even considered yet. If he has removed more than 100% of his original risk, his new risk must be less than zero. It just doesn't add up.

Of course, there's a very basic flaw here. You don't just add up percentage risk reductions to find the new risk. When our man has halved his risk by giving up smoking, it is this new, lower risk that is halved again by his exercise programme.

When it comes to *increasing* your risks, mind you, by changing your lifestyle for the worse, you might end up with a coronary risk six times the one you started with! It's quite simple to *add* more than 100% to your risk; you might add 500%.

When you follow the advice in this book and reduce your coronary risk, your new risk may be a small fraction of the risk you started with, but it will never get down to zero. No matter how radically you change your lifestyle, there will always be some risk attached to being alive.

◆ Simple risk scores are based on the top risk factors – cholesterol, blood pressure, smoking and diabetes

◆ A big reduction in risk may mean a big change in lifestyle but, once you've adapted, your new lifestyle can be more satisfying

◆ You can reduce your risk dramatically, but not down to zero

Chapter 25

If you already have heart disease

'Youth is a period of missed opportunities.'

Cyril Connolly, *Journal 1928–1937*, ed. D. Pryce-Jones, 1983

◆ If you have heart disease already, you have even more to gain by reducing your risk of a future heart attack

◆ Every part of this book will help you to reduce that risk

◆ There is now evidence that, if the right changes are made, narrowed arteries can get wider again; heart disease can be reversed!

It's too late now, isn't it?

If you have already had a heart attack, or suffer from angina, what has a book on *preventing* heart disease got to offer you? Isn't it like offering a breastplate to a man who's been stabbed through the heart?

The truth is that every part of this book – from the bits on chipping away at your relative risk to the chapters on cutting it down dramatically – every part, is vital for you if you have heart disease already.

When disease in the coronary arteries has already made itself known, by a previous heart attack or the onset of angina, the chances of a future heart attack are greatly increased. Because the absolute risk of a heart attack or coronary death is so high, cutting it down by, say, 30% is *even more worthwhile* than it is for someone without heart disease!

You are no longer dealing with the risk that you might one day get heart disease – but, then again, you might not; you are dealing with the certainty that you have heart disease and there is something you can do to halt its progress – or even send it into reverse.

The cynic may think that I'm offering a ray of hope to the desperate (like William Spooner's cousin who thought that a ray of hope was a rope of hay and that he'd just be clutching at straws). No, the information in this book could be your lifeline; it's up to you whether you grasp it or not.

Doctors once thought that the best you could hope for was to slow down the growth of fatty plaques that clog up arteries. We now have good evidence that atheroma can be reversed and arteries can get wider again – especially when the blood cholesterol level is brought down really low. For many people with established heart disease, drug treatment is needed as well as lifestyle changes and I shall deal with that in this chapter.

◆ Drugs can often control the symptoms of angina

◆ In some cases angioplasty is needed to widen a narrowed coronary artery with a balloon

◆ Sometimes a bypass operation is required to get round the blocked sections of the coronary arteries

◆ After surgery, the cholesterol should be kept below 5 mmol/l to reduce the chances of the blockage recurring

Dealing with angina

You may remember from Chapter 1 how angina occurs when the heart's oxygen supply is limited by narrowed coronary arteries.

Drug treatment is used to reduce the workload of the heart while relaxing the coronary arteries, if possible, to improve the balance between work and blood supply. The aim is to control the symptoms as well as possible even if a combination of drugs is needed to achieve this.

Sometimes angina is not controlled adequately by drugs – even when three or four of them are used together. This calls for a change to the plumbing.

Angioplasty involves passing a special catheter into the coronary artery and inflating a balloon at the narrow point to widen it. Usually a stent, which is a short tube made of stainless steel mesh, is inserted to keep the artery open.

In some cases, major surgery is needed to get round the problem. A coronary artery bypass graft gives the blood another route. A length of vein from the leg or an artery inside the chest wall is used to bypass the blockage in the coronary artery. Often several blockages have to be bypassed.

When balloon angioplasty goes to plan, there is not much to recover from and no need to stay in hospital. (Just occasionally, it has to be followed by emergency surgery.) Coronary artery bypass surgery, on the other hand, involves cutting open the chest wall; it's followed by a few days in the intensive care unit and several weeks of convalescence.

If you are seriously disabled by angina, having a balloon angioplasty or a bypass operation can make a huge difference, but these procedures are not a complete solution. Indeed, angioplasty often has to be repeated and it's very common for bypass grafts to become blocked like the original coronary artery. It is essential to protect the plumbing with the right diet and lifestyle, and to get the cholesterol level right down – below 5 mmol/l. And, of course, this will reduce your chances of having a heart attack too.

◆ After a heart attack, gentle walking is usually increased gradually during the first week

◆ It is essential to stop smoking and adopt a healthy lifestyle

◆ Many people make a full recovery from a heart attack

◆ Sometimes drugs are used to control angina or heart failure, or to reduce the chances of a further heart attack

After a heart attack

Long gone are the days when doctors put people on bed rest for several weeks after a heart attack! We now understand how important it is to get moving again. You would normally be sitting out of bed on the second or third day after admission with a heart attack. Gentle walking is gradually increased and, before the first week is up, you may be climbing a few stairs. Of course, some heart attacks are bigger than others and some people must take it more slowly than others.

Over the next few weeks, your exercise should be stepped up gradually and a continuing exercise routine, pitched at the right level, is very important. Don't rush it. Ease up if there are any symptoms such as chest pain or nausea.

Join a rehabilitation programme if you possibly can. A well run programme is invaluable, not just for supervising your exercise plan, but also for education and confidence-building, which are so important for getting back to normal.

Here are a few tips:

Smoking
If you were a smoker before your heart attack, you must stop now. Those who continue to smoke are much more likely to have another heart attack (and that may well be the last). Don't imagine that it will take years to reap the risk reduction after giving up: some of the risk is cut very quickly because smokers are more likely to have a thrombosis.

Weight control
Losing flab reduces the strain on your heart and lowers your blood pressure. The weight control plan in this book will improve your cholesterol too.

Why me?
If you are a slim non-smoker, you are probably asking why you had a heart attack. I'm sure your doctor will want to check your blood lipid levels but that will need to wait for three months after the attack (unless it was done in the first 24 hours). Whatever the result, you are clearly at increased risk and the diet and lifestyle explained in these pages will reduce that risk.

Feelings

You don't laugh off a heart attack. You're bound to take it to heart and it will shake your confidence. It's hardly surprising that anxiety is a normal response and it can give way to depression. The support of those close to you is so important but it's often hard for families to understand the emotional chaos that follows a heart attack. Some people wear their heart on their sleeve while others bottle it up. Sharing emotions and using relaxation techniques will help (see Chapter 22).

Sex

As emotional turmoil settles and life becomes a little more normal, victims of a heart attack and their partners often worry about the safety of becoming sexually active again. One night stands and secret liaisons are a serious coronary hazard. But, if climbing a couple of flights of stairs is no problem, or you can happily walk a mile in 20 minutes, there is no reason why you shouldn't enjoy making love to your partner. Don't be too adventurous to start with.

Driving

Don't drive for one month after a heart attack. If you have made a good recovery and you feel ready to drive at that stage, you may do so and you need not inform the DVLA at Swansea. You should check that your insurance policy doesn't impose any restrictions after a heart attack. On the other hand, if you have angina at rest or at the wheel, you should see your doctor, inform the DVLA, and avoid driving until it's sorted out. However fit and confident you feel, start with short, local journeys and take a passenger. Professional drivers holding LGV and PCV licences (which have replaced HGV and PSV licences) should inform the DVLA and follow their instructions.

Flying

Flying (in an aeroplane) will not be a problem for most survivors of a heart attack – following a recovery period of at least two or three weeks (but six weeks would be better). A pressurised cabin is equivalent to an altitude of about 6000 feet (1830 m) and those who are not fully recovered could become breathless. If you can walk 100 metres on the flat without any symptoms, it should be safe to fly (as a passenger, not a pilot). Of course, stresses at the airport are often more significant than those in the air and many can be avoided by good planning: leave plenty of time, use a porter for heavy baggage, and don't smuggle.

Work

Don't rush back to work before you feel ready. This may be as soon as six weeks after a heart attack but you may need some months to build up your stamina first. Some jobs are flexible enough to allow a gradual return, while others demand 'all or nothing'. If your job is not physically taxing, you are likely to be able to go back sooner than someone returning to heavy manual work.

Successful recovery – or failure?

Many people who survive a heart attack go on to make a full recovery and the small scar in the heart muscle causes no trouble at all. Some others suffer from persistent breathlessness that cannot be improved by fitness training. This is because more extensive damage to the heart muscle has reduced its pumping power and this 'heart failure' can be improved with drugs.

What drugs are used for coronary heart disease?

Drugs are used to treat heart failure, to control angina and to prevent future heart attacks. Most of the drugs were described in the chapter on blood pressure, so I won't go into detail about them here.

Treating heart failure

When your heart fails to pump at the proper pace, your legs and lungs can become waterlogged and diuretics relieve this.

Research has shown that using ACE inhibitors in heart failure makes you live longer. In the light of this, the argument for using diuretics alone for heart failure, except in the mildest of cases, no longer holds water. In fact, when a heart attack upsets the heart's main pumping chamber (the left ventricle) – even mildly and temporarily – your prognosis is improved by using an ACE inhibitor.

Of course, ACE inhibitors aren't suitable for everyone. When your doctor decides to use one, an ACE inhibitor would normally be started between three and ten days after a heart attack.

Controlling angina

The beta-blockers and calcium channel blockers that are so often used to reduce high blood pressure are also effective against angina.

In addition, nitrate drugs bring relief to many angina sufferers. Glyceryl trinitrate (GTN) is a quick-acting drug that is absorbed from a tablet or spray under the tongue; it can be used to relieve an attack once it's started, or to prevent an attack (e.g. before climbing a hill or seeing your bank manager). Nitrates can cause headaches in some people, but frequent use may solve the problem; some sufferers find that a GTN tablet under the tongue relieves their angina so quickly that they can spit it out before a headache starts. Nitrates can also be used – in skin patches or tablets – as long-acting angina preventers.

A new class of drugs has recently been introduced for controlling angina – potassium channel activators. Nicorandil works by widening arteries and veins; it can be added to more established drug therapy when this proves inadequate.

Preventing future heart attacks

ACTION POINT

◆ If you have had a heart attack or suffer from angina, you should take a low dose of aspirin unless there is a good reason not to (such as aspirin allergy)

Drug treatment can be used to 'prevent' future heart attacks in those who have already had a heart attack or those who are known to be at increased risk because of coronary artery disease. Please don't misunderstand me here. It is accurate, though misleading, to say that certain drugs can prevent heart attacks: they prevent some heart attacks but not others. Taking such a drug can reduce your risk of having a heart attack but it can never guarantee that you won't have one.

Aspirin is top of the list. If you have had a heart attack or suffer from angina, you should be taking a low dose of aspirin (such as 75 mg daily) unless there is a good reason not to. Good reasons would include having a stomach ulcer, haemophilia or genuine aspirin allergy. Discuss it with your doctor if you're uncertain. A drug called clopidogrel is a suitable alternative in some cases (but it, too, can irritate the stomach). All doctors have patients whom they would like to put on aspirin, in view of current evidence for its benefit, but who have 'slipped through the net'.

Talking of fishing nets, you probably remember that aspirin helps to prevent clots in the circulation in a similar way to fish oil – by making platelets less ready to stick together. While we would strongly recommend consumption of oily fish (e.g. two meals a week) both to those with heart disease and those without, we cannot recommend aspirin as a preventive measure for the healthy population at large. The small risk of serious bleeding from the stomach is overshadowed by the coronary protection for those with heart disease – but not necessarily for those at low coronary risk.

The doses of aspirin used to make platelets less 'sticky' are much lower than the 300–600 mg used to treat pain. These low doses are less likely to upset the stomach. Preventive aspirin is normally taken as a dispersible tablet in water, with or straight after food. Some people get on better with 'enteric-coated' tablets, which are sealed in a coating to protect the stomach.

Beta-blockers are used to reduce the risk of a further heart attack (unless there's a good reason to avoid this group of drugs, such as a history of asthma).

It has become clear that one of the most effective ways to cut down heart attacks among those with coronary heart disease is to tackle cholesterol – with drugs if necessary.

Drug treatment of raised cholesterol

The Lifestyle Heart Trial published in the *Lancet* in 1990 showed that with far-reaching lifestyle changes (very low-fat vegetarian diet, stopping smoking, stress management training, and moderate exercise) it was possible to improve coronary atherosclerosis – even in severe cases – within one year, without the use of cholesterol-lowering drugs.

Sceptics please note: this was a properly controlled trial in which the control group received conventional advice and made moderate lifestyle changes; their atherosclerosis got worse within the year! Although no cholesterol-lowering drugs were used, the cholesterol reductions in the experimental group were better than those often seen after drugs have been prescribed. Do you want figures? OK: in the experimental group, total cholesterol fell by 24.3% and LDL-cholesterol by 37.4%. The reductions were achieved even though these people had already reduced their fat intake to 31.5% of calories and their cholesterol consumption to 213 mg/day (on average) *before baseline testing.*

Sadly, the common experience of doctors is that most people with heart disease fail to make such radical lifestyle changes as the experimental group made in this study. I am convinced that many of them fail because they are not given the necessary information or incentive, and I hope this book will play some part in putting that right.

Trials and triumphs

Recently, several major trials using the powerful 'statin' drugs (HMG Co-A reductase inhibitors) have been published. They must be powerful because they have transformed the thinking of the medical profession. Even doctors who were sceptical about the value of lowering cholesterol levels accept that these drugs have a vital role in the prevention of coronary deaths among those with established heart disease – so-called 'secondary prevention'.

The Scandinavian Simvastatin Survival Study (4S), published in the *Lancet* in 1994, studied 4444 people with coronary heart disease (stable angina or previous heart attack). These were men and women with total cholesterol levels ranging from 5.5 mmol/l to 8.0 mmol/l. They were divided (at random) into a treatment group who were given simvastatin tablets and a control group who were given placebo (inactive) tablets. After 5.4 years' follow-up, the main findings were that treatment with simvastatin had:

- Reduced the death rate (all causes) by 30%;
- Reduced the coronary death rate by 42%.

Like the WOSCOPS study mentioned in Chapter 3, this trial helped to reassure doctors that lowering cholesterol levels could reduce the total death rate and not just deaths from heart disease; there had previously been fears that an increase in deaths from other causes might cancel out the benefit.

It was very helpful that this trial included women as well as men, and this is now the trend. So many earlier studies on heart disease had been restricted to men.

I am now going to explain something that might seem a little technical at first but has important implications for millions of people. The starting dose of simvastatin in the 4S study was 20 mg and this was adjusted to keep the cholesterol level between 3.0 and 5.2 mmol/l. Virtually all the people ended up on 20 or 40 mg; only two were on 10 mg! This is often not appreciated by those quoting this study. Countless people in the real world are taking just 10 mg of simvastatin daily although it has not reduced their cholesterol levels into the target range for the 4S trial. It would be quite unreasonable to expect the same relative risk reduction among these people as was achieved with 20–40 mg in the 4S study. There is a good argument for raising their doses.

So, how much were cholesterol levels lowered by these higher doses in the 4S study? Simvastatin reduced the average total cholesterol by 25% and the LDL-cholesterol by 35% – remarkably similar numbers to those in the Lifestyle Heart Trial that used no lipid-lowering drugs at all. I must point out that there is no comparison between the *numbers of people* in the Lifestyle Heart Trial (48) and the 4S study (over 4000). If you have undergone coronary angiography yourself, you will understand why a trial involving repeated angiography could hardly recruit thousands of subjects. The experimental group in the Lifestyle Heart Trial was clearly a small, highly motivated group whereas the 4S study was more representative of the general population. If they were really put in the picture, many more people could be motivated and successful.

Some years after publication of the original 4S study, follow-up indicates that the participants continuing to take simvastatin are still deriving benefit from it.

The lowest of the low

Another landmark trial was the Cholesterol and Recurrent Events (CARE) study published in the *New England Journal of Medicine* in 1996. This involved 4159 men and women who had suffered a heart attack in the previous 20 months. The age range was 21–75 but all the women were past the menopause. The novel thing about this trial was that the people had 'normal' cholesterol levels – the average being 5.4 mmol/l (well below our population average). You might pause to take that in: they had cholesterol levels that our population regards as normal; they had all had a heart attack; apparently, men in their 20s were included!

The CARE study randomly divided the people into two groups: the treatment group received 40 mg of pravastatin daily and the control group took placebo tablets. (A cholesterol-lowering resin called cholestyramine was added to pravastatin or placebo if the LDL-cholesterol level remained above 4.5 mmol/l.)

The central finding was similar to that in the 4S study: there was a 24% reduction in heart attacks (fatal and non-fatal) in the pravastatin group.

It seems that if you get heart disease despite having an average cholesterol level, you benefit from reducing the level below average. Perhaps it is somewhere near the truth to say: if you get heart disease, whatever your blood cholesterol concentration is, it's too high for you.

Looking closely at the figures from the CARE study gives us a clue that there may be a limit to this. Unlike the 4S study, the higher the LDL-cholesterol level at the start of the trial, the bigger the relative risk reduction produced by treatment. In fact, treatment did not seem to be of any benefit at all when the LDL-cholesterol was below 3.2 mmol/l to begin with. (Some of those who have heart attacks despite low levels of LDL-cholesterol may be at risk because of low HDL-cholesterol and high triglycerides – not to mention a low intake of antioxidants that makes any level of LDL more dangerous.)

More light was thrown on this by a colossal study published in the *Lancet* in 2002. The Heart Protection Study included 20,536 men and women aged between 40 and 80 (who already had heart disease or other arterial disease or diabetes) with a **total** cholesterol level of at least 3.5 mmol/l. Taking simvastatin (40 mg) produced the expected 25% reduction in heart attacks and strokes; the same benefit was seen even in those who started off with the lowest cholesterol levels. So, if you have diseased arteries or diabetes, perhaps you will benefit from taking a statin no matter how low your cholesterol is.

Other drugs

Statins are not the only lipid-lowering drugs available as you can see from Table 25. The fibrates are particularly useful for people who have very raised triglycerides. Anion-exchange resins are

sometimes used with statins in people with severely raised cholesterol levels (such as those with familial hypercholesterolaemia).
They are taken as a drink and not everyone finds them palatable.
These resins are not absorbed into the body but they can cause
constipation and they interfere with the absorption of fat-soluble
vitamins. Nicotinic acid is interesting because it was promoted as
an over-the-counter d.i.y. cholesterol remedy some years ago –
partly on the basis that it's 'just a vitamin'. The doses used to
lower cholesterol are vastly greater than the quantities obtained
from food; it's actually one of the more toxic lipid-lowering drugs
we use and calls for careful medical supervision. Ironically, the
slow-release versions (designed to reduce the common side effect
of flushing) that were sold over the counter appeared to be even
more toxic!

A new class of drugs, selective cholesterol absorption
inhibitors, was launched in 2003 with the introduction of
ezetimibe. Blocking the absorption of cholesterol from the intestine
gets rid of some of the cholesterol made in the liver as well as
cholesterol from food (see page 48). Ezetimibe can be added to a
statin to achieve a further reduction in blood cholesterol.

The stars

The statins have stolen the show. Massive trials using simvastatin
and pravastatin have convinced doctors that many more people
with heart disease should be taking these drugs. With the widespread use of other statins (Table 25), confidence has grown over
the past few years that they share the beneficial effects of simvastatin and pravastatin.

Impressive cholesterol reductions can usually be achieved with
atorvastatin and now there is good evidence from trials that it, too,
saves lives. In the GREACE study (GREek Atorvastatin Coronary-
heart-disease Evaluation) published in 2002, LDL-cholesterol was
reduced to below 2.6 mmol/l with atorvastatin (usually 20 mg),
producing a massive 47% reduction in deaths from heart disease;
the atorvastatin group also had 47% fewer strokes and enjoyed a
drop of 43% in total mortality.

What would happen if you gave atorvastatin to people with
high blood pressure, in addition to the drugs to lower their blood
pressure? That was one of the questions asked by the Anglo-Scan-
dinavian Cardiac Outcomes Trial (ASCOT). Some people received

Table 25 Lipid-lowering drugs

Class:	Main actions:
Statins (HMG CoA reductase inhibitors) Atorvastatin Fluvastatin Pravastatin Rosuvastatin Simvastatin	Reduce cholesterol production in liver *Lower LDL-cholesterol levels* (May lower triglycerides and raise HDL-cholesterol)
Fibrates Bezafibrate Ciprofibrate Clofibrate Fenofibrate Gemfibrozil	*Lower triglycerides* Lower LDL-cholesterol Raise HDL-cholesterol
Anion-exchange resins Cholestyramine Colestipol	Bind bile acids in gut *Lower LDL-cholesterol* (can *raise* triglycerides)
Nicotinic acid group Acipimox Nicotinic acid	Lower LDL-cholesterol Lower triglycerides Raise HDL-cholesterol
Fish oils	Lower triglycerides (reduce platelet 'stickiness')
Soluble fibre Ispaghula husk	Increases excretion of bile acids Lowers LDL-cholesterol
Selective cholesterol absorption inhibitors Ezetimibe	Block cholesterol uptake from gut Lower LDL-cholesterol

atorvastatin 10 mg daily while others were given placebo (dummy) tablets to take with their treatment for blood pressure. This part of the trial was stopped early when it became clear that atorvastatin was saving lives by preventing strokes and heart attacks.

All drugs can produce side effects in some people; side effects can be trivial or catastrophic. Theoretically, the statins could cause liver or muscle problems. The small risk of a serious reaction in the muscles increases when statins are combined with fibrates; one statin (cerivastatin) was withdrawn when it became apparent that combining it with gemfibrozil was particularly hazardous. If you are taking a statin and have unexplained muscle pains or weakness, your doctor can arrange a simple blood test (creatine kinase) to make sure that there is no significant inflammation in your muscles.

Big studies such as the Heart Protection Study, together with the widespread use of statins in recent years, have provided considerable reassurance that these drugs are generally well tolerated and safe. Even so, remember that we are talking about lifetime treatment and, so far, those treated in the large clinical trials have been followed up only for a number of years rather than several decades.

What are we waiting for?

We've seen the evidence. Why aren't doctors prescribing statin therapy for more people with heart disease? This is the question that many specialists and enthusiasts are asking.

GPs are right to be cautious and cost-conscious, but the evidence supporting statins in secondary prevention is overwhelming.

When I was writing the first edition, results of the LIPID trial (Long-term Intervention with Pravastatin in Ischaemic Disease) had just become available. Conducted in Australia and New Zealand, this huge study recruited 9014 men and women with heart disease – many of them with 'normal' cholesterol levels. Cholesterol levels ranged from just 4 mmol/l to 7 mmol/l and these people had either had a heart attack or were admitted to hospital with unstable angina. Pravastatin treatment reduced the total death rate by 23% and deaths due to heart attack by 29%. There was also a 20% reduction in strokes. Unlike the CARE study, the benefit seemed to be just as big in those with the lowest cholesterol levels.

In the light of all this evidence, current guidelines recommend that if you have heart disease, you should reduce your cholesterol level below 5 mmol/l (LDL-cholesterol below 3 mmol/l) using a statin if necessary. Indeed, if you know your arteries are clogged with atheroma, there is a good argument for taking a statin (and aiming for a cholesterol reduction of 30%) even if your cholesterol level is already below 5 mmol/l. People with heart disease look set to consume tons of these drugs in the coming years. This will cost a lot of money. But it will save expensive bypass grafts, much misery, and many lives.

'We have saved five pence. (*Pause*) But at what cost?'
_____

Samuel Beckett (1906–89)
All That Fall, 1957, p. 25

◆ Statin drugs can reduce the death rate by about 30% in people
with heart disease

◆ Most people with heart disease will need a statin to bring
cholesterol down to the target level – below 5 mmol/l
(LDL-cholesterol below 3 mmol/l)

◆ Statins should be considered for people with heart disease or
other arterial disease (e.g. stroke, claudication) or diabetes, even
if the cholesterol level is below 5 mmol/l

◆ Lifestyle changes can bring remarkable benefits but marginal
adjustments yield marginal results

◆ The nation is set to consume many tons of statins

Finding your freedom

Chapter 26

Looking forward

'When people are free to do as they please, they usually imitate each other.'

Eric Hoffer,
The Passionate State of Mind, 1955

You are free – free to choose the way you eat and the way you live. Oh, I know that some are more limited than others by lack of money or by circumstance. But there's only one person who can decide whether you smoke, or take exercise, or control your weight. There is a vast range of foods available, and there are many different ways to cook. You can choose. You are free to follow fashion – to imitate those afflicted by a lethal epidemic.

You are free – free to get fit and to flourish on a first-class diet. You can be liberated and live, or you can be a lemming.

In the last chapter, we saw how dramatically statin drugs can reduce the risk of future heart attacks in people who already have heart disease (secondary prevention). If you don't have heart disease – and, of course, you're reading this book because you want to keep it that way – you may be saying: "What about me?"

Perhaps you're thinking: "A good diet and healthy lifestyle are all very well but, if this statin stuff is so good, why should I wait to have a heart attack before taking it? How about a bit of primary prevention? In any case, my first heart attack might kill me!"

Do you remember the WOSCOPS study? This showed that by giving the drug pravastatin to middle-aged men who had *not* had a heart attack (but who had an average cholesterol level of 7 mmol/l) you could reduce their risk of coronary death significantly. In fact, the *relative* risk went down as much as it does when you give a statin drug to people who already have heart disease.

Remember, though, that the *absolute* risk is much lower in those without heart disease, so you have to treat many more people, and spend much more money, before you save one life.

"Surely it's worth it," I hear you say: "it could save *my* life."

How do you decide how many people should be drugged, and how much money should be spent, to save one life? After all, for most of us, the answers to such questions will depend on whose life is being discussed.

The *National Service Framework (NSF) for Coronary Heart Disease* published in 2000 set out standards for prevention as well as treatment of heart disease. Those who do not yet have heart disease, but whose risk of developing it in the next ten years is about 30%, are to be offered lifestyle advice. In addition, statin drugs are to be used to lower cholesterol levels below 5 mmol/l (LDL-cholesterol below 3 mmol/l).

Consider the case of a man aged 70 who doesn't have diabetes but who smokes; he has a 'normal' cholesterol level of 5.1 mmol/l with an HDL-cholesterol of 1.0 mmol/l; his blood pressure is moderately raised with a systolic of 160 mmHg. Like most men of his age who smoke, this man has a heart disease risk above 30% over ten years (see Figure 16) despite his 'normal' cholesterol. As his GP, I am required by the NSF to prescribe a statin to take his cholesterol below 5 mmol/l.

If we fully implement these standards, a huge proportion of the population will be taking statins. And the idea is that once we've dealt with the people who have a 30% ten-year risk, we can move on to those with a 15% risk – as resources allow. Of course, the NSF also states that lifestyle advice is to be given. The trouble is that brief advice about lifestyle in consultations isn't very effective.

As a reader of this book, you have a detailed guide telling you which changes are worthwhile and how to make them. But being told in a consultation to improve your diet (perhaps with a few supplementary instructions such as 'reduce saturates' and 'increase polyunsaturates') is a bit like being told to go and fly an aeroplane – and being left to work out the practical details for yourself. I'm not blaming doctors; they don't have enough time to practise medicine, let alone give flying lessons.

Because dietary advice makes little difference, some health professionals have been duped: they think that *diet* makes little difference. The evidence confirms that when people make the right changes, the impact is dramatic.

Those who changed their diets in the *Lyon Diet Heart Study* enjoyed a 70% reduction in coronary events and cardiac deaths – a much bigger risk reduction than seen in any statin trial.

If we are to spend more and more millions on statins in the hope of preventing people from developing heart disease, should we not put some serious resources into helping them change the way they eat and live? Do we really want to put statins in the water supply to fight a plague produced by faulty lifestyles?

When it comes to deciding who should receive statins first, faced with a whole population at risk, the NSF is quite right to give priority to those at highest risk.

How low can you get?

"That's not fair!" you might protest. "Why should I be disqualified from taking this marvellous stuff because my risk is not quite high enough?"

In the first edition, I predicted that statins would be prescribed for people at lower and lower levels of risk. This has certainly come to pass (although there are still lots of people at very high risk who are not yet taking a statin and should be).

But before you go to your doctor, demanding a statin – on the basis that, as a taxpayer, you're entitled, no matter how low your coronary risk – you should reflect that really long-term safety has yet to be established. I am optimistic that statins will prove to be safe, but only time will tell.

In the meantime, I choose to reduce my own coronary risk (by a bigger percentage than many are managing with drugs) by enjoying a deliciously varied diet and an invigorating, healthy lifestyle.

Whether you take a statin or not, whether you have a 'normal' cholesterol or not, don't forget that the impact of a good diet and lifestyle goes far beyond cholesterol. Don't forget the reduced risk of cancer, the anti-ageing effects, the protection against oxidation of LDL, the reduced risk of thrombosis, the control of blood pressure and, incidentally, the sense of wellbeing.

◆ You are free to reduce your risk, or to follow harmful customs

◆ Statin drugs have less to offer those at low risk, and really long-term safety has not yet been established

◆ Statins should be prescribed first for those with heart disease, and next for those at very high risk of getting heart disease

◆ Your lifestyle remains crucial, whether you take a drug to lower cholesterol or not

◆ There is only one person who can change your lifestyle

I have a deep concern. I see our nation gripped by an epidemic – a scourge that strikes at its very heart. Yet some populations, with their simple, natural ways of life, whatever else they lack, they lack the heartache of this scourge.

I am concerned that we doctors (who have little time to dwell upon our own nutrition, let alone on yours), in our eagerness to treat this epidemic with potent statin drugs, may overlook a simple truth: you have the power to change; you can improve the way you eat and live – and, yes, enjoy life all the more.

It's your life. It's up to you.

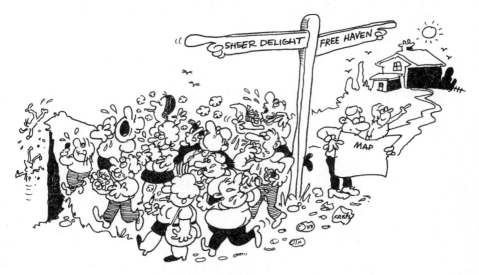

It's your life. It's up to you.

Chapter 27

Let's get cooking!

'The discovery of a new dish does more for the happiness of mankind than the discovery of a new star.'

Anthelme Brillat-Savarin (1755–1826)
Physiologie du Goût, 1826

Don't be a slave

Don't be a slave to tradition that calls for oodles of redundant fat. Don't be a slave to recipes that say: measure this and weigh that.

Always be well stocked with vegetables, grains, pulses and pasta. Never run short of fruit – fresh, dried, canned and frozen. Buy fish, poultry and low-fat dairy products as required. Create dishes to suit the mood and occasion. How can you go wrong?

So, what you'll find in this chapter is not a comprehensive catalogue of coronary-conscious cuisine but, rather, a few signposts along your path of discovery.

Note:

- Unless otherwise stated, recipes serve 4.

- All spoon measures are level; tsp = teaspoon; tbsp = tablespoon.

- All oven cooking times are for a preheated oven.

- Microwave cooking times are a guide for using a 650-watt appliance.

Casseroles

It's not so much what you put in it as what you put it in that qualifies a creation to be called a casserole. Take what you have from the four major food groups, add some liquid, cook gently in a deep, lidded pot, and it will live up to the name.

The convenience of casseroles lies in the fact that they look after themselves and can be made in advance. Make sure they don't dry out: add water, wine, stock, or even white sauce but remember that some vegetables, such as tomatoes, also yield a lot of liquid during cooking. Pulses can be precooked, and it is often convenient to buy them, ready to use, in cans. Look out for those without added salt or sugar. Grains and pasta, too, are best added to the casserole ready-cooked, towards the end of the cooking time. Casseroles are great for using up leftover cooked pulses, grains and pasta.

Here are some suggested ingredients:

- cooked rice, barley, cracked wheat or bulgar wheat
- cooked or part-cooked potato
- cooked pasta
- vegetables, e.g. tomatoes, celery, peppers, mushrooms, onion, cabbage, carrot, aubergine
- cooked pulses or beans, e.g. kidney beans, mung beans, blackeye beans, haricot beans, soya beans, lentils, split peas, chickpeas, peas.

You can add fish, poultry or other meat but vegetarian casseroles can also be delicious; the mixture of pulses and grains will provide all the protein you need. Throw in fruit (such as apple or dried fruit) if you wish. Season with plenty of pepper, herbs, spices and garlic. Useful toppings include breadcrumbs, a little grated Parmesan cheese or chopped nuts such as walnuts or almonds. Sprinkle these on top after cooking and grill until brown and crisp.

Of course, if you don't yet feel confident about setting off into the unknown, you can simply modify a traditional recipe.

Here is a typical ingredients list for chicken casserole:

2 medium or large onions, chopped
2 celery sticks, sliced
100 g (4 oz) mushrooms, sliced
15 ml (1 tbsp) cooking oil

25 g (1 oz) butter
salt and pepper
50 g (2 oz) rindless bacon, chopped
4 chicken joints
45 ml (3 tbsp) plain flour
400-g (14-oz) can chopped tomatoes
300 ml (½ pint) chicken stock

Without being too adventurous, you might make simple changes to the above ingredients, such as cutting out the butter, selecting skinned chicken breasts, using smoked turkey rashers instead of bacon and increasing the vegetable content just a little. Reduce the stock to allow for liquid from the courgettes added to the following recipe.

Chicken and vegetable casserole

I would recommend making this without adding salt but, if your palate's sodium sensor is still set very high, you could use a little LoSalt or Solo. Salt is actually being added in the smoked turkey rashers, and if your stock comes from a chicken stock cube, you'll get plenty of salt that way!

This simple adaptation of a recipe will give you a delicious casserole. You can also make perfectly good casseroles without first browning any meat or vegetables in a frying pan. If you aren't used to breaking away from set recipes, the confidence and the freedom will come with practice and you'll soon be managing without recipes at all.

2 large onions, chopped
2 celery sticks, sliced
3 medium courgettes, thickly sliced
100 g (4 oz) mushrooms, sliced
20 ml (4 tsp) olive oil
2 garlic cloves, crushed
black pepper
4 carrots, sliced
50 g (2 oz) smoked turkey rashers, chopped
4 skinless, boneless chicken breasts, cut into chunks
45 ml (3 tbsp) plain flour
150 ml (¼ pint) chicken stock
400-g (14-oz) can chopped tomatoes
dried herbs: ¼ tsp sage; 1 tsp rosemary; ½ tsp oregano

Here's what to do:

Fry the onions, celery, mushrooms and courgettes in the olive oil over high heat, stirring frequently, until lightly browned. Add the garlic and pepper to taste. Enjoy the aroma. Use a slotted spoon to transfer these vegetables to a large ovenproof casserole, leaving as much of the oil in the pan as possible. Add the carrots and turkey rashers to the casserole.

Brown the chicken in the oil remaining in the pan, then transfer it to the casserole. Stir the flour into the small amount of oil remaining in the pan. Gradually stir in the stock and bring to the boil, stirring, to make a thick sauce. Add the tomatoes, stir and then transfer to the casserole. Mix in the herbs.

Cover the casserole and cook in the oven at 180°C (350°F, gas 4), for 45–60 minutes.

Pedro's pie

Here is a successful, quick dish that my father knocked up, inspired simply by what was available at the time.

Tasty though this is, notice how salt creeps in with the soy sauce, Worcestershire sauce and even in the tomato purée.

100 g (4 oz) mushrooms, sliced
5 ml (1 tsp) rapeseed oil
400-g (14-oz) can chopped tomatoes
5 ml (1 tsp) dried mixed herbs
5 ml (1 tsp) dry mustard
5 ml (1 tsp) Worcestershire sauce
5 ml (1 tsp) tomato purée
5 ml (1 tsp) dark soy sauce
100 g (4 oz) cooked pasta
1 garlic clove, crushed
100 g (4 oz) fresh wholemeal breadcrumbs

Heat half the oil in a saucepan. Add the mushrooms and cook for 1–2 minutes, stirring frequently. Add all the remaining ingredients except the garlic, breadcrumbs and remaining oil. Bring to the boil, stirring continuously and then pour the mixture into a lasagne dish.

Top with the breadcrumbs. Mix the crushed garlic with the remaining oil and 'dot' this over the breadcrumbs. Bake at 200°C (400°F, gas 6), for 25 minutes, until the breadcrumbs are golden brown.

Microwave chinese chicken and mushrooms

This is another of my father's creations. The chicken is always beautifully tender, but it is important to cut it into cubes just large enough to cover a standard postage stamp. Such tender meat in only 6½ minutes is a success story for the microwave. These ingredients give a subtle, delicate flavour but you can always add fresh root ginger and garlic for more zing.

These quantities will make four small portions; serve with plenty of rice and stir-fried vegetables as accompaniments.

2 skinless, boneless chicken breasts
1 egg white (or dried egg white)
10 ml (2 tsp) cornflour
20 ml (4 tsp) rapeseed oil
300-g (11-oz) can chopped mushrooms, drained
227-g (8-oz) can water chestnuts, drained and thinly sliced
2 or 3 spring onions, cut into short lengths
½ red pepper, deseeded and diced
5 ml (1 tsp) light soy sauce
15 ml (3 tsp) extra dry vermouth

Trim any sinews or remains of soft bone from the chicken breasts and cut them into small cubes. Place in a microwaveproof dish. Mix the egg white, cornflour and 5 ml (1 tsp) of the oil to a smooth, thin paste. Add the egg white mixture to the chicken and stir thoroughly.

Cook in the microwave on medium power for 3 minutes, stirring well, first after 1 minute and then after 2 minutes. Add the remaining ingredients and stir well. Cook on full power for 3–3½ minutes, stirring twice.

Tip: Dried egg white is very convenient: simply mix the dry powder equivalent for one egg white with the cornflour, then add a little water to make a paste, and stir in the 5 ml (1 tsp) oil (see page 131).

Avoiding cross-contamination
Remember to wash the spoon used to stir the part-cooked mixture before serving the cooked chicken, to avoid the possibility of salmonella contamination.

Variations
Add frozen peas or sweetcorn. Fresh button or closed-cap mushrooms can be used in place of canned mushrooms.

Cooking rice to perfection

Microwave and freezer technology make it possible to produce perfect rice in a jiffy. Plain boiled rice can be kept in the freezer for up to two months. You can then defrost and thoroughly reheat it in the microwave just when you need it. It's convenient to cook about 450 g (1 lb) of long-grain or basmati rice in one batch and freeze it in two or three portions for future use.

Bring plenty of water to the boil in a large saucepan. Meanwhile, wash the rice thoroughly in a large, fine wire sieve until the water runs clear. Add the rice to the boiling water and stir well until it comes back to the boil. Boil for exactly 10 minutes, stirring occasionally. Drain the rice in a sieve and rinse thoroughly under cold running water. Drain well.

The drained rice can now be frozen or reheated in the microwave when required.

A few more poultry suggestions

Low-fat turkey lasagne

This is what my wife does with leftover turkey. Of course, if you add skin and fatty bits, it won't be a low-fat dish at all!

If you want to cut corners, you can use one of the excellent ready-made tomato sauces. There are several available with a fat content of less than 1% (1 g fat per 100 g) but they will contain more salt than a home-made sauce.

350–450 g (12–16 oz) cooked turkey, chopped
1 pepper (red, green or yellow – or use a mixture),
deseeded and thinly sliced
6–8 sheets no-precook lasagne (wholemeal, white or green)
1 oz Parmesan or pecorino cheese, grated
2 oz fresh, wholemeal breadcrumbs

Tomato Sauce:
5 ml (1 tsp) olive oil
1 onion, finely chopped
1 garlic clove, crushed (add more if you like!)
400-g (14-oz) can chopped tomatoes
50 ml (2 fl oz) vegetable stock (or cooking water from vegetables)

15 ml (1 tbsp) tomato purée
dried herbs: ½ tsp basil and ½ tsp oregano

White Sauce:
250 g (9 oz) quark or skimmed milk soft cheese
100 ml (4 fl oz) skimmed milk

First make the tomato sauce. Heat the olive oil in a small saucepan. Add the chopped onion and cook for 2–3 minutes until softened slightly. Add the garlic and toss over the heat briefly, but don't allow the garlic to brown. Remove the pan from the heat and stir in the tomatoes, stock, tomato purée, basil and oregano. If you want to use this tomato sauce for other recipes, cook it for longer until it has reduced slightly. Add the turkey and peppers to the tomato sauce.

To make the white sauce, mix the quark and skimmed milk, stirring until smooth.

Lightly grease an oblong ovenproof dish measuring about 23×18×5 cm (9×7×2 inch) with olive or rapeseed oil to prevent the pasta from sticking. Pour half the tomato sauce mixture into the dish. Arrange a single layer of lasagne on top, breaking it if necessary so that it fits snugly.

Pour half the white sauce over the lasagne, spreading it evenly with a spoon to cover the pasta completely. Pour the remaining tomato sauce mixture on top and add a second layer of pasta, pressing it down if necessary. Spread the remaining white sauce on top to cover the lasagne completely. Mix the cheese with the breadcrumbs and sprinkle this over the sauce. Cover loosely with foil and stand dish on a baking tray, then cook in the oven at 180°C (350°F, gas 4) for 20 minutes. Remove the foil and cook for a further 20 minutes until the topping is crisp and brown.

STOCK ANSWERS

Recipes frequently call for stock. If your answer is a stock cube, you'll be adding a lot of salt (and some fat). Vegetable bouillon powders, too, may have salt as the top ingredient. The ideal solution is a home-made broth consisting of the ingredients you have in stock – vegetable scraps, chicken bones and so on. Water drained from cooked vegetables is always a good start. For chicken stock you might use meaty chicken bones, celery, onion, carrot, garlic, coriander, lemon grass and pepper. Cover with liquid, bring to the boil, skim off any scum, then simmer for a couple of hours. It's useful to make big batches of stock and keep some in the freezer.

Many supermarkets have ready-made refrigerated stocks (e.g. vegetable, chicken, fish) that are not salty and simply need to be diluted. Of course, if you're a bit short of stock, whether you make your own or buy it, you can always dilute it with wine, vermouth or sherry!

Coq au vin

This is always a hit at dinner parties, unless you invite vegetarians. It's an ideal dish for the slow cooker (and also for the slow cook as everything's done in advance so there's no last-minute panic).

30 ml (2 tbsp) olive or rapeseed oil
4 skinless, boneless chicken breasts
about 16 button onions, peeled
1 garlic clove, crushed
6 smoked turkey rashers, cut into strips
50 g (2 oz) plain flour
150 ml (¼ pint) chicken stock
300 ml (½ pint) red wine
30 ml (2 tbsp) brandy
100 g (4 oz) button mushrooms
2 bay leaves
1 bouquet garni
pinch of grated nutmeg
black pepper

To cook the casserole in a slow cooker, preheat the cooker according to the manufacturer's instructions. Heat the oil in a large frying

*pan and brown the chicken breasts on both sides, then place them in
the slow cooker.*

*Cook the onion and garlic in the oil, without browning the garlic.
Stir in the flour. Gradually add the stock, red wine and brandy.
Bring to the boil, stirring, and add the remaining ingredients. Pour
the sauce mixture over the chicken and cook on the low setting for
6–8 hours. Remove the bouquet garni and bay leaves before serving.*

*To cook coq au vin in the oven, add an extra 150 ml (¼ pint) liquid
(preferably wine!). Cover and cook at 180°C (350°F, gas 4) for 1 hour.*

Turkey-breast roll

Slices of turkey-breast roll make an attractive addition to a platter
of cold meats on a buffet. You can equally well use chicken breasts
for this recipe and, generally, chicken is more tender.

4 turkey breast fillets
225 g half-fat cottage cheese
225 g young spinach leaves, chopped

*Using a meat mallet or rolling pin, beat the turkey fillets into
submission until they are evenly thin and well flattened. Spread a
layer of cottage cheese evenly over the turkey and add a topping of
spinach. Roll up each steak like a Swiss roll.*

*Wrap each roll in a piece of muslin to hold it neatly together and
brush with rapeseed or olive oil. You can use foil instead of muslin,
in which case brush the turkey with oil before wrapping in foil,
and remove the foil towards the end of cooking to brown the poultry.*

*Place in a roasting tin or ovenproof dish and bake at 190°C
(375°F, gas 5) for 35 minutes. Leave the turkey to cool in its
wrapping, replacing the foil removed at the end of cooking.
When cold, unwrap, slice the rolls and serve with salad.*

A salt course for beginners

If you are used to traditional food, with loads of fat and salt, you
should have no difficulty switching to low-fat cuisine. Very low-fat
dishes are not necessarily any less delicious than high-fat ones and they
can even be served to the uninitiated at dinner parties.

However, I don't recommend taking a sudden leap to very low-salt
cooking at the same time. If you suddenly present your family with
a low-sodium meal, they may well demand the saltcellar and this

could create an obstacle to further progress. It is better to reduce the salt content of your food gradually, allowing the palate a period of time for adjustment. During this time, increase your skill in the use of herbs, spices and other flavourings.

Remember, though, that when using ingredients such as soy sauce, stock cubes and smoked turkey rashers you are adding salt and this should be quite enough to satisfy the average palate.

Spice power

The power of herbs, spices and similar ingredients to complement the flavour of your dishes cannot be overstated – especially when the salt content is reduced.

Use fresh herbs when you can, and in some cases, perhaps treble the quantity you would use of dried herbs. Of course, you'll always need dried herbs to fall back on; store them in tightly sealed containers or jars in a cool place out of the light.

Spices are aromatic or pungent parts of a plant – often seeds, roots or bark – used to flavour food. Store them carefully as for dried herbs. Buy both dried herbs and spices in modest quantities that you will use up over a few months as they lose their flavour when stored for years.

Garlic, of course, has earned itself a whole chapter in this book. Use as much as your social life, or your partner, can stand. Fresh root ginger is also a delight to use: peel it first and then grate it.

Peppercorns freshly ground from a peppermill give a better flavour than bought ready-ground pepper. Mixed whole peppercorns (green, black, white and pink) are an agreeable alternative to black pepper.

In the end, sensitive seasoning comes with experience, but a simple book on herbs and spices is a useful source of basic information while you are experimenting with flavours.

Game for a laugh

Frisky, frolicking animals that run (or hop) wild have far leaner, healthier bodies than sedentary residents of a farm. Anything from the ostrich to the kangaroo seems fair game these days and such creatures certainly provide a lower-fat meat and an entertaining change from regular fare.

Stewed venison

Venison, the meat of the red deer, can be a bit tough. Hanging
meat tenderises it and brings out the flavour; traditionally, venison
is hung until slightly 'high'. It will be improved by marinating for
12 hours before cooking.

90 ml (6 tbsp) plain flour
700 g (1½ lb) stewing venison, cubed
45 ml (3 tbsp) olive or rapeseed oil
stock (see method)
1 bouquet garni

Marinade:
1 celery stick, chopped
2 onions, chopped
2 carrots, chopped
2 bay leaves
1 blade of mace
pepper
400 ml (14 fl oz) red wine

*Put all the ingredients for the marinade, except the wine, into a
dish large enough to hold them and the venison. Add the venison
and pour in enough wine to cover the meat; drink the rest.
Leave for about 12 hours, turning the meat a couple of times.*

*Drain the meat, reserving the liquid and other marinade
ingredients, then pat it dry on absorbent kitchen paper.
Make up the marinade liquid to 400 ml (14 fl oz) with stock.*

*Season the flour with pepper and toss the venison in it.
Heat the oil in a frying pan, and fry the meat until browned.
Transfer the venison to an ovenproof casserole, leaving as much oil
in the pan as possible. Stir the flour remaining from coating the
venison into the oil in the pan and cook gently, stirring occasionally
for a few minutes. Take the pan off the heat and gradually stir in
the wine mixture. Bring to the boil and continue stirring until
the sauce thickens.*

*Add the vegetables, bay leaves and mace from the marinade to
the casserole, then pour in the sauce. Add the bouquet garni.
Cover the casserole and cook in the oven at 160°C (325°F, gas 3)
for 2½ hours. Serve with potatoes and plenty of vegetables.*

Absurdly simple

It's vital to have a variety of simple, quick meals in your repertoire. Here's a taster:

Sardines on toast

This makes a snack for one or two people. While it's going down, write a letter to the canned sardine manufacturer explaining that you'd rather buy sardines without added salt.

> 1 can sardines in olive oil, drained
> 2 slices wholemeal toast
> malt vinegar
> black pepper
>
> *I won't tell you how to cook toast, but remember that you don't need any spread. Simply place the sardines on the toast and gently flake the fish with a fork, spreading them out to cover the toast up to the edges. Place under the grill until the sardines are piping hot, but don't burn the edges of the toast. Remove from the grill, add vinegar and black pepper to taste.*

Baked beans on toast

Another snack for one or two people.

> 425-g (15-oz) can baked beans (reduced sugar and salt)
> 2 slices wholemeal toast
> Worcestershire sauce (optional)

Need I say more? No spread on the toast again, of course. Add a little Worcestershire sauce to the beans if you wish.

Quick spaghetti with tuna sauce

Select a very low-fat brand of tomato sauce intended for making bolognese sauce, for example, Dolmio.

> 300 g (11 oz) wholewheat spaghetti
> 2×200-g (7-oz) cans tuna in water (not brine)
> 500-g (17½-oz) jar tomato sauce
>
> *Bring a large saucepan of water to the boil. Gradually lower fistfuls of spaghetti into the boiling water (keeping your fist out). As the spaghetti softens, coil it around in the pan, so it is completely*

immersed. Boil briskly for 10 minutes, or according to the packet instructions until tender but not soft. Meanwhile, drain the tuna and empty it into a smaller saucepan. Add the tomato sauce and heat gently, stirring to flake the tuna into the sauce. Drain the spaghetti in a colander or large sieve and transfer it to plates using tongs or a spoon and fork. Top the spaghetti with the tuna sauce and serve at once.

Microwave salmon pasta

The bones in canned salmon can be removed but they are edible and are a good source of calcium. Don't overheat the fish sauce as this makes the bones become harder.

300 g (11 oz) pasta twists or garlic-flavoured tagliatelle
250 g (9 oz) quark or skimmed-milk soft cheese
25 g (1 oz) grated Parmesan or pecorino cheese
75 ml (2½ fl oz) skimmed milk
5 ml (1 tsp) onion, very finely chopped (optional)
200 g (7 oz) canned salmon (pink or red)
freshly ground mixed peppercorns or pepper
chopped parsley to garnish (optional)

Bring a large saucepan of water to the boil and boil the pasta for 10 minutes or according to the packet instructions, until tender but not soft.

Meanwhile, mix the quark, Parmesan or pecorino cheese, skimmed milk and onion in a microwaveproof jug or bowl. Cook in the microwave on medium power for 1 minute, until just warm. If overheated the mixture will curdle and separate. Carefully stir in the salmon, without breaking it up too much, and warm the sauce gently in the microwave again.

Drain the pasta, return it to the saucepan and stir in the salmon sauce. Serve immediately, garnished with parsley and seasoned with freshly ground pepper. Salad or colourful vegetables, such as a big pile of peas, go very well with the pasta.

Variations

Notice that, when served with vegetables, this very quick meal provides the four important food groups. There are variations of course. If you leave out the salmon altogether, you will need to use a little more Parmesan or pecorino cheese for flavour. Another option, again adding more Parmesan, is to use 4–6 lightly grilled and chopped, smoked turkey rashers instead of the salmon.

Feasting on fish

Fish can be baked, braised, poached, steamed, smoked, fried and, as in Japanese cuisine, eaten uncooked. It is important not to over-cook fish.

The microwave oven is ideal for everyday fish cookery. Salmon steaks or whole trout cook to perfection in minutes with lemon juice, garlic pepper and herbs. If you have a sophisticated microwave, you don't even have to think about timing; the sensor stops it automatically when the food is ready. This is real conve-nience food and there's no need for any recipes – you just clean the fish, put it in a microwaveproof dish, add your chosen seasonings and cover. Then place it in the microwave and press the buttons, following the manufacturer's instructions.

Trout, apple and apricot rolls

When you have a few more minutes available, you might like to try this. It can be cooked equally well in the microwave, in which case halve the quantity of liquid given below.

4 small trout, heads and tails removed
227-g (8-oz) can apricots in fruit juice
1 apple, cored and chopped
1 onion, chopped
5 ml (1 tsp) grated fresh root ginger
50 g (2 oz) fresh wholemeal breadcrumbs
5 ml (1 tsp) white wine vinegar
dried herbs: ½ tsp dill and ½ tsp rosemary
black pepper
45 ml (3 tbsp) ginger wine

Place the trout on a chopping board, skin side up. Press firmly along the backbone. Turn the fish over and gently lift the backbone away from the flesh: it should come away completely with most of the smaller bones. Remove any stray bones and cut the fins from the fish.

Chop 4–5 apricots and reserve the remaining apricots and juice. Mix the apple, chopped apricots, onion, ginger, breadcrumbs and vinegar. Mix in a little of the reserved fruit juice to moisten the ingredients and bind them into a stuffing consistency. Season with herbs and pepper and divide into four.

Lay a trout skin side down on the board. Place a portion of stuffing at the wider (head) end of the fish, and roll up fairly snugly. Place the rolled fish in an ovenproof dish and repeat with the remaining trout and stuffing. Add the ginger wine and about 45 ml (3 tbsp) of the reserved fruit juice to the dish. Cover tightly and cook in the oven at 180°C (350°F, gas 4) for 30 minutes.

Meanwhile, thinly slice one or two more of the remaining apricots and use them to garnish the trout rolls.

Salmon and almond (S almon D)

Here's a higher-fat way of cooking salmon steaks, for those who are determined to put on weight.

4 salmon steaks
juice of ½ lemon
pinch of dried dill
1 egg white
50 g (1¾ oz) ground almonds
15 ml (1 tbsp) olive oil
1 garlic clove, finely chopped

Wash the salmon steaks and place them in a microwaveproof dish. Pour the lemon juice over the salmon and sprinkle with dill. Cover and cook in the microwave on full power for about 6 minutes, turning and rearranging the salmon steaks halfway through cooking. Leave the cooked salmon to cool.

Remove the skin from the salmon steaks and brush them with egg white, then coat in ground almond. Heat the oil in a frying pan, adding the fish and the garlic at the same time. Cook until the almond coating is golden brown, turning once. Serve immediately.

Smoked mackerel pâté

Traditional recipes for this add dollops of unnecessary saturated fat in the form of butter. We have found that this coronary-friendly pâté is equally acceptable to guests.

Quantities are not critical, but I prefer the pâté made with plenty of lemon juice. If you want a really smooth pâté, purée the mackerel in a food processor, but we find the texture of this version more interesting. You can use other smoked fish, such as trout.

225 g (8 oz) smoked mackerel
250 g virtually fat-free fromage frais, quark,
or very low-fat yoghurt (or use a mixture of these)
30 ml (2 tbsp) horseradish sauce
(not creamed horseradish)
juice of 1 or 2 lemons
black pepper
lemon wedges to garnish

*Skin the mackerel and use a fork to flake the fish in a large bowl.
Add the other ingredients, adjusting the lemon juice to taste and mix
to form a pleasantly coarse pâté. Serve garnished with lemon wedges.
Offer matzos, crispbreads or toasted triangles of wholemeal pitta
bread with the pâté.*

Tipsy fish casserole

Fish like cider, wine and vermouth. You can try endless variations
to this simple recipe.

700 g (1½ lb) white fish, e.g. cod, haddock or coley
2 onions, chopped
225 g (½ lb) tomatoes, sliced
150 ml (¼ pint) dry cider or white wine
5 ml (1 tsp) dried mixed herbs
black pepper
60 ml (4 tbsp) fresh breadcrumbs

*Wash the fish and remove the skin if you prefer. Either cut the
fillets into four portions or into bite-sized cubes and place them in
an ovenproof casserole. Sprinkle the onion over the fish and cover
with the tomato slices. Gently pour in the cider or wine and season
with the mixed herbs and black pepper.*

*Cover and cook in the oven at 160°C (325°F, gas 3) for
20–30 minutes. Remove the lid and sprinkle the breadcrumbs over
the fish. Brown the breadcrumb topping under the grill and serve.*

Fish and chips

Traditional battered fish and fried chips are very high-fat foods
and, when you don't cook it yourself, you have no control over the type
of fat used.

If you don't have a problem with your weight, it's reasonable to have fried fish occasionally, as long as it's shallow-fried in a suitable oil. To coat the fish in flour or cornmeal, dip it in a plate of skimmed milk or egg white first before laying each side on a plate of the coating. Use as little olive oil or rapeseed oil as possible and get it sizzling hot before adding the fish. Cook over medium heat and turn the fish over as soon as the first side is golden brown.

Baked chips

And the chips? Of course, you can buy oven chips and they are very much lower in fat than deep-fried chips. However, it is possible to produce your own version of oven chips. Don't expect them to be exactly like the chips you're used to, but proper potatoes do taste infinitely better than the majority of re-formed frozen varieties.

> *3 large potatoes*
> *5–10 ml (1–2 tsp) rapeseed oil*
>
> *Peel the potatoes, cut them into chips, and boil them for just 2–4 minutes, depending on size, until very lightly cooked but not tender. Meanwhile, pour the oil on to a baking tray and heat it in the oven at 220°C (425°F, gas 7). Thoroughly drain the chips, and dry them on absorbent kitchen paper. Spread them on the baking tray, then turn them over a few times to make sure they are very lightly coated with oil on all sides.*
>
> *Bake the chips for 40 minutes, turning a couple of times, until they are crisp and golden. Serve immediately, while still crisp.*

Making the most of a roast

The principle used to bake chips can be used to make excellent roast potatoes, too, just as acceptable to everyone as the lard-laden ones that disgrace the traditional English roast.

Roast potatoes

> *8 potatoes (depending on size of potato and appetites of people)*
> *15 ml (1 tbsp) rapeseed oil*
>
> *Peel the potatoes if you wish, but they're delicious unpeeled. Cut them into large chunks (not too small) and boil for about 10 minutes.*

Meanwhile, pour the oil on to a baking tray and heat it in the oven at 220°C (425°F, gas 7). Drain the potatoes, return them to the pan and place over a low heat or on the warm hotplate for a few minutes, shaking the pan to slightly 'fluff' them.

Working quickly, transfer the potatoes to the baking tray, turning them with a spatula to ensure they are coated very lightly with hot oil. Bake the potatoes for about 1 hour, turning them a couple of times to keep them coated with oil, until golden brown and crisp.

Variations

Parsnips, too, are wonderful roasted this way; don't cut them too small, and parboil for only 5 minutes or they'll go mushy.

In fact, just between ourselves, my wife and I sometimes have a feast of assorted roast root vegetables cooked like this, in a really tiny amount of rapeseed oil, liberally seasoned with freshly ground mixed peppercorns. The children are happy to eat them too. Carrots and turnips need parboiling for even less time than parsnips.

Weight for me!

If you're overweight, you may be fed up with reading recipes that suggest adding oil. Of course, a dish that has low-fat ingredients and adds just a quarter of a tablespoon of rapeseed oil per person, is still far lower in fat than most traditional cooked food. All the same, I take the point.

When you're concerned about every calorie, by all means do most of your cooking without adding any fat at all. Make casseroles without browning any ingredients; they'll be fine. Grill, bake, boil or steam but don't fry. Make sure you choose widely from the first four food groups, including plenty of whole grains as well as pasta and potatoes. Keep up your minimum of five portions of fruit and vegetables a day. Use very low-fat dairy products freely (less than 1 g fat per 100 g). Include fish in your diet at least twice a week and use plenty of pulses. You might consider supplementing your vitamin E intake, but remember that we cannot be certain that high doses are safe, or that they will actually prevent heart disease (see page 96).

Oat cuisine

Oats get votes in all sorts of popular dishes, savoury and sweet. They also provide soluble fibre. If you feel so inclined, you can slip some oat bran – which is a particularly good source of soluble fibre – into most moist recipes.

Muesli

Here are the basic ingredients for mundane muesli, but the possibilities for exciting variations – with grains, seeds, dried fruit and nuts – are endless.

2 cups porridge oats
2 cups barley flakes
2 cups rye flakes
1 cup wheat bran or oat bran (optional)
2 cups sultanas, raisins and/or other dried fruit
1 cup walnuts, hazelnuts and/or almonds

Mix the ingredients and store them in an airtight container. Sugar can be added, but it's better simply to increase the dried fruit content if the muesli is not sweet enough for your taste. Serve with skimmed milk.

Flapjack

This is a high-fat recipe but at least you are spared all the butter of traditional flapjack and all the trans fatty acids of manufactured products. This recipe makes a crisp and crumbly flapjack. Eat in small quantities!

90 ml (3 fl oz) rapeseed oil
30 ml (2 tbsp) golden syrup
225 g (8 oz) rolled oats

Warm the syrup in a large saucepan and mix in the oil and oats. Line the bottom of a straight-sided, shallow 18-cm (7-in) square tin with non-stick baking parchment. Transfer the mixture to the tin and press it down well. Bake at 180°C (350°F, gas 4) for about 45 minutes, until golden brown. Cut into small squares while warm, but leave it in the tin until cold.

Kids' stuff

Kids stuff with sweets and crisps, but will they eat that sumptuous dish so lovingly prepared? The most appealing meals will sometimes be rejected. Often, it is the simplest ideas that find favour with the younger gourmet. Here are a few.

Cheese and chive potato scones

As we saw in Chapter 15, children are more likely to eat food when they've had a hand in its preparation, but do make sure it's a clean hand. Cutting the scones into animal shapes makes them much more appealing to children – especially when they've done it themselves.

Adults (and children who've already got used to highly-salted processed foods) will find these bland without salt. It is far better to bring young children up appreciating low-salt foods.

> *450 g (1 lb) potatoes*
> *50 g (2 oz) cheddar cheese, grated*
> *100 g (4 oz) plain flour, sifted*
> *15 ml (1 tbsp) olive or rapeseed oil*
> *45 ml (3 tbsp) chives, chopped*
> *black pepper to taste*

> *Cook the potatoes in a saucepan of boiling water for 20 minutes. Drain them thoroughly and mash them in the saucepan. Add the flour, oil and chives. Season with pepper, and mix to a dough with a wooden spoon. Call the children and make sure they wash their hands thoroughly. Roll out the dough on a floured surface to a thickness of just 5 mm (¼ in) – no thicker or they'll be stodgy. Preheat a heavy-bottomed pan over a medium heat. Let the children cut the dough into farm animal shapes with the cutters of their choosing.*
> *Cook the scones in the hot pan for ten minutes or so until crisp and golden brown on both sides. Serve immediately with sweetcorn haystacks and broccoli trees.*

Tip: next time the children ask for that takeaway burger, remind them that Old MacDonald had a farm, as well as a chain of fast food outlets.

Egg soldiers

Here's an even simpler idea. Make sure the children have washed, ready to help when the soldiers need egging on. They need to be closely supervised or you'll end up with egg on your face. As soon as they've finished dipping the bread soldiers in egg, it's important that they wash their hands again before they lick raw egg from their fingers.

Quantities suitable for two children:
15 ml (1 tbsp) rapeseed oil
1 egg, beaten
15 ml (1 tbsp) milk
pepper to taste
1 slice of bread (medium thickness)

Put the oil in a heavy-bottomed pan and pre-heat over a medium heat. Cut the bread into soldiers. Add the milk and pepper to the egg and whisk with a fork. Pour the egg mixture onto a suitably deep plate and help the children dunk each soldier until well soaked with egg. Cook the soldiers thoroughly in the pan until crisp and brown on both sides and cooked right through. Serve immediately with battalions of carrot sticks and sugarsnap peas (raw or lightly cooked).

Snow White and the Seven Dwarfs

Fairy tales can help children discover the magic of food. In this little pudding, the dwarfs look so attractive, with their bright green kiwi feet and their strawberry red hats, that adults can't resist them either. Of course, for the child with a smaller tummy, especially one too young to count, a couple of dwarfs can always be on holiday or working late.

Quantities for one child:
1 kiwi fruit, peeled
1 banana peeled
7 strawberries
1 scoop of vanilla ice cream

Slice the kiwi fruit and arrange seven slices (feet) in a ring round the plate. Cut seven lengths of banana – approximately 25 mm (1 inch) – and stand these little bodies on the kiwi feet. (The height of the dwarfs can be varied according to appetite.) Wash the strawberries and cut off the stalk end to form a flat base; place the cut surface of each strawberry securely onto a piece of banana. The seven dwarfs complete, enter Snow White – a scoop of vanilla ice cream in the centre.

Some afters thoughts

Many puddings can be adapted to make something much less destructive but just as delicious.

Christmas pudding

Traditional Christmas pudding is loaded with saturated-fat-sodden suet. With this very low-fat version you can celebrate with peace of mind – and delight your guests. It's the custom to store Christmas puddings for at least a month; we've never been that organised and this version doesn't protest about being made on Christmas Eve.

The following quantities make a large, 1.5 litre (2¾ pint) pudding.

450 g (16 oz) fresh wholemeal breadcrumbs
1 eating apple, chopped (no need to peel)
1 banana, peeled and chopped
100 g (4 oz) walnuts, chopped
25 g (1 oz) almonds
225 g (8 oz) currants
225 g (8 oz) sultanas
225 g (8 oz) muscovado sugar
15 ml (3 tsp) ground mixed spice
3 eggs or egg replacer (see page 131)
grated rind and juice of 1 lemon
dash of gravy browning
up to 150 ml (¼ pint) skimmed milk (less if bread less dry)
a good slosh of brandy

The breadcrumbs, apple, banana, walnuts and almonds can be processed together in a food processor. Transfer to a large mixing bowl. Add all the remaining ingredients, except the milk and brandy. Pour in milk and brandy slowly, while stirring, until a good pudding consistency, dropping but not sloppy, is achieved. The darker the sugar, the darker the mix but a little gravy browning brings it to a satisfying rich colour.

Put into a 1.5 litre (2¾ pint) greased pudding basin. Cover with grease-proof paper and then foil, folding a pleat in each to allow for expansion, and fasten with string or an elastic band around the rim of the basin. Boil the pudding for 5 hours, topping up the water as necessary. Alternatively cook for 1½ hours in a pressure cooker,

*following the manufacturer's instructions. Remove the covering
and allow the pudding to cool completely. Cover with fresh paper
and foil (never foil alone as the acid from the fruit in the pudding
causes it to disintegrate).*

*Reheat the pudding on Christmas Day by boiling for 1 hour
(or 20 minutes in a pressure cooker), although it's just as delicious
on any other day of the year. Serve doused with flaming brandy.*

Brandy sauce

I'm dreaming of a white . . . sauce.

There's nothing like steaming brandy sauce to go with your
Christmas Pudding.

We've seen how white sauce for savoury dishes can be as simple
as quark with skimmed milk, varying the amount of skimmed milk
according to the consistency required. White sauce can also be
made with skimmed milk and cornflour (instead of making a fat
and flour paste known as a roux) for both savoury and sweet
recipes.

45 ml (3 tbsp) cornflour
15 ml (1 tbsp) sugar
600 ml (1 pint) skimmed milk
brandy or white rum

*Mix the cornflour and sugar in a saucepan off the heat. Slowly add
the milk, stirring continuously to avoid having lumps. Gently heat
the cold mixture, stirring continuously, until the sauce boils.
Cook gently for 2–3 minutes, then remove from the heat while
stirring. This gives a smooth, thick sauce. Stir in plenty of brandy
or white rum, to taste (brandy turns the sauce an off-white colour).*

Summer pudding

Not wishing to be seasonist, I must include something for a hot
summer's day.

450 g (1 lb) mixed soft fruit
(e.g. blackcurrants and blackberries)
30 ml (2 tbsp) water
sugar to taste
150 g (5 oz) thinly sliced bread

Wash the fruit. Heat the water and sugar until the sugar has dissolved, then bring to the boil while stirring. Add the fruits to the syrup and poach them gently for a few minutes, until they become soft without losing their shape.

Cut the crusts off the bread and line a 900 ml (1½ pint) pudding basin with the slices, overlapping them neatly. Empty the fruit into the bread-lined basin and use more bread to cover the top. Press the top with a weighted saucer. Stand the basin in a shallow dish to catch any escaping juices and leave the pudding to meditate in the refrigerator overnight. By the time it turns out the next day, it should be in good shape and able to stand up for itself. To be safe, turn the pudding out just when you are ready to serve it; this avoids any sagging disasters. Serve with vanilla-flavoured, virtually fat-free fromage frais. In winter, you might prefer hot custard, made with skimmed milk.

Afternoon tea

If you have room for afternoon tea, a piece of fruit cake is very tempting. Sadly, that piece of fruit cake, like most traditional baked goods, is likely to contain a good helping of saturated fat.

I mentioned earlier in the book that, in many recipes for baked foods, you can simply replace the fat with prune purée, and fruit cake is an ideal example. In fact, we could have made our Christmas pudding according to a traditional recipe, merely replacing the suet with the same weight of prune purée.

Prune purée
To prepare 280 g (10 oz) prune purée, blend 225 g (8 oz) of ready-to-eat prunes with 90 ml (6 tbsp) water to form a smooth paste, in a food processor or blender. Replace fat in a traditional recipe with an equal weight of prune purée.

Very rich fruit cake
This is as delicious as any fruit cake and none of your friends will believe it's made without fat. Who says you can't have your cake and eat it?

280 g (10 oz) currants
200 g (7 oz) sultanas
110 g (4 oz) raisins
70 g (2½ oz) glacé cherries, cut into quarters
70 g (2½ oz) almonds, chopped
70 g (2½ oz) cut mixed peel
grated rind of 1 lemon
30 ml (2 tbsp) brandy
200 g (7 oz) plain wholemeal flour
1 tsp ground mixed spice
½ tsp grated nutmeg
60 g (2 oz) ground almonds
175 g (6 oz) soft brown sugar
175 g (6 oz) prune purée
15 ml (1 tbsp) black treacle
8 egg whites or dried equivalent (see page 131)

Mix the dried fruit, cherries, almonds, peel, lemon rind and
brandy in a bowl. This may be left to stand, covered, overnight.

Sift the flour, spice and nutmeg into another bowl and
add the ground almonds. Replace any bran sifted from the flour.
Line a 20-cm (8-in) round or 18-cm (7-in) square tin with grease-
proof paper and wipe the paper with rapeseed oil.

Mix the sugar and prune purée together in a large mixing
bowl and beat in the treacle. Add the egg whites in stages, beating
thoroughly after each addition. Fold in the flour mixture and
the prepared fruit alternately, bit by bit, beating well until all the
ingredients are well mixed. Transfer the mixture into the prepared
tin. Smooth the top with the back of a wetted metal spoon and
bake the cake at 150°C (300°F, gas 2) for 3 hours or until firm to
the touch and cooked through.

To test if the cake is cooked through, insert a clean metal skewer
into the middle; if the skewer comes out free of any sticky mixture,
the cake is cooked. If there are distinct smears of mixture sticking to
the skewer, replace the cake in the oven and test it again after about
15 minutes. If the cake looks slightly dark on top before it is cooked
through, lay a square of foil loosely over the tin before returning it
to the oven. Once cooked, leave the cake to cool in the tin for about
1 hour, then turn it out onto a wire rack to cool completely.

Chapter 28

Action plan

Where do you start? You want to tackle all your important risk factors. You know it's not very effective to put all your energy into one risk factor and ignore the others.

That doesn't mean it's practical to tackle everything at once. Then again, if you start with one risk factor, you have to be careful not to forget about the others and lose your motivation as time goes by. You need ... ACTION PLAN! (Cue theme music.)

You need to answer these questions:

- What is my level of risk now?

- What changes do I need to make?

- What is my timetable for change?

If you know your average blood pressure and cholesterol level, you could use Figure 16 in Chapter 24 as a ready reckoner of your risk. You also need to take into account the other factors like family history, lack of exercise and poor diet that could increase your risk further – even if your blood pressure and cholesterol level seem OK.

Use the action plan (Table 26) to see what changes you need to make. Every tick in the **NO** column shows you that action is needed. Don't be overwhelmed if you've ticked every box! You've got a lot to sort out but you can take six months to do it if you want.

It's a good idea to tick the boxes with a pencil – then you can rub out your tick under **NO** and place one under **YES** when you've put something right. How satisfying it will be to see the **NO** column empty and the **YES** column fill up! This will signify a huge reduction in your coronary risk. You could make your own progress chart based on this table, leaving room for a magnificent gold star by each goal.

Setting a timetable is important – even if you have to adjust it. The beauty of this system is that you don't lose track of what you've achieved and what remains to be tackled.

It's a good idea to enter an annual review date in your calendar or diary, to make sure you haven't slipped back. You could link this to getting your blood pressure checked every year.

It's only once a week, Doc

Of course, if your **NO** column is empty because you have high-fat dairy products, eat salted snacks, and polish off a pound of chocolate almost once a week, there's a lot of room for improvement!

Perhaps your tradition of a cooked breakfast on Sunday morning is important to you. Fair enough. At least use a good pan, requiring the minimum of rapeseed oil or olive oil; have mushrooms, tomatoes, baked beans and smoked turkey rashers or lean bacon – not sausage, streaky bacon, egg and greasy fried bread.

When it comes to such things as chocolate, full-fat cheese, cream and pork crackling, it's very much easier not to spend the week looking forward to the one day when these will be allowed. Otherwise, not only do you end up with a 'moderate diet' that has disappointing results, but you also enjoy your food less – always hankering after forbidden fruits. Simply fill your menu with an appetising abundance of helpful foods; you will then feel free to enjoy those other items on rare occasions that are genuine exceptions to your routine.

Priorities, practicalities and precautions

If you are a smoker, giving up should be your top priority. There's little point in fine tuning your dairy products while smoking 30 a day. Read Chapter 20 again and work out your timetable for Ready, Steady, Stop.

If you regularly eat lunch in a staff canteen, it's worth meeting the catering staff to make sure something suitable is always available. In restaurants, too, be specific: why shouldn't you have your fish cooked in olive oil instead of butter?

Don't forget that the positive goals (such as eating more pulses and fish) are just as important as the negative ones (such as eating less processed meat). In fact, they go hand in hand: processed meat will be replaced by pulses and fish.

If your only regular exercise at the moment is lifting a knife and fork, remember to increase very gradually, starting with gentle walking before you get too frisky. Read Chapter 19 again. Make out a timetable, perhaps reaching half an hour's brisk walking a day over a three-month period.

Unless you live in splendid isolation, this living and eating business is a family affair. It's hard to give up smoking in a household of smokers; it's hard to eat a good diet when the cupboards are crammed with high-fat processed foods. Have you prepared your shopping list from Chapter 12? Chapter 27 will get you started in the kitchen, but further help with low-fat cookery can be found in *Useful publications* at the end of the book.

REVERSING HEART DISEASE

There is strong evidence for the benefit of statin drugs in people who have heart disease even when the cholesterol level is not raised.

If you've had a heart attack or suffer from angina, the narrowing of your coronary arteries has made itself known. Fatty deposits gradually build up in our arteries for many years before we find out there's a problem. Unfortunately, we can't just have a quick look in our arteries to see how they're getting on. (Perhaps it would be too frightening if we could.) Wouldn't it be good if you could have a 'decoke'?

The Lifestyle Heart Trial published in the *Lancet* in 1990 showed that a big enough change in lifestyle could actually reverse heart disease without drugs. Those who were given routine advice made moderate lifestyle changes and their coronary arteries continued to get narrower. But a programme that involved a big change in diet, stopping smoking, managing stress and taking exercise resulted in some widening of the coronary arteries after just one year. Think how much more might be achieved in ten years!

The programme in this book is carefully balanced. It isn't a gimmick; it brings together all the ways of protecting your arteries that are firmly backed up by scientific research. Focusing your efforts on one 'cure' (whether it's fish oil or exercise) while ignoring everything else, isn't likely to be very effective. So use the Action Plan to put the whole programme into effect and start unblocking those arteries right now!

Table 26 Action Plan Chart for you to fill in.

	Action Needed (NO)	OK (YES)
Am I a non-smoker?	☐	☐
Was my last blood pressure reading:		
Within the last year?	☐	☐
Normal?	☐	☐
Have I had my urine checked (for diabetes)?	☐	☐
Have I had a cholesterol check?	☐	☐
Was my total cholesterol below 5.0 mmol/l? (Or LDL-cholesterol below 3.0 mmol/l)	☐	☐
Is my Body Mass Index below 25?	☐	☐
Do I have 20 minutes continuous exercise a day? (Or 30 minutes 5 days a week)	☐	☐
Have I got stress under control?	☐	☐
Have I discussed drug therapy (e.g. aspirin, statin) with my doctor in the last year?	☐	☐
Do I eat several portions of wholegrain foods each day? (Cereals, bread, rice, pasta)	☐	☐
Do I choose carbohydrate foods with a low glycaemic index? (Pastas, pulses, mixed grain breads, etc.)	☐	☐
Do I eat at least 5 portions of fruit and vegetables a day?	☐	☐
Do I regularly eat good sources of folic acid: Brussels sprouts, spinach, kale, blackeye beans?	☐	☐
Have I considered whether I want to take one 0.4 mg folic acid tablet daily?	☐	☐

	Action Needed (NO)	OK (YES)
Do I avoid fatty red meat or always trim off visible fat?	☐	☐
Do I avoid fatty minced meat or always drain off the fat?	☐	☐
Do I have sausages, meat pies, pâtés or other processed meat products less than once a week?	☐	☐
Do I avoid fatty poultry (e.g. goose; duck with skin)?	☐	☐
Do I always remove skin from chicken and turkey?	☐	☐
Do I eat fish at least twice a week?	☐	☐
Do I eat oily fish once a week (or take fish oils)?	☐	☐
Do I eat at least 5 servings of pulses (peas, beans, lentils, chickpeas, etc.) a week?	☐	☐
Do I eat less than 3 egg yolks a week?	☐	☐
Do I avoid butter, and fat spreads that are not high in mono-unsaturates or fortified with stanol/sterol?	☐	☐
If using a reduced-fat spread, do I make sure it's just a scraping?	☐	☐
Do I avoid full-fat mayonnaise, salad dressing or sauces?	☐	☐
Do I avoid cooking oils/fats high in saturates?	☐	☐
When baking, do I avoid butter, lard, suet or unsuitable shortening?	☐	☐
Do I eat bought cakes and biscuits less than once a week? (The alternative is home-made, not stolen)	☐	☐
Do I eat chocolate/fudge/toffee etc. less than once a week?	☐	☐
Do I eat high-fat puddings/ice cream less than once a week?	☐	☐

	Action Needed (NO)	OK (YES)
Do I use skimmed milk instead of whole milk?	☐	☐
Do I have higher-fat dairy products less than once a week? (e.g. full-fat yoghurts, cream)	☐	☐
Do I have cheese (other than cottage cheese, quark, etc.) less than once a week?	☐	☐
Have I stopped adding salt in the kitchen and at the table?	☐	☐
Do I check the sodium content of processed foods?	☐	☐
Do I have salted snacks (nuts, crisps, etc.) less than once a week?	☐	☐
Do I avoid regular use of soy sauce/other salty seasonings?	☐	☐
Do I have fried food less than once a week?	☐	☐
Do I make sauces with skimmed milk and without a roux (butter and flour)?	☐	☐
Do I drain off meat/poultry fat before making gravy?	☐	☐
Do I eat in a canteen/restaurant (without knowing about fat and salt used) less than once a week?	☐	☐
Do I eat takeaway food (other than chicken kebab) less than twice a month?	☐	☐
Do I avoid having cafetière coffee every day?	☐	☐
Do I drink 6 glasses or more of water a day? (or other low-fat, low-sugar drink)	☐	☐
Do I drink less than 3 units of alcohol a day?	☐	☐
Do I have a wide variety of delicious low-fat recipes?	☐	☐

Glossary

ACE inhibitors A class of drugs (which act on the renin–angiotensin system) used to treat high blood pressure and heart failure.

aerobic exercise Repetitive movement of large muscles (e.g. running) resulting in an increased supply of oxygen to the muscles.

alpha-blockers A class of drugs that lower blood pressure by relaxing muscle in artery walls. They can be used to relieve prostate symptoms by relaxing muscle round the bladder outlet.

alpha-linolenic acid An essential polyunsaturated fatty acid in the omega-3 family that can be converted by the body to other omega-3 fatty acids (such as EPA and DHA which are found in fish). Walnuts are a rich source.

anaerobic exercise Muscles straining against resistance for short periods (e.g. tug of war), without an increased supply of oxygen.

aneurysm An abnormally wide section of an artery, resulting from a weakness in the artery wall.

angina (or angina pectoris) A 'tight' or 'heavy' pain and/or breathlessness caused by an inadequate supply of oxygen to the heart muscle – often triggered by exercise, stress or cold weather. Pain is typically felt across the chest, but may occur in the jaw, shoulder or arm. Unlike a heart attack, it doesn't damage the heart muscle and pain settles quickly.

angiogram An X-ray examination of blood vessels, after injecting a substance opaque to X-rays. Coronary angiography examines the coronary arteries supplying the heart.

antioxidant A chemical that neutralises the damaging effects of free radicals. Notable examples are vitamins C, E, and beta-carotene.

aorta The main artery that carries oxygen-rich blood from the heart to all the other arteries.

arrhythmia Any abnormal rhythm of the heartbeat.

arteriole A small artery that leads to capillary blood vessels.

artery A blood vessel that carries blood *away* from the heart.

atheroma Fatty deposits that build up on the lining of arteries.

atherosclerosis The process in which fatty and fibrous deposits cause narrowing and hardening of arteries.

beta-blockers A class of drugs that slow the heart and lower blood pressure.

biofeedback A technique in which a signal feeds back information to a person about some unconscious body function (such as blood pressure). With training, it is possible to exert control over the function (e.g. to lower the blood pressure).

blood pressure The pressure of the blood in the arteries expressed as the maximum (systolic) over the minimum (diastolic) pressure in millimetres of mercury (mmHg).

body mass index (BMI) Your body weight in kilograms divided by the square of your height in metres. A BMI between 20 and 25 is considered normal.

brachial artery The major artery in the arm, used for measuring blood pressure.

C-reactive protein A protein in the blood which is found in higher concentrations during inflammation. Raised levels are linked with an increased risk of coronary heart disease.

calcium channel blockers A class of drugs used to treat angina and high blood pressure. These drugs relax artery walls by blocking the passage of calcium through cell membranes.

capillaries The smallest blood vessels, which allow oxygen to pass from the blood to body cells (and waste products from cells to the blood).

cardiac arrest A complete halt in the pumping action of the heart.

cardiomyopathy A disease of the heart muscle that reduces the heart's pumping efficiency. There are various causes but often the cause is unknown.

cardiovascular disease A disease of the heart or circulation (such as coronary heart disease or stroke).

carotid arteries The major arteries in the neck.

CHD Coronary heart disease.

cholesterol A lipid – or fatty substance – found in the blood and cells of animals but not found in plants.

cilia (pronounced "sillier") Microscopic, hair-like structures. Movement of cilia in the lungs results in a cleansing flow of mucus that is brought to a standstill by smoking.

claudication Pain in the leg(s) on walking as a result of inadequate blood flow to the exercising muscles; it is relieved by rest.

climacteric The 'change of life', also known as the perimenopause; the time around the menopause during which a woman has symptoms due to falling oestrogen levels.

clinical trial A scientific experiment to test the value of a medical treatment. The best clinical trials are controlled, randomised, and double-blind. For example, if an active drug is being compared with a placebo (control), whether a patient receives the drug or the placebo is decided at random (like tossing a coin) and both patient and doctor are 'blind' to the truth until the end of the trial. In a single-blind trial, the doctor knows which patients are having active treatment; results may be affected by bias.

coronary arteries The arteries supplying blood to the heart.

coronary heart disease Heart disease resulting from atheroma of the coronary arteries; it may cause angina, a heart attack, or sudden death.

coronary thrombosis Formation of a blood clot in a coronary artery – a heart attack.

CRP C-reactive protein.

DHA Docosahexaenoic acid.

diabetes (diabetes mellitus) The medical condition in which blood glucose levels rise as a result of inadequate production of (or response to) insulin.

diastole The period in which the heart muscle relaxes between beats.

diastolic blood pressure The pressure of blood in the arteries during diastole.

It is the minimum pressure and is written underneath the systolic when blood pressure is recorded.

diuretic A drug that stimulates production of urine.

docosahexaenoic acid An omega-3 polyunsaturated fatty acid notably found in fish oil.

eicosapentaenoic acid An omega-3 polyunsaturated fatty acid notably found in fish oil.

embolus (plural: emboli) An abnormal particle, usually a blood clot, that is carried along in the circulation. A fragment of blood clot may move downstream until it lodges in a narrower part of the blood vessel, causing an obstruction (embolism).

endometrium The layer of tissue lining the uterus (womb).

EPA Eicosapentaenoic acid.

essential hypertension High blood pressure for which no specific cause is found.

extrinsic sugar Sugar that has been extracted from the plant cells in which it occurs naturally.

familial hypercholesterolaemia An inherited condition causing very high blood cholesterol levels; it affects about 1 in 500 people. Fatty lumps (xanthomas) may develop under the skin, especially round tendons. Drug treatment (in addition to lifestyle management) is essential to prevent early death from heart disease.

familial hyperlipidaemia Any of several inherited disorders causing high levels of blood lipids (e.g. cholesterol and/or triglycerides).

fatty acids The chemical units that make up a fat, usually in combination with glycerol to form triglycerides.

fatty streaks Fatty deposits on the lining of artery walls that can lead on to atheroma.

fibrinogen A protein (in the blood) involved in the formation of blood clots; high levels of fibrinogen increase the risk of a heart attack.

flavonoids A group of over 3000 antioxidant compounds occurring in apples, onions, coloured fruits and vegetables, red wine, and tea.

foam cell A scavenging white blood cell that has become laden with cholesterol and may contribute to the development of fatty streaks.

folic acid A B vitamin that helps to lower blood homocysteine levels. Rich sources are: green, leafy vegetables; Brussels sprouts; blackeye beans.

free radical An unstable chemical that causes damage (e.g. to lipids, proteins, DNA) by oxidation.

gamma-linolenic acid A polyunsaturated fatty acid in the omega-6 family, abundant in evening primrose oil.

GI Glycaemic index.

glycaemic index A number indicating how fast the carbohydrate in a food is converted to blood glucose.

HDL-cholesterol High-density lipoprotein cholesterol. Cholesterol in this form is being transported away from artery walls. It is often called 'the good cholesterol' because higher levels of HDL-cholesterol are linked with lower risk of heart disease.

heart attack Blockage of a coronary artery resulting in death of an area of heart muscle.

heart block A fault in the heart's natural pacemaker causing the heart to beat abnormally slowly (e.g. 30 beats per minute).

homocysteine A breakdown product of the amino acid methionine. There is a link between high blood levels of homocysteine and coronary heart disease. Homocysteine may play a part in atherosclerosis and thrombosis.

hormone replacement therapy Replacement of the female hormone oestrogen (with or without progestogen) after output from the ovaries has declined or stopped.

HRT Hormone replacement therapy.

hypercholesterolaemia High level of cholesterol in the blood.

hyperlipidaemia Raised levels of blood lipids (e.g. cholesterol, triglycerides).

IHD Ischaemic heart disease.

infarction The death of body tissue (e.g. brain, heart muscle) that occurs when the blood supply is cut off (e.g. by a clot or embolus).

intrinsic sugar Sugar that is still in the plant cell where nature put it (e.g. the sugar in an apple).

ischaemia Inadequate blood flow to an area of the body.

ischaemic heart disease Another term for coronary heart disease.

larynx The 'voice box' in the neck. You can feel the carotid pulse to one side of the larynx.

LDL-cholesterol Low-density lipoprotein cholesterol. Cholesterol in this form is sometimes called 'bad cholesterol' because it can be deposited in plaques, and higher levels are linked with higher death rates from coronary heart disease.

linoleic acid An omega-6 polyunsaturated fatty acid abundant in oils such as safflower oil, corn oil, and sunflower oil.

lipids Fatty substances such as cholesterol and triglycerides. Lipids do not dissolve in water but are more soluble in organic solvents.

lipoprotein lipase An enzyme that releases triglycerides from the lipoproteins which transport them; it also raises HDL levels. The rise in HDL-cholesterol that occurs with regular exercise may be the result of increased lipoprotein lipase activity in trained muscles.

lipoproteins Lipid particles linked with protein. This is the form in which cholesterol is transported in the bloodstream.

maximum heart rate The number of heartbeats per minute given by subtracting your age in years from 220. At age 50, the maximum heart rate would be 170 beats per minute; the *target* range for exercise could be 65–75% of the maximum (110–127 at age 50).

menopause A woman's last menstrual period.

metabolism All the complex chemical processes within the human body (or other organisms) necessary to maintain life – including the chemical reactions that convert food into energy for movement.

MI Myocardial infarction.

mmol/l A measure of concentration – the number of millimoles (mmols) of a substance in one litre (1l) of a fluid. A millimole is the molecular weight (or atomic weight) in milligrams (mg). In the UK, cholesterol levels are expressed as millimoles of cholesterol in one litre of serum. In the USA, they measure mg/dl – milligrams per decilitre (one-tenth of a litre). To convert a cholesterol measurement in mmol/l to mg/dl you multiply by 39. A cholesterol level of 5.2 mmol/l is just over 200 mg/dl.

mono-unsaturated fatty acids (mono-unsaturates) Fatty acids in which only one area of the molecule is not saturated with hydrogen. Replacing saturates with mono-unsaturates helps to lower LDL-cholesterol without reducing HDL-cholesterol.

myocardial infarction A heart attack.

myocardium The heart muscle.

oesophagus (or gullet) The muscular tube that carries food and drink from the throat to the stomach.

oestrogen The major female hormone (or, strictly, group of hormones) produced by the ovaries before the menopause. Natural oestrogens (e.g. oestradiol) are used for HRT but synthetic versions are available (such as ethinyl oestradiol which is used in the contraceptive pill).

omega-3 fatty acids Polyunsaturated fatty acids such as EPA and DHA that are particularly abundant in fish oils.

omega-6 fatty acids Polyunsaturated fatty acids such as linoleic acid found, for example, in vegetable oils and nuts.

pacemaker The group of cells in the heart (or an electronic device) that starts off the electrical wave which causes a heartbeat. The heart's natural p-acemaker (sinoatrial node) normally regulates the heart rate. When this system fails, an artificial, electronic pacemaker is sometimes used.

placebo A 'dummy' drug containing no active ingredients but designed to pass off as the real thing. Administering a placebo normally has some benefit. For example, giving a placebo painkiller to someone in pain usually produces some relief (the 'placebo effect'). Placebos used in clinical trials should look, smell and taste like the real drug so no one can tell who's having the active treatment until the code is broken at the end of the trial.

plaque A deposit (consisting of fatty substances such as cholesterol, hardened with fibrous matter and calcium) in an artery affected by atherosclerosis.

platelets (thrombocytes) The smallest of the blood cells. Platelets plug damaged areas in blood vessels and are a vital part of the blood-clotting system.

polyunsaturated fatty acids (polyunsaturates) Fatty acids in which more than one area of the molecule is not saturated with hydrogen. Replacing saturates with polyunsaturates lowers LDL-cholesterol, but HDL-cholesterol falls as well.

pravastatin One of the statin drugs. Pravastatin was used to lower cholesterol in the WOSCOPS and CARE studies.

primary prevention Measures taken to prevent someone developing a disease (e.g. changing your lifestyle to reduce your coronary risk, before there are any signs of heart disease).

progesterone The female hormone produced by the ovaries in the second half of the menstrual cycle (after ovulation). Synthetic versions (progestogens) are used with oestrogen when HRT is prescribed for women who still have a uterus.

radial pulse The pulse in the radial artery, which can be felt on the thumb side of the wrist.

renin An enzyme in the kidney that sets off a chain reaction to produce angiotensin II and raise blood pressure.

saturated fatty acids (saturates) Fatty acids in which the molecule has no room for any more hydrogen atoms. A diet high in saturated fatty acids raises blood cholesterol levels and increases the risk of thrombosis.

sclerosis Hardening of some part of the body (as in atherosclerosis).

secondary hypercholesterolaemia High blood cholesterol levels caused by an underlying medical condition (such as thyroid or liver disease).

secondary prevention Measures taken to limit the effects or progress of a disease once it has occurred (e.g. giving a statin drug to someone with heart disease).

serum the clear yellowish fluid that is left after extracting all the solid components (e.g. red and white cells) from blood.

simvastatin A statin drug used to lower blood cholesterol levels. Simvastatin was used in the 4S study.

sphygmomanometer An instrument used to measure blood pressure.

stanols Substances derived from sterols which, like plant sterols, can be added to fatty foods to reduce absorption of cholesterol from the intestine.

statins A class of drugs used to lower blood cholesterol levels. The formal name for statins (HMG CoA reductase inhibitors) describes the way they work, which is to block the activity of an enzyme involved in cholesterol production.

sterols A group of naturally occurring compounds which includes cholesterol – a sterol found only in animals. Plant sterols can be added to a fat spread to lower blood cholesterol by reducing cholesterol absorption in the intestine.

stroke Damage to part of the brain resulting from a breakdown in the blood supply (which can be caused by a thrombus, an embolus or a bleed). The consequences reflect the area of brain damaged and may include defects of speech, vision, sensation and movement.

systole The period in which a heart chamber is contracting. With every heartbeat, the upper chambers (atria) contract first, squeezing blood into the ventricles below them. This 'atrial systole' is followed immediately by contraction of the main pumping chambers (ventricular systole).

systolic blood pressure The maximum pressure in the arteries as blood is forced out of the heart in ventricular systole. The systolic pressure is written above the diastolic.

target range The heart-rate range (such as 65–75% of your maximum rate) that you aim to stay within during a session of aerobic exercise.

thrombosis The formation of a blood clot within the circulation. Thrombosis in an artery can result in a heart attack or stroke; deep vein thrombosis can send an embolus to the lungs (pulmonary embolism).

thrombus A blood clot that develops *within* the circulation (unlike the blood clot that develops *outside* the circulation when you graze your knee).

trans fatty acids Unsaturated fatty acids in which the molecule is 'twisted' into a different shape from the normal (cis) form. (In the cis isomer, the two hydrogen atoms on each side of the double bond are on the same side of the molecule; in the trans isomer they are on opposite sides, as shown on page 34.) Trans fatty acids have the same unwanted effects as saturated fatty acids. Hard margarines and hydrogenated vegetable oils are likely to contain high levels of trans fatty acids.

triglycerides Fats in which three fatty acids are bonded to a glycerol molecule. The fat in our food and the fat we store in our bodies is generally in this form. The blood triglyceride concentration is measured in a fasting lipid test but is less clearly linked with heart disease than cholesterol levels are. Very high blood triglyceride levels raise the risk of pancreatitis.

xanthelasmas (or xanthelasmata) Yellowish, fatty deposits in the eyelids that are *sometimes* linked with high levels of blood cholesterol.

xanthomas (or xanthomata) Fatty lumps under the skin, often associated with various types of hyperlipidaemia. In familial hypercholesterolaemia, xanthomas are typically on tendons (e.g. the Achilles tendon in the heel).

Useful organisations

If you write for information from any of these organisations, it is helpful to enclose a large self-addressed envelope.

Al-Anon Family Groups
61 Great Dover Street
London SE1 4YF
Tel: 020 7403 0888
Fax: 020 7378 9910
Website:
www.hexnet.co.uk/alanon/
World-wide organisation offering support to families and friends of problem drinkers; has nearly 1000 local groups. Alateen, part of Al-Anon, is dedicated to helping teenagers with an alcoholic relative.

Alcohol Concern
Waterbridge House
32–36 Loman Street
London SE1 0EE
Tel: 020 7928 7377
Fax: 020 7928 4644
Website:
www.alcoholconcern.org.uk
National charity working against alcohol misuse. Members receive regular magazine and have access to extensive information and training services.

Alcoholics Anonymous (AA)
Baltic Chambers
50 Wellington Street
Glasgow G2 6HJ
Helpline: 0845 769 7555
Tel: 0141 226 2214
Website:
www.alcoholics-anonymous.org.uk
Northern office of worldwide charity which offers information and support, via local groups, to people with an alcohol problem who want to stop drinking.

Alcoholics Anonymous (AA)
PO Box 1
Stonebow House
Stonebow
York YO1 7NJ
Helpline: 0845 769 7555
Tel: 01904 644 026
Fax: 01904 629 091
Website:
www.alcoholics-anonymous.org.uk
Headquarters of worldwide organisation which offers information and support, via local groups, to people with alcohol problems who want to stop drinking.

ASH (Action on Smoking and Health)
102 Clifton Street
London EC2A 4HW
Helpline: 0800 169 0169
Tel: 020 7739 5902
Fax: 020 7613 0531
Website: www.ash.org.uk
National organisation with local branches. Campaigns on antismoking policies. Offers free information on website or for sale from H.Q. Catalogue on request.

ASH in Wales
220C Cowbridge Road East
Canton
Cardiff CF5 1GY
Helpline: 0800 1690 169
Tel: 02920 641 101
Fax: 02920 641 045
Website: www.ash.org.uk
National organisation with local branches. Campaigns for antismoking policies. Has free leaflets plus range of publications and videos for sale.

ASH Northern Ireland
Ulster Cancer Foundation
40–42 Eglantine Avenue
Belfast BT9 6DS
Tel: 02890 663 281
Fax: 02890 660 081
Website: www.ulstercancer.org
National organisation with local groups. Campaigns for antismoking policies. Range of publications and videos for sale

ASH Scotland
8 Frederick Street
Edinburgh EH2 2HB
Helpline: 0800 169 0169
Tel: 0131 225 4725
Fax: 0131 220 6604
Website: www.ashscotland.org.uk
National organisation with local branches.Campaigns for antismoking policies. Free information on website and for sale from HQ. Catalogue on request.

British Association For Cardiac Rehabilitation (BACR)
c/o British Cardiac Society
9 Fitzroy Square
London W1T 5HW
Tel: 020 7383 3887
Fax: 020 7383 5961
Website: www.bcs.com/bacr
Holds national register of cardiac rehabilitation programmes. Health professionals and non-professionals with bona fide interest in rehab of cardiac patients can become members of the BACR.

British Cardiac Patients Association (BCPA)
2 Station Road
Swavesey
Cambridge CB4 5QJ
Helpline: 0800 479 2800
Tel: 01954 202 022
Fax: 01954 202 020
Website: www.bcpa.co.uk
Supports heart patients and their carers. Publishes regular magazine.

British Heart Foundation (BHF)
14 Fitzhardinge Street
London W1H 6DH
Helpline: 08450 708070
Tel: 020 7935 0185
Fax: 020 7486 5820
Website: www.bhf.org.uk
*Funds research, promotes education
and raises money to buy equipment to
treat heart disease. List of publications,
posters and videos; send stamped
addressed envelope Their helpline,
HeartstartUK, can arrange training in
emergency life-saving techniques for
lay people.*

British Hypertension Society
Website: www.hyp.ac.uk/bhsinfo

British Nutrition Foundation
High Holborn House
52–54 High Holborn
London, WC1V 6RQ
Fax: 020 7404 6747
Website: www.nutrition.org.uk
*Professional association. Authoritative
publications and information sheets
available on request: stamped addressed
envelope requested as no telephone
advice is available.*

Cardiomyopathy Association
40 The Metro Centre
Tolpits Lane
Watford
Herts WD18 9SB
Helpline: 0800 0181 024
Tel: 01923 249977
Fax: 01923 249987
Website: www.cardiomyopathy.org
*Offers information for health
professionals; also support and
information for people with
cardiomyopathy and their families.*

**Chest, Heart and Stroke
Association (N. Ireland)**
21 Dublin Road
Belfast BT2 7HB
Helpline: 08457 697 299
Tel: 02890 320 184
Fax: 02890 333 487
Website: www.nichsa.com
*Funds research and provides
information on chest, heart and stroke-
related illnesses.*

Chest, Heart and Stroke Scotland
65 North Castle Street
Edinburgh EH2 3LT
Tel: 0131 225 6963
Fax: 0131 220 6313
Website: www.chss.org.uk
*Funds research and provides
information on chest, heart and stroke-
related illnesses.*

**Citizens Advice (National
Association – NACAB)**
Myddleton House
115–123 Pentonville Road
London N1 9LZ
Tel: 020 7833 2181
Fax: 020 7833 4371
Website: www.citizensadvice.org.uk
*HQ of national charity offering a wide
variety of practical, financial and legal
advice. Network of local branches
throughout the UK listed in phone
books and in Yellow Pages under
Counselling and Advice.*

Consumers' Association
2 Marylebone Road
London NW1 4DF
Helpline: 0845 307 4000
Tel: 020 7486 5544
Fax: 020 7770 7600
Website: www.which.net
*Campaigns on behalf of consumers and
produces reports on products including
foods.*

Coronary Prevention Group (CPG)
London School of Hygiene and
Tropical Medicine
2 Taviton Street
London WC1H 0BT
Tel: 020 7927 2125
Fax: 020 7927 2127
Website: www.healthnet.org.uk
First British charity devoted to
prevention of coronary heart disease.
Produces booklets and fact sheets
available on the website or by post.
Please send stamped addressed
envelope.

Department of Health (DoH)
PO Box 777
London SE1 6XH
Helpline: 0800 555 777
Tel: 020 7210 4850
Fax: 01623 724 524
Textphone: 020 7210 5025
Website: www.doh.gov.uk
Produces literature about health issues,
available via helpline. A more technical
site with National Service Frameworks
available from internet e.g.
www.doh.gov.uk/nsf/

Diabetes UK
10 Parkway
London NW1 7AA
Helpline: 020 7424 1030
Tel: 020 7424 1000
Fax: 020 7424 1001
Textline 020 7424 1888
Website: www.diabetes.org.uk
Provides advice and information on
diabetes; has local support groups.

Diabetes UK, Distribution Centre
PO Box 3030
Swindon SN3 4WN
Helpline: 0800 585 088
Part of Diabetes UK, separate from
London HQ for ordering publications.

Drinkline (National Alcohol Helpline)
Essentia Group
Lower Ground, Sky Park
72 Finneston Square
Glasgow G3 8ET
Helpline: 0800 917 8282
Fax: 0141 568 4001
Funded by Department of Health,
provides educational material for
schools, health professionals and
general information on drink, sex and
drugs issues. Refers to local agencies for
support.

Health Development Agency
Holborn Gate
330 High Holborn
London WC1V 7BA
Helpline: 0870 121 4194
Tel: 020 7430 0850
Fax: 020 7061 3390
Website: www.hda-online.org.uk
Formerly Health Education Authority;
now only deals with research.
Publications on health matters can be
ordered via helpline.

Heart UK
7 North Road
Maidenhead SL6 1PE
Tel: 01628 628 638
Fax: 01628 628 698
Website: www.heartuk.org.uk
Will help anyone at high risk of heart
attack, but specialises in inherited
conditions causing high cholesterol (i.e.
familial hypercholesterolaemia). (Was
Family Heart Association.)

Irish Heart Foundation
4 Clyde Road
Ballsbridge
Dublin 4
Tel: 00353 1 668 5001
Fax: 00353 1 668 5896
Website: www.irishheart.ie
*Offers information, publications,
training and support in prevention of
heart disease. Collaborates with other
heart-related organisations and has
some local support groups.*

**MIND (National Association for
Mental Health)**
Granta House
15–19 Broadway
London E15 4BQ
Helpline: 0845 766 0163
Tel: 020 8519 2122
Fax: 020 8522 1725
Website: www.mind.org.uk
*Mental health organisation working for
a better life for everyone experiencing
mental distress. Offers support via local
branches. Publications available on 020
8221 9666.*

NHS Direct
Helpline: 0845 4647
Tel: 020 8867 1367
Website: www.nhsdirect.nhs.uk
*NHS Direct is a 24-hour helpline
offering confidential healthcare advice,
information and referral service 365
days of the year. A good first port of call
for any health advice. Textphone for
people with a hearing impairment 0845
606 4647.*

Quit
211 Old Street
London EC1V 9NR
Helpline: 0800 002200
Tel: 020 7251 1551
Fax: 020 7251 1661
Website: www.quit.org.uk
*Offers advice to stop smoking in
English and Asian languages; also to
schools, and on pregnancy. Runs
training courses for health
professionals. Can put people in touch
with local support groups.*

Relate (Marriage Guidance)
Herbert Gray College
Little Church Street
Rugby CV21 3AP
Helpline: 0845 130 4010
Tel: 01788 573 241
Fax: 01788 535 007
Website: www.relate.org.uk
*Offers relationship counselling via local
branches. Relate publications on health,
sexual, self-esteem, depression,
bereavement and remarriage issues
available from bookshops, libraries or
via website.*

Sport England
16 Upper Woburn Place
London WC1H 0QP
Tel: 020 7273 1500
Fax: 020 7273 1868
Website: www.sportengland.org
*Government agency promoting sport in
England with a wide variety of activity
programmes.*

Sport Scotland
Caledonia House
1 Redheughs Rigg
South Gyle
Edinburgh EH12 9DQ
Tel: 0131 317 7200
Fax: 0131 317 7202
Website: www.sportscotland.org.uk
*Government agency in Scotland
promoting sport with a wide range of
activity programmes.*

**Sports Council for Northern
Ireland**
House of Sport
Upper Malone Road
Belfast BT9 5LA
Tel: 02890 381 222
Fax: 02890 682 757
Website: www.sportni.com
*Government agency promoting sport in
Northern Ireland with a wide variety of
activity programmes.*

Sports Council for Wales
Sophia Gardens
Cardiff CF1 9SW
Tel: 02920 300 500
Fax: 02920 300 600
Website:
www.sports-council-wales.co.uk
*Headquarters for national network of
local clubs who arrange integrated
projects to bring disabled and able-
bodied people together. Promotes sport
in Wales and distribute lottery funding.
Supports Paralympic athletes.*

Stroke Association
Stroke House
240 City Road
London EC1V 2PR
Helpline: 0845 303 3100
Tel: 020 7566 0300
Fax: 020 7490 2686
Website: www.stroke.org.uk
*Funds research and provides
information now specialising in stroke
only. Publications can be ordered from
01604 623 933.*

**Vegetarian Society of the United
Kingdom**
Parkdale
Dunham Road
Altrincham
Cheshire WA14 4QG
Tel: 0161 925 2000
Fax: 0161 926 9182
Website: www.vegsoc.org
*Offers information on the vegetarian
way of life, day and residential training
courses at own Centre. Provides
literature for GCSE projects, advice to
school caterers. Food manufacturers
and restaurants can apply for
vegetarian accreditation.*

Womens Health
52 Featherstone Street
London EC1Y 8RT
Helpline: 0845 125 5254
Tel: 020 7251 6333
Fax: 020 7250 4152
Minicom: 020 7490 5489
Website:
www.womenshealthlondon.org.uk
*Provides information on gynaecological
and sexual issues to help women make
informed decisions about their health.
Range of publications and quarterly
newsletter. To use reference library,
please telephone first.*

Women's Health Concern (WHC)
PO Box 2126
Marlow SL7 2RY
Helpline: 01628 483 612
Tel: 01628 488 065
Fax: 01628 474 042
Website:
www.womens-health-concern.org
National charity that offers help to women, particularly on questions of hormone health, HRT and gynaecology.

Yorktest Laboratories Ltd
Murton Way
Osbaldwick
York YO19 5US
Tel: 0800 074 6185
Website:
www.homocysteinetest.com
Yorktest supply testing kits by mail order. A kit to check blood homocysteine levels has now been added to their range.

Useful publications

Cooking and Eating

Cooking for a Healthy Heart,
by Jacqui Lynas, published by
Hamlyn (2002)
ISBN 0 600 60570 1

The Everyday Diabetic Cookbook,
by Stella Bowling, published by
Grub Street/British Diabetic
Association (1995)
ISBN 1 898697 25 6

The Everyday Light-Hearted Cookbook,
by Anne Lindsay, published by
Grub Street/British Heart
Foundation (1994)
ISBN 0 948817 78 X

*The Light-Hearted Cookbook:
Recipes for a Healthy Heart*,
by Anne Lindsay, published
by Grub Street/British Heart
Foundation (1999)
ISBN 1 902304 15 2

*Low Fat, Low Cholesterol: recipes for a
healthy heart*, by Christine France,
published by Southwater (2000)
ISBN 1 84215 093 6

*The Parentalk Guide to Your Child and
Food*, by Dr Derrick Cutting,
published by Hodder & Stoughton
(2001)
ISBN 0 340 78540 3

Quick Children's Meals, by Annabel
Karmel, published by Ebury Press
(1997)
ISBN 0 09 185189 0

*Sue Kreitzman's Complete Low-Fat
Cookbook*, by Sue Kreitzman,
published by Piatkus (1996)
ISBN 0 7499 1661 3

*The Ultimate Low Fat Low Cholesterol
Cookbook*, by Christine France,
published by Lorenzo Books (1996)
ISBN 1 859672 37 X

Stopping Smoking

*Allen Carr's Easy Way to Stop
Smoking*, by Allen Carr, published
by Penguin (1999)
ISBN 0 14 027763 3

*How to Stop Smoking and Stay
Stopped for Good*, by Gillian Riley,
published by Vermilion (2003)
ISBN 0 09 188776 3

Stop Smoking for Good, by Robert
Brynin, published by Hodder &
Stoughton (1995)
ISBN 0 340 63240 2

General Health

*Diabetes – the 'at your fingertips'
guide*, (Fifth edition) by Professor
Peter Sönksen, Dr Charles Fox and
Sue Judd, published by Class
Publishing (2003)
ISBN 1 85959 087 X

The New Glucose Revolution, by
Dr Anthony Leeds, Assoc. Prof.
Jennie Brand Miller, Kaye Foster-
Powell and Dr Stephen Colagiuri,
published by Avalon Publishing
Group (2003)
ISBN 1 56924 506 1

*Heart Health – the 'at your fingertips'
guide*, (Third edition) by Dr Graham
Jackson, published by Class
Publishing (2004)
ISBN 1 85959 097 X

*High Blood Pressure – the 'at your
fingertips' guide* (Third edition),
by Dr Tom Fahey, Professor Deidre
Murphy with Dr Julian Tudor Hart,
published by Class Publishing
(2004)
ISBN 1 85959 090 X

Stress

Understanding Stress, by Professor
Greg Wilkinson, published by
Family Doctor Publications (2000)
ISBN 1 898205 91 4

The Family Doctor Series covers
around 27 titles including
cholesterol, stress and high blood
pressure. Published by FDP,
10 Butchers Row, Banbury, Oxon
OX16 8JH (Tel: 01295 276627)

Many of the organisations listed
in the previous section publish
advisory leaflets, which are
available on application.

Index

**Have you found *Stop that heart attack!* useful and practical?
If so, you may be interested in other books from Class Publishing.**

Heart Health – the 'at your fingertips' guide
NEW THIRD EDITION   £14.99
Dr Graham Jackson
This practical handbook, written by a leading cardiologist, answers all your questions about heart conditions. It tells you all about you and your heart; how to keep your heart healthy, or if it has been affected by heart disease – how to make it as strong as possible.

Diabetes – the 'at your fingertips' guide
FIFTH EDITION   £14.99
Professor Peter Sönksen, Dr Charles Fox and Sue Judd
Over 460 questions on diabetes are answered clearly and accurately – the ideal reference book for everyone with diabetes.
'I have no hesitation in commending this book . . .' – *Sir Steve Redgrave, Vice President, Diabetes UK*

Parkinson's – the 'at your fingertips' guide
SECOND EDITION   £14.99
Dr Marie Oxtoby and Professor Adrian Williams
Full of practical help and advice for people with Parkinson's disease and their families. This book gives you the information and the confidence to tackle the challenges that PD presents.

Dementia: Alzheimer's and other dementias – the 'at your fingertips' guide
SECOND EDITION   £14.99
Harry Cayton, Dr Nori Graham and Dr James Warner
At last – a book that tells you everything you need to know about Alzheimer's and other dementias. An invaluable contribution to understanding all forms of dementia.

High Blood Pressure – the 'at your fingertips' guide
NEW THIRD EDITION   £14.99
Dr Tom Fahey, Professor Deirdre Murphy with Dr Julian Tudor Hart
The authors use all their years of experience as blood pressure experts to answer your questions on high blood pressure.
'Readable and comprehensive information' – *Dr Sylvia McLaughlan, Director General, The Stroke Association*

Stroke – the 'at your fingertips' guide
£14.99
Dr Anthony Rudd, Penny Irwin and Bridget Penhale
This essential guidebook tells you all about strokes – most importantly how to recover from them. As well as providing clear explanations of the medical processes, tests, and treatments, the book is full of practical advice, including recuperation plans; you will find it inspiring.

Asthma – the 'at your fingertips' guide
THIRD EDITION   £14.99
Dr Mark Levy, Professor Sean Hilton and Greta Barnes
This book shows you how to keep your asthma – or your family's asthma – under control, making it easier to live a full, happy and healthy life.

Cancer – the 'at your fingertips' guide
THIRD EDITION   £14.99
Val Speechley and Maxine Rosenfield
This invaluable reference guide gives you clear and practical information about cancer. Whether you have cancer yourself, or are caring for someone who does, you will find in this book the information you need to reassure yourself, and enable you to take control.

PRIORITY ORDER FORM

Cut out or photocopy this form and send it (post free in the UK) to:

Class Publishing Priority Service,
FREEPOST, London W6 7BR

Please send me urgently (tick boxes below)

Post included price per copy (UK only)

☐ **Stop that heart attack!** (ISBN 1 85959 096 9) £17.99

☐ **Heart Health – the 'at your fingertips' guide** (ISBN 1 85959 097 7) £17.99

☐ **High Blood Pressure – the 'at your fingertips' guide** ISBN 1 85959 090 X) £17.99

☐ **Diabetes – the 'at your fingertips' guide** (ISBN 1 85959 087 X) £17.99

☐ **Stroke – the 'at your fingertips' guide** (ISBN 1872362 98 2) £17.99

☐ **Parkinson's – the 'at your fingertips' guide** (ISBN 1 872362 96 6) £17.99

☐ **Asthma – the 'at your fingertips' guide** (ISBN 1 85959 006 3) £17.99

☐ **Dementia: Alzheimer's and other dementias – the 'at your fingertips' guide** (ISBN 1 85959 075 6) £17.99

☐ **Cancer – the 'at your fingertips' guide** (ISBN 1 85959 036 5) £17.99

TOTAL _____

Easy ways to pay

Cheque: I enclose a cheque payable to Class Publishing for £ _____

Credit card: Please debit my ☐ Mastercard ☐ Visa ☐ Amex ☐ Switch

Number _____ Expiry date ____ / ____

Name _____

My address for delivery is _____

_____

Town _____ County _____ Postcode _____

Telephone number (in case of query) _____

Credit card billing address (if different from above) _____

_____

Town _____ County _____ Postcode _____

Class Publishing's guarantee: remember that if, for any reason, you are not satisfied with these books, we will refund all your money, without any questions asked. Prices and VAT rates may be altered for reasons beyond our control.

☐ *Please send me details of other Class Publishing titles that may be of interest to me*